Post-Authorization Safety Studies of Medicinal Products

Post-Authorization Safety Studies of Medicinal Products

The PASS Book

Edited by

Ayad K. Ali
Eli Lilly and Company, Indianapolis, IN, United States

Abraham G. Hartzema
University of Florida, Gainesville, FL, United States

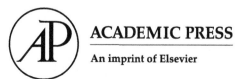

ACADEMIC PRESS

An imprint of Elsevier

Library of Congress Cataloging-in-Publication Data
A catalog record for this book is available from the Library of Congress

British Library Cataloguing-in-Publication Data
A catalogue record for this book is available from the British Library

ISBN: 978-0-12-809217-0

For information on all Academic Press publications visit our website at
https://www.elsevier.com/books-and-journals

  Working together
to grow libraries in
developing countries

www.elsevier.com • www.bookaid.org

Publisher: John Fedor
Acquisition Editor: Erin Hill-Parks
Editorial Project Manager: Jennifer Horigan
Production Project Manager: Punithavathy Govindaradjane
Cover Designer: Victoria Pearson

Typeset by TNQ Technologies

Contents

LIST OF CONTRIBUTORS xi

FOREWORD xiii

CHAPTER 1   **Introduction** 1

Ayad K. Ali, Abraham G. Hartzema

Risk Management and Benefit–Risk Evaluation 4

Transparency 5

About This Book 6

References 7

CHAPTER 2   **Risk Management Process** 9

CHAPTER 2.1   Risk Assessment 11

Emil Cochino

Disclaimer/Acknowledgments 11

Introduction 11

Safety Specification 13

Pharmacovigilance Plan 14

References 18

CHAPTER 2.2   Risk Minimization 20

Giampiero Mazzaglia, Sabine Straus

Disclaimer/Acknowledgments 20

Introduction 20

Risk Minimization Methods 22

Effectiveness of Risk Minimization 32

References 42

CHAPTER 3   **Data Sources for PASS** 47

CHAPTER 3.1   Health Insurance Administrative Claims 49

Beth L. Nordstrom, Kathy H. Fraeman, Dimitra Lambrelli

Introduction 49

Contents of Claims Databases 50
Strengths and Limitations of Claims Databases........................52
Methodological Considerations 55
Claims-Based Post-Authorization Safety Studies.....................57
References 60

CHAPTER 3.2   Electronic Medical Records 63

Beth L. Nordstrom, Kathy H. Fraeman, Dimitra Lambrelli

Introduction 63
Contents of Electronic Medical Record Databases....................63
Strengths and Limitations of Electronic Medical Record
Databases 66
EMR-Based Post-Authorization Safety Studies.........................68
PASS Using EMR Linked to Other Data 70
References 72

CHAPTER 3.3   Registries... 74

Stella Blackburn

Introduction 74
European Registries 75
Registry-Based Post-Authorization Safety Studies...................76
References 78

CHAPTER 3.4   Big Data 79

Jeremy Rassen, Sebastian Schneeweiss

Introduction 79
Big Data for Post-Authorization Safety Studies 79
Creation of "Bigness" 81
Methodological Considerations 85
Modern Methods for Post-Authorization Safety Studies
Employing Big Data 87
References 88

CHAPTER 3.5   Social Media 92

Andrew Paul Cox, Evie Merinopoulou

Introduction 92
Social Media Sources 93
Social Media and Pharmacovigilance 94
Challenges With Social Media Listening.....................................95
Methodological Considerations 98
Ethical Considerations 99
References 102

CHAPTER 4   **Study Designs for PASS** 105

CHAPTER 4.1   Drug Utilization and Prescription-Event Monitoring Studies 107

Massoud Toussi, Deborah Layton

Introduction 107
Methodological Considerations 108
Data Source for Drug Utilization Studies 110
Prescription-Event Monitoring Studies.........................111
Modified Prescription-Event Monitoring Studies 114
Specialist Cohort-Event Monitoring Studies................116
References 117

CHAPTER 4.2   Self-Controlled Studies 120

Shirley V. Wang, Ayad K. Ali

Introduction 120
Assumptions and Data Requirements 121
Types of Self-Controlled Designs.................................125
Methodological Considerations 132
References 137

CHAPTER 4.3   Cohort and Nested Case—Control Studies 139

Beth L. Nordstrom

Introduction 139
Cohort Studies 139
Nested Case—Control Studies 144
References 148

CHAPTER 4.4   Enriched Studies 150

Jennifer B. Christian, Nancy A. Dreyer

Introduction 150
Strengths and Limitations of Enriched Studies 152
Evaluation of Secondary Data Sources for Enriched Studies 153
Operationalizing Enriched Studies 154
Methodological Considerations 154
References 156

CHAPTER 4.5   Prospective Studies 158

Alejandro Arana, Anne Fourrier-Reglat, Massoud Toussi

Introduction 158
Prospective Interventional Studies..............................158
Prospective Noninterventional Studies........................160
Methodological Considerations 161
References 162

CHAPTER 5   **Analytical Approaches for PASS**...................165

CHAPTER 5.1   Exposure Propensity Scores.............................. 167

John D. Seeger

Introduction 167
Confounding by Indication..169
Development of Exposure Propensity Scores 171
Strengths of Exposure Propensity Scores..................173
Applications of Exposure Propensity Scores..............175
Transparency 179
References 180

CHAPTER 5.2   Disease Risk Scores 182

*Richard Wyss, Robert J. Glynn, Justin Bohn, Charles Poole,
Joshua J. Gagne, Ayad K. Ali*

Disclaimer/Acknowledgments.....................................182
Introduction 182
Development of Disease Risk Scores 183
Methodological Considerations 186
Disease Risk Scores Versus Exposure Propensity Scores 188
Empirical Example 190
Future Directions...192
References 193

CHAPTER 5.3   Instrumental Variables.................................. 197

Joseph A.C. Delaney, Ayad K. Ali

Introduction 197
Instrumental Variable in Noninterventional Post-
Authorization Safety Studies.......................................198
Methodological Considerations 198
Limitations of Instrumental Variable 200
References 201

CHAPTER 5.4   Data Analytic Platforms 203

Stephanie Reisinger, Javier Cid, Ayad K. Ali

Introduction 203
Common Data Models and Modular Analysis Programs 204
Data Analytic Platforms and Transparency.................205
Limitations of Data and Analysis Standardization 207
References 207

CHAPTER 5.5   Proactive Safety Surveillance 209

Joshua J. Gagne, Sengwee Toh, Ayad K. Ali

Introduction 209
Vaccine Safety Datalink...210

Sentinels 213
The Canadian Network for Observational Drug
Effect Studies 215
The Asian Pharmacoepidemiology Network 217
References 218

CHAPTER 6   **Benefit-Risk Evaluation ....** 223

CHAPTER 6.1   Benefite—Risk Evaluation Frameworks 225

Lesley Wise

Introduction 225
Stakeholders 226
Benefit Information..227
Risk Information 229
Impact of Uncertainty..232
Preferences and Values 233
Risk Minimization Measures...233
Overall Benefit—Risk Assessment 235
Role of Post-Authorization Safety Studies in Benefit—Risk
Assessment 236
Ongoing Benefit—Risk Evaluation....................................237
References 239

CHAPTER 6.2   Post-Authorization Effectiveness Studies 242

Stella Blackburn, Ayad K. Ali

Introduction 242
PAES in Europe...244
PAES in United States 246
Examples of Required PAES..246
Future Directions..247
References 248

CHAPTER 7   **PASS for Specialty Products.........................** 251

CHAPTER 7.1   Post-Authorization Safety Studies for Biosimilars
and Interchangeable Biologic Products.........................253

Jaclyn L.F. Bosco, Nancy A. Dreyer, Ayad K. Ali

Introduction 253
Biologics and Biosimilars Regulation 255
Safety Concerns With Biologics and Biosimilars......................256
Special Considerations for Biosimilars 258

Post-Authorization Safety Studies Designs for Biologics
and Biosimilars 261
Methodological Considerations 265
References 273

CHAPTER 7.2   Post-Authorization Safety Studies for Medical
Devices and Combination Products 277

*Jessica J. Jalbert, Theodore C. Lystig, Mary E. Ritchey,
Ayad K. Ali*

Introduction 277
Safety Concerns With Medical Devices 278
Methodological Considerations 279
References 290

CHAPTER 7.3   Post-Authorization Safety Studies for Vaccines 293

*Priscilla Velentgas, Roger Baxter, Philip Bryan,
Mendel Haag, Lorna Hazell, Rachel Jablonski,
Alena Khromova, Ombretta Palucci, Saad Shakir,
Walter Straus, Robert P. Wise, Ayad K. Ali*

Disclaimer/Acknowledgments 293
Introduction 293
Special Considerations for Vaccine Post-Authorization
Safety Studies 295
Vaccine Safety Surveillance Programs 297
Regulatory Requirements for Vaccine Post-Authorization
Safety Studies 298
Enhanced Passive Safety Surveillance for Vaccines 300
Designs for Vaccine Post-Authorization Safety Studies 304
Methodological Considerations 318
References 324

CHAPTER 8   **The European Union Post-Authorization
Study Register** 329

Thomas Goedcke, Xavier Kurz

Disclaimer/Acknowledgments 329
Introduction 329
References 335

INDEX **337**

List of Contributors

Ayad K. Ali   Eli Lilly and Company, Indianapolis, IN, United States

Alejandro Arana   RTI Health Solutions, Barcelona, Spain

Roger Baxter   Kaiser Permanente, Oakland, CA, United States

Stella Blackburn   IQVIA, Durham, NC, United States

Justin Bohn   Brigham and Women's Hospital and Harvard Medical School, Boston, MA, United States

Jaclyn L.F. Bosco   IQVIA, Durham, NC, United States

Philip Bryan   Medicines and Healthcare Products Regulatory Agency, London, United Kingdom

Jennifer B. Christian   IQVIA, Durham, NC, United States

Javier Cid   Evidera, Bethesda, MD, United States

Emil Cochino   European Medicines Agency, London, United Kingdom

Andrew Paul Cox   Evidera, Bethesda, MD, United States

Joseph A.C. Delaney   University of Washington, Seattle, WA, United States

Nancy A. Dreyer   IQVIA, Durham, NC, United States

Anne Fourrier-Reglat   University of Bordeaux, Cedex, France

Kathy H. Fraeman   Evidera, Bethesda, MD, United States

Joshua J. Gagne   Brigham and Women's Hospital and Harvard Medical School, Boston, MA, United States

Robert J. Glynn   Brigham and Women's Hospital and Harvard Medical School, Boston, MA, United States

Thomas Goedcke   European Medicines Agency, London, United Kingdom

Mendel Haag   Seqirus, Amsterdam, The Netherlands

Abraham G. Hartzema   University of Florida, Gainesville, FL, United States

Lorna Hazell   Drug Safety Research Unit, Southampton, United Kingdom

Rachel Jablonski   IQVIA, Cambridge, MA, United States

Jessica J. Jalbert   LASER Analytica, New York, NY, United States

Alena Khromova   Sanofi Pasteur, Toronto, Canada

Xavier Kurz   European Medicines Agency, London, United Kingdom

Dimitra Lambrelli Evidera, Bethesda, MD, United States
Deborah Layton IQVIA, London, United Kingdom
Theodore C. Lystig Medtronic, Minneapolis, MN, United States
Giampiero Mazzaglia European Medicines Agency, London, United Kingdom
Evie Merinopoulou Evidera, Bethesda, MD, United States
Beth L. Nordstrom Evidera, Bethesda, MD, United States
Ombretta Palucci IQVIA, Cambridge, MA, United States
Charles Poole University of North Carolina at Chapel Hill, Chapel Hill, NC, United States
Jeremy Rassen Aetion, Inc., New York, NY, United States
Stephanie Reisinger Evidera, Bethesda, MD, United States
Mary E. Ritchey RTI Health Solutions, Durham, NC, United States
Sebastian Schneeweiss Aetion, Inc., New York, NY, United States; Brigham and Women's Hospital and Harvard Medical School, Boston, MA, United States
John D. Seeger Optum, Eden Prairie, MN, United States
Saad Shakir Drug Safety Research Unit, Southampton, United Kingdom
Sabine Straus Medicines Evaluation Board, Utrecht, The Netherlands
Walter Straus Merck and Co., Inc., Kenilworth, NJ, United States
Sengwee Toh Harvard Medical School and Harvard Pilgrim Health Care Institute, Boston, MA, United States
Massoud Toussi IQVIA, Cedex, France
Priscilla Velentgas IQVIA, Cambridge, MA, United States
Shirley V. Wang Division of Pharmacoepidemiology and Pharmaco-economics, Department of Medicine, Brigham and Women's Hospital and Harvard Medical School, Boston, MA, United States
Lesley Wise Takeda Pharmaceuticals, London, United Kingdom
Robert P. Wise AstraZeneca, Gaithersburg, MD, United States
Richard Wyss Brigham and Women's Hospital and Harvard Medical School, Boston, MA, United States

Foreword

When the "five rights" of therapeutics are obeyed—the right patient, the right medicinal product, the right time, the right dose, and the right route—modern medicinal products are among the most valuable health-care interventions that we have. Yet, if only things were so simple, the value of a product depends crucially on how it is applied, and as any pharmacoepidemiologist should know all too well, medicinal products are no more inherently good or bad than a hammer or chisel. Many challenges prevent the optimal use of medicinal products, including risks that are all too often discovered only after large populations have been exposed, leaving regulators, manufacturers, payers, policymakers, and other stakeholders to figure out how we can design systems to improve the safe use of medicinal products.

Because of these challenges, it is an exciting time to be working in pharmacoepidemiology and pharmacovigilance. The world of therapeutics continues to rapidly evolve, and the demand for rigorous post-authorization safety studies (PASS) has never been greater. This demand, in turn, increases the value of information regarding the history, design, execution, and interpretation of PASS. This book serves just such a role.

The opportunity to work in medicinal product safety is an opportunity to affect the care of populations, thus improving the lives of mothers and fathers, brothers and sisters, sons and daughters millions at a time. This work is also inherently multidisciplinary, as the field of pharmacoepidemiology draws from pharmacology, medicine, and epidemiology alike. The conduct of well-designed PASS requires multiple skills, ranging from mastery of data sources, study designs, and analytic approaches to control for bias to knowledge of benefit–risk evaluation and risk management as it is exercised by regulators. Thus, "everybody has something to bring to the picnic."

Although there is a steady demand for rigorous assessments of the safety of authorized products, pharmacoepidemiology is an evolving field, with new methods, data sources, and directions. 10 or 20 years ago, concepts or categories such as "digital health" or "biosimilars" were nascent concepts—now they are common parlance. These and other emerging frontiers will continue to push the boundaries of our field, forcing us to develop new methods and frameworks for the host of challenges and opportunities that they present. For example, how can digital technologies be optimized to enhance surveillance for adverse events postlaunch? How must models that we have developed to examine chemical medicinal products be modified to evaluate cellular therapies, where no two batches are exactly identical, and where complex product−host−environment interactions may ultimately determine their safety? And such lessons do not stop with medicinal products alone, given the insights and methods from the field that can be applied to vaccines, devices, and diagnostics.

Ultimately, decisions about products come down to a benefit−risk balance, though this appraisal may be performed quite differently by different stakeholders. Regulators must decide whether evidentiary thresholds for market access or a relabeling of a product have been met. Payers must decide whether a product is medically necessary, whether it should be covered, and if so, how it should be reimbursed. Hospitals must decide whether to include a product within their formulary. Manufacturers must decide whether to pursue an optional study that might illuminate additional information regarding a product's benefits but which might also identify new risks. Providers must device with patients whether a treatment should be used, and if so, which one.

These decisions have real consequences, and while the considerations of regulators differ from those of clinicians, patients, or caregivers, at the end of the day, these decisions inevitably combine facts with judgments and must often be revisited iteratively over time, as information regarding a product's risks, benefits, and value accrues.

Many of us may not remember a time when it was otherwise, yet modern pharmaceutical regulation, including the imperative of well-done PASS, is relatively young. Although the value of such studies may be self-evident, their execution is hardly straightforward. Thus, the importance of this novel contribution that carefully reviews not only the history and conceptual foundations of the field but also data sources, study designs, analytic approaches, and study implementation. Yogi Berra once said, "It is tough to make predictions, especially about the future." Although there may be some truth to this perspective, it is safe to say that the importance of PASS is unlikely to diminish anytime soon.

Caleb Alexander, MD, MS
Johns Hopkins Bloomberg School of Public Health, Baltimore, MD, United States

CHAPTER 1

Introduction

Ayad K. Ali[1], Abraham G. Hartzema[2]

[1]Eli Lilly and Company, Indianapolis, IN, United States; [2]University of Florida,
Gainesville, FL, United States

On submission of the marketing authorization application (MAA), regulatory agencies review the submitted evidence with the aim to learn as much as possible about the efficacy and safety of the medicinal product during the pre-authorization phase, which assists in making marketing authorization decision to allow patients to have timely access to efficacious and safe medicinal products. However, studies conducted in the preauthorization phase of product development have inherent limitations that prevent characterization of all adverse events (Table 1.1 lists the main limitations of typical preauthorization clinical trials). The full safety profile of medicinal products can be determined after exposure by relatively large number of patients of diverse demographics and medical histories, and by those who are treated for extended periods. Pre-authorization studies are sufficient to elucidate and characterize adverse events that are more frequently occurring and those that are detected in short follow-ups. Thus, other uncommon, rare, and serious adverse events are increasingly gone undetected during the preauthorization phase of product development.

Post-authorization studies (PAS)—including post-authorization safety studies (PASS) and post-authorization effectiveness studies (PAES)—are intended to fill the knowledge gap about the safety and effectiveness of medicinal products in the postmarket setting; they are more commonly used to better delineate the benefit–risk profile of medicinal products during their life cycle. These studies are optimal for the detection and evaluation of adverse events that are uncommon, rare, and serious; those that occur after prolonged exposure; and those that increase in frequency and severity with time. Table 1.2 describes the categories of adverse events according to frequency of occurrence (CIOMS, 1999).

Using real-world data, PASS are studies conducted to evaluate the benefit–risk profile of medicinal products after marketing, which also provide support to regulatory decision-making. From regulatory standpoint, any study with safety

CONTENTS

Risk Management and Benefit–Risk Evaluation 4

Transparency 5

About This Book....6

References 7

1

Post-Authorization Safety Studies of Medicinal Products. https://doi.org/10.1016/B978-0-12-809217-0.00001-5

Table 1.1 Common Limitations of Preauthorization Studies

Component	Description
Objectives	Investigate the efficacy and characterize the most common adverse events of the medicinal product. Usually do not have safety objectives.
Size	Not of sufficient size to detect uncommon and rare adverse events of the medicinal product.
Target	Results are not generalizable to patients who will use the medicinal product in the usual health-care setting.
Setting	Highly controlled environment that may not reflect the real-world setting. Protocol-mandated treatment and testing, and scheduled patient visit with high patient adherence.
Duration	Short treatment duration that prevents the detection of adverse events with long latency periods.
Analyses	Focus on efficacy endpoints rather than safety.

Table 1.2 Frequency Categories of Adverse Events

Category	Frequency of Occurrence (%)
Very rare[a]	<0.01
Rare[a]	0.01 to <0.1
Uncommon (infrequent)[a]	0.1 to <1
Common (frequent)	1 to <10
Very common	≥10

[a]*Possible to be detected by post-authorization safety studies.*

objectives are considered PASS, which include those that aim to identify (i.e., signal detection), characterize (i.e., signal clarification), or quantify product-related risks (e.g., establish the likelihood of risk occurrence and investigate missing information); confirm the safety profile of medicinal products (i.e., signal evaluation); or measure the effectiveness of risk minimization activities (EMA, 2018). Additionally, PASS can speed up the marketing authorization process by being added as a conditional requirement for approval in the new MAA or can be required when the medicinal product is marketed and new questions about its safety arise. The main purpose of PASS is to establish the safety profile of medicinal products as early as possible in their life cycle.

PASS have gained much interest over the last decade, especially after the enactment of the European Pharmacovigilance Legislation in 2010 and subsequent implementation in 2012 (EMA, 2012a), which was described as the biggest change in the regulation of medicinal products in the European Union (EU) since early 1990s, as it added legal requirements for the planning and conduct of pharmacovigilance activities—including PASS by marketing authorization holders (MAH) (Engel et al., 2017). Regulatory guidelines have been developed to guide the design, implementation, and reporting of PASS in the EU, including the guideline on good pharmacovigilance practices (GVP) (EMA, 2012b), which includes a specific module on PASS (Module VIII) that highlights regulatory classifications, and format and content of study protocols and final study reports (EMA, 2012c, 2013; 2017).

The European Medicines Agency (EMA) and the United States Food and Drug Administration (FDA) use different nomenclatures to refer to safety studies that are voluntarily or mandatorily conducted by MAH in the postmarket setting. For the FDA, the Food and Drug Administration Amendments Act of 2007 may require MAH to conduct postmarketing studies to assess known serious risks or signals of serious risks related to the use of medicinal products or identify an unexpected serious risk when available data indicate that a potential for such risks exits (FDA, 2011). The FDA makes a distinction between postmarketing commitments (PMC) and postmarketing requirements (PMR). PMC are voluntary agreements between the FDA and the MAH to conduct studies; on the other hand, PMR are studies that are obligatory to be conducted by the MAH. Although all PASS in the pharmacovigilance plan are considered legally enforceable, the EU regulators classify them in three categories based on the expected impact of their results on the post-authorization benefit−risk evaluation (EMA, 2018). For imposed PASS (Category 1 and 2), noninterventional PASS have specific legislative requirements for the protocol submission and final results assessment, under the supervision of the EMA's Pharmacovigilance Risk Assessment Committee (PRAC). Although the protocol submission to the competent authority is not mandatory for required PASS (Category 3), unless specifically requested, the final study results are required to be submitted within the agreed due dates as variations to the marketing authorization. Furthermore, the EMA uses the term MAH or license holders for those companies responsible for the marketing of the medicinal product; the FDA uses the term sponsors and may use the term applicants for those responsible for conducting the PMR or PMC. Similarly, as the EMA uses the term post-authorization phase, the FDA uses the term postapproval to indicate the postmarketing phase in the life cycle of the product. In this book, we adopt terms that are used by the EU regulators.

Plans for PASS may be submitted with the original MAA or subsequently as a stand-alone submission. They can be part of the new application dossier and proposed by the MAH in support of the new application, may be required by the regulatory authority at the time of authorization of the product, or by post-authorization as new safety questions emerge. These can be related to any medicinal products intended for human use, including pharmaceuticals, biologics, vaccines, devices, and combination products.

RISK MANAGEMENT AND BENEFIT—RISK EVALUATION

Risk identification and assessment is key for successful planning of PASS. Data from multiple sources are evaluated to provide a list of safety concerns for the particular medicinal product. The safety concerns may be important identified risks, important potential risks, or areas of missing information that could impact patient treatment. These safety concerns form the basis for subsequent planning of PASS.

At the time of authorization, many risks of the medicinal products would have been identified as part of the assessment of the MAA. The ones deemed important for the benefit—risk balance of the products might require further characterization to confirm if they are real or not, or to establish their severity, frequency, and risk factors. Often such research takes form of PASS. In addition, PASS might also be able to identify new safety concerns, investigate missing information, or measure the effectiveness of risk minimization activities established for the products.

Risk management is an iterative process that involves the identification, characterization, evaluation, and minimization of risks associated with medicinal products. It also includes assessing the effectiveness of risk minimization activities. Some of these components have existed for many years—even if not being formally recognized as risk management—but the Pharmacovigilance Planning E2E guideline of the International Conference on Harmonization (ICH) provided a framework for pharmacovigilance planning, which encompassed the first three components (ICH, 2004). Risk minimization was not included in the ICH E2E guideline but is an essential part of maximizing benefit—risk balance of medicinal products both for the individual patient and for the target population as a whole.

In the context of the life cycle approach to risk management, risk minimization is aimed to prevent or reduce the probability of the occurrence of adverse events with the exposure to medicinal products or to reduce their severity should they occur. For all medicinal products, an EU risk management plan includes routine risk minimization measures (RMM), which are related to the summary of product characteristics, the package leaflet, the product labeling, the pack size, and the legal status of the product. However, for some products it may be necessary to implement additional RMM, such as educational programs for health-care professionals and patients. The impact of additional RMM requires careful assessment not only to ensure that their objectives are fulfilled but also to evaluate if the measures in place are proportionate or further improvement is warranted.

Benefit—risk evaluations take place throughout the product life cycle, and different stakeholders may have different views on some parts of any particular evaluation. There may also be the need to communicate benefit—risk evaluations outside of the immediate stakeholder audience to aid transparency over assumptions and decision-making. Benefit—risk evaluation frameworks have evolved over the last decade from purely descriptive to structured descriptive frameworks with some quantitative information, through to frameworks that are in essence fully quantitative assessments with some descriptive text. Apart from any regulatory requirements, MAH will use the increasing heterogeneity of patients in the post-authorization phase to perform PAES to identify "benefit factors," i.e., predictors of positive response to the medicinal products. This will enable targeted prescribing, which will increase the benefit—risk balance of the products, increase the likelihood that an individual patient will beneficially respond to the treatment, and increase value for payers. Safety objectives can be added to PAES making them classified as PASS from regulatory perspective.

TRANSPARENCY

Since 2010, the European Network of Centers for Pharmacoepidemiology and Pharmacovigilance (ENCePP) was set up with the aim of further strengthening the monitoring of medicinal products in Europe, by facilitating high-quality, independent studies, and if required, cooperation between centers for multi-center studies. One of the key concepts in promoting quality is transparency. The ENCePP provides a portal (the EU PAS Register) for the registration of PASS, including protocols and study results (ENCePP, 2018).

In contrast to clinical trials, the legal obligation to register noninterventional studies in the EU applies only to PASS imposed as an obligation by a regulatory authority (Category 1 and Category 2 PASS). The EU PAS Register has been developed with the aim of filling this obligation. Registration is also recommended in the GVP for all PASS. More generally, the EU PAS Register is open for registration of pharmacoepidemiologic studies—including clinical trials—regardless of whether they are initiated, managed, or sponsored by MAH, or whether they are conducted by research centers, and regardless of the countries where they are conducted. Registration of PASS can be done at any stage (i.e., from planning to completion). The EU PAS Register contains information on the study objectives; the main methodological aspects; administrative details, including study timelines and sources of funding; and associated key documents, including study protocols and study results where available. Yet, the availability of full-text protocols in the register is not satisfactory, and MAH and regulators can increase the availability of protocols and review results to assist in the improvement of the design and implementation of future PASS (only half of the protocols submitted to PRAC are registered, and nearly one-third of PRAC reviews to MAH are publically published) (Engel et al., 2017).

ABOUT THIS BOOK

PASS have become an important impetus to enhance the safety profile of newly launched products. Nonetheless, there are many challenges in study design, application, and interpretation of findings, and failure to apply good practice recommendations could yield misleading interpretations with potentially adverse impacts on individual patients and the public health. A recent review of PASS protocols submitted to the EU PAS Register showed that more than one-third of protocols evaluated by PRAC had design-related concerns (Engel et al., 2017), which reflects the need for more thoughtful PASS designs and analytics to ensure high-quality studies are being planned and implemented according to good practice guidelines in pharmacoepidemiology, pharmacovigilance, and outcomes research.

The value of real-world findings from PASS stem from the pharmacoepidemiologic principles applied in the choice of appropriate data sources, study designs, and analytical approaches. Well-designed and conducted PASS have increasingly important clinical, regulatory, and public health implications. There are many resources on methodological standards in product safety research, particularly Module VIII of GVP (EMA, 2017), and the ENCePP Guide on Methodological Standards in Pharmacoepidemiology (EMA, 2010). However, a PASS-specific textbook is not available.

Important considerations about the design, implementation, and interpretation of PASS are discussed in this book. We divided the book into seven main chapters following the introduction chapter. In Chapter 2, the risk management process is introduced, which includes chapters that describe the processes involved in risk assessment and different tools of risk minimization. It also shows how PASS are important for assessing the effectiveness of risk minimization activities. Data sources and study designs that are commonly used in PASS are discussed in Chapters 3 and 4, respectively. Corresponding chapters cover strengths, challenges, and applications of health insurance administrative claims; electronic medical records; registries; big data; social media; drug utilization studies; prescription event monitoring studies; self-controlled designs; cohorts; nested case–control designs; enriched studies; and prospective designs, including pragmatic trials.

Most important analytical approaches to account for confounding and bias in PASS are highlighted in Chapter 5, which discusses exposure propensity scores; disease risk scores; instrumental variables technique; and data standardization and analytic platforms. Such platforms bring together strong pharmacoepidemiologic designs, analyses, speed, and quality needed to plan and run PASS in support of effective clinical and regulatory decision-making using big, real-world data. Furthermore, the past decade has witnessed the proliferation of proactive safety surveillance systems built on electronic health-care data. Chapter 5 will also describe the current and future roles of these systems in PASS. The benefit—risk evaluation process in the context of PASS is introduced in Chapter 6 with special emphasis on benefit—risk evaluation frameworks and PAES.

The majority of PASS are planned for pharmaceutical products, but similar design and analysis concepts can be applied to other medicinal products. Thus, PASS for specialty products are discussed in Chapter 7, including chapters about biosimilars and interchangeable biologics; medical devices and combination products; and vaccines. Special considerations are given to aspects of biologics and biosimilars manufacturing and why they pose special challenges for safety assessments; exposure and outcome identification in medical device PASS; and for vaccine PASS, challenges around the variability in batches and the widespread use in healthy populations. Finally, as a means of promoting quality through transparency in the planning, implementation, and reporting of PASS, the EU PAS Register is introduced in Chapter 8.

The safe airplane is the one that stays on the ground, and the safe medicinal product is the one that stays in its original package! There are risks in taking medications, just as there are risks in flying; on the other hand, there are risks in not taking medications, just as there are risks in not using airplanes for transportation when needed. Whenever a medicinal product is given a risk is taken, but risk prevention and mitigation can be accomplished with the help of valid results from properly designed and conducted PASS. This textbook serves as source of information about methodological considerations for PASS, including data sources, study designs, and analytical approaches, which are commonly applied in pharmacoepidemiologic research.

References

Council for International Organizations of Medical Sciences (CIOMS), 1999. Guidelines for Preparing Core Clinical-Safety Information on Drugs. Report of CIOMS Working Groups III and V, second ed. Geneva, Switzerland.

The European Network of Centers for Pharmacoepidemiology and Pharmacovigilance (ENCePP), April 2018. The European Union Electronic Register of Post-Authorization Studies (EU PAS Register). Available from: http://www.encepp.eu/encepp_studies/indexRegister.shtml.

Engel, P., Almas, M.F., De Bruin, M.L., Starzyk, K., Blackburn, S., Dreyer, N.A., 2017. Lessons learned on the design and the conduct of Post-Authorization Safety Studies: review of 3 years of PRAC oversight. Br. J. Clin. Pharmacol. 83 (4), 884–893.

European Medicines Agency (EMA), 2010. The European Network of Centers for Pharmacoepidemiology and Pharmacovigilance (ENCePP). Guide on Methodological Standards in Pharmacoepidemiology (Revision 6). Available from: http://www.encepp.eu/standards_and_guidances/documents/ENCePPGuideofMethStandardsinPE_Rev6.pdf.

European Medicines Agency (EMA), 2012a. Implementation of the Pharmacovigilance Legislation. Available from: http://www.ema.europa.eu/ema/index.jsp?curl=pages/regulation/general/general_content_000520.jsp&mid=WC0b01ac05804fa031.

European Medicines Agency (EMA), 2012b. Good Pharmacovigilance Practices. Available from: http://www.ema.europa.eu/ema/index.jsp?curl=pages/regulation/document_listing/document_listing_000345.jsp&mid=WC0b01ac058058f32c.

European Medicines Agency (EMA), September 2012. Guidance for the Format and Content of the Protocol of Non-interventional Post-authorisation Safety Studies. Available from: http://www.ema.europa.eu/docs/en_GB/document_library/Other/2012/10/WC500133174.pdf.

European Medicines Agency (EMA), July 2013. Guidance for the Format and Content of the Final Study Report of Non-interventional Post-authorisation Safety Studies. Available from: http://www.ema.europa.eu/docs/en_GB/document_library/Regulatory_and_procedural_guideline/2013/01/WC500137939.pdf.

European Medicines Agency (EMA), October 2017. Guideline on Good Pharmacovigilance Practices (GVP). Module VIII-Post-authorisation Safety Studies (Rev 3). Available from: http://www.ema.europa.eu/docs/en_GB/document_library/Scientific_guideline/2012/06/WC500129137.pdf.

European Medicines Agency (EMA), 2018. Post-authorisation Safety Studies (PASS). Available from: http://www.ema.europa.eu/ema/index.jsp?curl=pages/regulation/document_listing/document_listing_000377.jsp&mid=WC0b01ac058066e979.

Food and Drug Administration (FDA), April 2011. Guidance for Industry: Postmarketing Studies and Clinical Trials—Implementation of Section 505(o)(3) of the Federal Food, Drug, and Cosmetic Act. Available from: https://www.fda.gov/downloads/Drugs/GuidanceComplianceRegulatoryInformation/Guidances/UCM172001.pdf.

International Conference on Harmonization (ICH), November 2004. ICH Harmonized Tripartite Guideline: Pharmacovigilance Planning E2E. Available from: https://www.ich.org/fileadmin/Public_Web_Site/ICH_Products/Guidelines/Efficacy/E2E/Step4/E2E_Guideline.pdf.

2

Risk Management Process

2.1 Risk Assessment 11
2.2 Risk Minimization 20

Risk Assessment

Emil Cochino

European Medicines Agency, London, United Kingdom

DISCLAIMER/ACKNOWLEDGMENTS

The views expressed in this chapter are the personal views of the author and may not be understood or quoted as being made on behalf of or reflecting the position of the European Medicines Agency or one of its committees or working parties.

INTRODUCTION

A medicinal product is authorized on the basis that in the specified indication(s), at the time of authorization, the benefit-risk balance is judged to be positive for the target population. Generally, a medicinal product will be associated with adverse reactions and these will vary in terms of severity, likelihood of occurrence, effect on individual patients, and public health impact. However, not all adverse reactions and risks will have been identified at the time when an initial marketing authorization is granted and some will only be discovered and characterized in the post-authorization phase. The aim of risk management plan (RMP) is to document the risk management system (RMS) considered necessary to identify, characterize, and minimize the important risks of a medicinal product. The RMP contains safety specification, pharmacovigilance plan, and Risk Minimization Plan (RMiP). As knowledge regarding the safety profile of a medicinal product increases over time, so will the RMP change.

For medicinal products applying for a marketing authorization in the European Union (EU), either nationally or centralized, the applicants are required to submit for assessment and approval of an RMP describing the RMS, together with a summary thereof (European Commission, 2001). The content and format requirements for the European Union risk management plan are further detailed in the EU legislation (European Commission, 2010, 2012). The European

CONTENTS

Disclaimer/ Acknowledg ments 11

Introduction 11

Safety Specification 13

Pharmacovigilance Plan 14
Routine Pharmacovigilance Activities 15
Additional Pharmacovigilance Activities 16

References 18

Post-Authorization Safety Studies of Medicinal Products. https://doi.org/10.1016/B978-0-12-809217-0.00002-7

Medicines Agency (EMA) drafted and published in 2012 and updated in 2017 the good pharmacovigilance practices Module V—RMS and the RMP template (EMA, 2017a,b), a set of guideline documents describing the risk management requirements for applicants and Marketing Authorization Holders (MAH), and provision for submission and assessment of RMP to/by EU regulatory agencies.

The safety information for a new medicinal product is described in the application dossier submitted by the MAH to the EMA (for centrally authorized products) or to the national competent authorities (for medicinal products approved through national, decentralized, or mutual recognition procedures) (European Commission, 2016). The safety data are assessed by the competent authority as part of the initial marketing authorization application procedure, and the risks of the product are assessed and put into context of the benefits. The identified risks of the product would therefore be included in the product information to be communicated to health-care professionals, patients, and consumers. The RMP further describes and documents the risks that are considered important for the benefit-risk balance of the product. Additionally, the RMP proposed measures to further characterize, minimize, or manage the risks that are likely to have the greatest impact on the product's use post-authorization.

Although the RMP includes all the identified risks of the medicinal product that are undesirable clinical outcomes and for which there is sufficient evidence that they are caused by the product, the focus of the document is on important identified risks that are likely to have an impact on the benefit-risk balance of the product. Similarly, for potential risks, the RMP focuses on those that, when further characterized and if confirmed, would have an impact on the benefit-risk balance of the medicinal product. The important identified and important potential risks would therefore warrant further evaluation as part of the pharmacovigilance plan (such as post-authorization safety studies [PASS] investigating the frequency, severity, seriousness, and outcome of the risks under normal conditions of use) or risk minimization activities.

In addition to the risks of the product, the RMP also describes the missing information—gaps in knowledge about the safety of a medicinal product for certain anticipated utilization or for use in particular patient population, for which there is insufficient product exposure to determine whether the safety profile differs from that characterized so far. Missing information safety concerns would also warrant pharmacovigilance activities, most often in the form of PASS, such as drug utilization studies (see Chapter 4.1 for details).

The RMP structure requirements are described in the EU legislation (European Commission, 2012). The three main parts mirror the essential activities in risk management: safety specification (Part II), pharmacovigilance plan (Part III), and RMiP (Part V) (Table 2.1.1). The content requirements for the RMP are risk-proportionate. The safety specification of a medicinal product containing

Table 2.1.1 Components of the European Risk Management Plan

Component	Description
Safety specification	The identification or characterization of the safety profile of the medicinal product, with emphasis on important identified and important potential risks and missing information, and also on which safety concerns need to be managed proactively or require further studies (e.g., PASS).
Pharmacovigilance plan	The planning of pharmacovigilance activities to characterize and quantify clinically relevant risks and to identify new adverse reactions.
Risk minimization plan	The planning and implementation of risk minimization measures, including the evaluation of the effectiveness of these activities.

a new active substance will include more information than one of a generic or hybrid product, as the uncertainty is greater at the approval of the first product containing an active substance. However, the list of safety concerns is determined by the risks associated with the substance or to the specifics of each product. Similarly, equal requirements apply for the post-authorization pharmacovigilance activities and risk minimization activities reflect the safety profile of the products and for common risks. The RMiP includes a detailed description for routine and additional risk minimization activities that are required to prevent, reduce, or mitigate the risks associated with the safety concerns included in the RMP. Further details on these activities are provided in Chapter 2.2.

SAFETY SPECIFICATION

The purpose of the safety specification is to provide an adequate discussion on the safety profile of the medicinal product, with focus on those aspects that need further risk management activities. It includes a summary of the important identified risks, important potential risks, and missing information. It also addresses the populations potentially at risk (where the product is likely to be used, both as authorized and off-label), and any outstanding safety questions that warrant further investigation to refine the understanding of the benefit-risk balance during the post-authorization period. The safety specification forms the basis for the pharmacovigilance plan and the RMiP. It consists of eight modules, of which RMP Modules SI–SV, SVII, and SVIII correspond to safety specification headings in the International Conference on Harmonization (ICH) Guideline on Pharmacovigilance Planning (E2E) (ICH, 2004). RMP Module SVI includes additional elements required to be submitted in the EU (Table 2.1.2).

Table 2.1.2 Components of the Safety Specification Part of the European Risk Management Plan

Component	Description
Epidemiology of the indication(s) and target population	Includes data relevant for the identification of the safety concerns related to the incidence, prevalence, and the natural history of the disease, demographics of the target population, including comorbidities and comedications, and existing treatment options.
Nonclinical data	Presents a high-level summary of the significant nonclinical safety findings related to toxicity, safety pharmacology, and drug interactions.
Clinical trial exposure	Includes summary information on the clinical trial exposure useful to assess the size and the limitations of the human safety database.
Populations not studied in clinical trials	Aims at identifying populations understudied in clinical trials, to evaluate if there is a scientific rationale for anticipating a different safety profile in the particular population/use.
Post-authorization experience	Relevant for postmarketing RMP updates, provides an overview of exposure in the post-authorization phase, to estimate the size of the safety database following the marketing of the product.
Additional EU requirements for safety specification	Presents the potential for misuse for illegal purposes and the measures needed to prevent or limit such occurrence.
Identified and potential risks	Describes the criteria used to identify important risks and provides a detailed presentation of the safety concerns. • For important risks, this includes potential mechanisms, evidence source and strength of evidence, characterization of the risk, risk factors and risk groups, preventability, impact on the benefit-risk balance of the product, and the public health impact. • For missing information, this includes evidence source, population in need for further characterization, and the anticipated risk/consequence of the missing information.
Summary of the safety concerns	Presents in tabular format the list of safety concerns for the product.

PHARMACOVIGILANCE PLAN

The purpose of the RMP pharmacovigilance plan is to discuss how the safety concerns will be further characterized by postmarketing and present an overview of activities. It provides a structured plan for the investigation of whether a potential risk is confirmed as an identified risk or refuted; further characterization of safety concerns, including severity, frequency, and risk factors; how missing information will be sought; and measuring the effectiveness of risk minimization measures. For a medicinal product approved in the EU, the RMS includes routine pharmacovigilance activities and, when warranted, additional pharmacovigilance activities, such as PASS.

Routine Pharmacovigilance Activities

Routine pharmacovigilance activities include for all products safety signal detection and adverse reaction reporting; although these two types of activities are not described in the RMP, as they are detailed in the pharmacovigilance system master file, they constitute essential tools for monitoring the safety profile of the product in postmarketing use. The requirements for signal management and adverse event reports management and reporting are described in EMA and ICH guidelines (EMA, 2012, 2014; ICH, 1994, 2003).

Signal management includes a set of activities performed to determine whether (based on an examination of individual case safety reports, aggregated data from proactive surveillance systems or studies, literature information, or other sources) there are new risks associated with a medicinal product or whether its known risks have changed. The steps for signal management are presented in Fig. 2.1.1. The impact of the risks identified during signal detection activities on the product benefit-risk balance will determine if they should be considered important and added in the RMP of the product and if a regulatory request for an RMP update will be part of the outcome recommendation. Routine pharmacovigilance activities that are described in the RMP include specific adverse reaction follow-up questionnaires that are used by the MAH to obtain structured information on reported suspected adverse reactions of special interest. They are usually sent to the reporter of the adverse reaction (such as health-care professionals or patients) to ask to provide information on the circumstances of the event, including data on the patient, disease, the severity and resolution of the event, and other potential factors that might have contributed to the occurrence of the event. Other routine activities are required for certain type of products (such as enhanced passive surveillance systems for seasonal influenza vaccines) or to investigate a safety

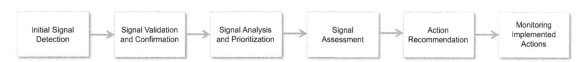

FIGURE 2.1.1
Signal management steps.

concern (using disproportionality analyses and cumulative reviews of adverse events of interest).

Additional Pharmacovigilance Activities

Additional pharmacovigilance activities are the focus of the pharmacovigilance plan in the RMP. They may include nonclinical studies, clinical trials, or non-interventional studies. In the EU, PASS is defined in the legislation as any study relating to an authorized medicinal product conducted with the aim of identifying, characterizing, or quantifying a safety hazard, or confirming the safety profile of the medicinal product or of measuring the effectiveness of risk minimization measures (European Commission, 2001). The EMA provides extensive guidance on conducting PASS, including the recommendations for study registration in the European Union post-authorization study Register (see Chapter 8 for more information), study protocol format and content, reporting to competent authorities, publication, data protection, quality systems, and the operation of the EU network regarding PASS approval, conduct, and assessment (EMA, 2016; ENCePP, 2017).

Depending on the type of marketing authorization application, most of the RMP modules and sections might have a reduced content or even omitted entirely (e.g., for generic applications, only the list of safety concerns needs to be included in the safety specification), the pharmacovigilance plan is always required in the RMP and should contain a discussion on the need of PASS. Important potential risks in the RMP are expected to lead to the conduct of PASS to further characterize the risks; important identified risks might also require PASS to measure the risks when the product is used outside the confines of clinical trials.

At the time of market authorization, the RMP would include a detailed justification on why PASS are needed, together with a short description of the study. The summary table of additional pharmacovigilance activities in the RMP includes the PASS name, objectives, safety concerns addressed, and milestones for reporting to competent authorities with due dates (e.g., interim reports, final clinical study reports). If available, the study protocols are assessed as part of the initial marketing authorization application and included in the RMP Annex 3. If protocols are not available in pre-authorization, they would be routinely submitted for assessment after approval but before the PASS start. Although all PASS in the pharmacovigilance plan are considered legally enforceable, the EU regulators classify them in three categories based on the expected impact of their results on the post-authorization benefit-risk balance evaluation (Table 2.1.3). For imposed PASS (Category 1 and 2), noninterventional PASS have specific legislative requirements for the protocol submission

Table 2.1.3 Regulatory Classification of Post-Authorization Safety Studies (PASS) in the European Union

Category	Class	Description
Category 1	Imposed PASS	Conditions to the marketing authorization holder because they are key to the benefit-risk profile of the medicinal product.
Category 2	Imposed PASS	Conditions to the marketing authorization holder because they are specific obligations in the context of a conditional marketing authorization or a marketing authorization under exceptional circumstances.
Category 3	Required PASS	Considered important for the benefit-risk evaluation.

and final results assessment, under the supervision of the EMA's Pharmacovigilance Risk Assessment Committee , regardless of route of authorization (European Commission, 2001, 2016). Although the protocol submission to the competent authority is not mandatory for required PASS (Category 3), unless specifically requested, the final study results are required to be submitted within the agreed due dates as variations to the marketing authorization.

With the exception of some patient registries, it is expected that over time the PASS will be completed and thus removed from the RMP. The results of the PASS in the RMP pharmacovigilance plan are expected to influence the safety profile of the product and lead to changes in the list of safety concerns. It may be that important identified or potential risks can be removed from the safety specification in the RMP. For example, when results of well-conducted PASS do not support the initial supposition or when the impact to the individual patient has been shown to be less than anticipated, resulting in the potential risk not being considered important. Equally, it may be that important potential risks need to be reclassified to important identified risks. For example, if scientific and clinical data strengthen the association between the risk and the product.

Given the overall aim of obtaining more information regarding the benefit-risk balance in certain patient populations excluded in the pre-authorization phase, it is expected that as the product matures, the classification as missing information might not be appropriate anymore once data from PASS become available, or when there is no reasonable expectation that the existing or future feasible pharmacovigilance activities could further characterize the safety profile of the product with respect to the areas of missing information.

Additionally, Part IV of the RMP presents briefly the plans for post-authorization effectiveness studies (PAES) required by regulators to assess efficacy or effectiveness concerns. Most of the PAES will also have safety component, but their assignment as PASS or PAES would be determined by the primary reason why the study is required by regulators. Chapter 6.1 discusses PAES with detail.

References

EMA, 2012. Guideline on Good Pharmacovigilance Practices (GVP) - Module IX — Signal Management. Available on EMA website at: http://www.ema.europa.eu/docs/en_GB/document_library/Scientific_guideline/2012/06/WC500129138.pdf.

EMA, 2014. Guideline on Good Pharmacovigilance Practices (GVP) Module VI — Management and Reporting of Adverse Reactions to Medicinal Products (Rev 1). Available on EMA website at: http://www.ema.europa.eu/docs/en_GB/document_library/Scientific_guideline/2014/09/WC500172402.pdf.

EMA, 2016. Guideline on Good Pharmacovigilance Practices (GVP) Module VIII — Post-authorisation Safety Studies (Rev 2). Available on EMA website at: http://www.ema.europa.eu/docs/en_GB/document_library/Scientific_guideline/2012/06/WC500129137.pdf.

EMA, 2017a. Guideline on Good Pharmacovigilance Practices: Module V — Risk Management Systems (Rev 2). Available on EMA website at: http://www.ema.europa.eu/ema/index.jsp?curl=pages/regulation/document_listing/document_listing_000345.jsp.

EMA, 2017b. Guidance on Format of the Risk-management Plan in the European Union (Rev.2) — in Integrated Format, Referred to as "RMP Template". Available on EMA website at: http://www.ema.europa.eu/ema/index.jsp?curl=pages/regulation/document_listing/document_listing_000360.jsp&mid=WC0b01ac058067a113.

ENCePP (2017) — European Network of Centres for Pharmacoepidemiology and Pharmacovigilance: The European Union electronic Register of Post-Authorisation Studies (EU PAS Register) can be Accessed at http://www.encepp.eu/encepp/studiesDatabase.jsp.

European Commission, 2001. Directive 2001/83/EC of the European Parliament and of the Council of 6 November 2001 on the Community Code Relating to Medicinal Products for Human Use. Available at: http://ec.europa.eu/health/files/eudralex/vol-1/dir_2001_83_cons/dir2001_83_cons_20081230_en.pdf.

European Commission, 2010. Regulation (EU) No 1235/2010 of the European Parliament and of the Council of 15 December 2010 Amending, as Regards Pharmacovigilance of Medicinal Products for Human Use, Regulation (EC) No 726/2004 Laying Down Community Procedures for the Authorisation and Supervision of Medicinal Products for Human and Veterinary Use and Establishing a European Medicines Agency, and Regulation (EC) No 1394/2007 on Advanced Therapy Medicinal Products [Online]. Available from: http://eur-lex.europa.eu/LexUriServ/LexUriServ.do?uri=OJ:L:2010:348:0001:0016:EN:PDF.

European Commission, 2012. Implementing Regulation (EU) No 520/2012 of 19 June 2012 on the Performance of Pharmacovigilance Activities provided for in Regulation (EC) No 726/2004 of the European Parliament and of the Council and Directive 2001/83/EC of the European Parliament and of the Council. Available from: http://ec.europa.eu/health//sites/health/files/files/eudralex/vol-1/reg_2012_520/reg_2012_520_en.pdf.

European Commission, 2016. EudraLex - Volume 2-Pharmaceutical Legislation on Notice to Applicants and Regulatory Guidelines for Medicinal Products for Human Use. Available at: http://ec.europa.eu/health/documents/eudralex/vol-2_en.

ICH, 1994. Harmonised Tripartite Guideline Clinical Safety Data Management: Definitions and Standards for Expedited Reporting E2A. Available at: http://www.ich.org/fileadmin/Public_Web_Site/ICH_Products/Guidelines/Efficacy/E2A/Step4/E2A_Guideline.pdf.

ICH, 2003. Harmonised Tripartite Guideline Post-Approval Safety Data Management: Definitions and Standards for Expedited Reporting E2D. Available at: http://www.ich.org/fileadmin/Public_Web_Site/ICH_Products/Guidelines/Efficacy/E2D/Step4/E2D_Guideline.pdf.

ICH, 2004. Harmonised Tripartite Guideline Pharmacovigilance Planning E2E. Available at: http://www.ich.org/fileadmin/Public_Web_Site/ICH_Products/Guidelines/Efficacy/E2E/Step4/E2E_Guideline.pdf.

Risk Minimization

Giampiero Mazzaglia[1], Sabine Straus[2]

[1]*European Medicines Agency, London, United Kingdom;* [2]*Medicines Evaluation Board, Utrecht, The Netherlands*

CONTENTS

Disclaimer/
Acknowledg
ments 20

Introduction 20

Risk Minimization
Methods 22
*Routine Risk
Minimization* 23
*Additional Risk
Minimization* 27
*Tools for Additional Risk
Minimization* 27

Effectiveness of Risk
Minimization 32
*Models for Risk
Minimization Evaluation
Post-Authorization
Safety Studies* 33
*Risk Minimization Tool
Coverage, Awareness,
and Usage* 35
*Risk Knowledge/
Comprehension* 36
Behavioral Modification .. 37
Safety Outcomes 41

References 42

DISCLAIMER/ACKNOWLEDGMENTS

The views expressed in this chapter are the personal views of the authors and may not be understood or quoted as being made on behalf of or reflecting the position of the European Medicines Agency or one of its committees or working parties.

INTRODUCTION

Knowledge of the full benefit-risk balance of a medicinal product is limited at the time of licensing and can change after approval. This is a consequence of the inherent limitations of pre-authorization clinical trials, such as the relatively homogeneous population to maximize the discriminatory power of drug effects and the limited size and duration for detecting potentially rare but serious adverse events in real-world patients (Singh and Loke, 2012; Vandenbroucke and Psaty, 2008). Therefore, benefits and risks need to be evaluated during the entire product life cycle because, when the product is marketed, the exposed population increases and becomes more heterogeneous with potential diminishing responsiveness to the beneficial effects and increasing likelihood to detect adverse drug effects (Eichler et al., 2011).

Risk management aims to ensure that the benefits of the product outweigh the risk by the greatest possible margin during the whole product life cycle. Definitions of risk management have been provided in the European Union (EU) and US regulatory guidelines (EMA, 2012a; FDA, 2005, 2009). In spite of the differences in wording, both definitions reflect the interrelated and reiterated nature of the risk management, which consists of the steps outlined in Table 2.2.1.

Risk quantification and characterization are fundamental pillars for risk management planning, but the final goal of risk management is to ensure

Table 2.2.1 Risk Management Steps

Step	Description
Risk quantification	The identification of the safety profile of the product is based on the current available data. The risk included in the RMP could have an impact on the benefit-risk balance of the product when further characterized and/or if not managed appropriately in daily clinical practice, thus requiring risk characterization and/or minimization.
Risk characterization	The planning of pharmacovigilance activities (routine and additional) to characterize known risks, to identify new risks, and to increase the knowledge in general about the safety profile of the product.
Risk minimization/ mitigation	The planning and implementing activities aimed to reduce the probability or severity of an adverse reaction associated with the exposure to a product or to reduce its severity should it occur.
Effectiveness evaluation	The planning of additional pharmacovigilance activities to assess whether risk minimization/mitigation measures address the risks of the product sufficiently to maintain positive benefit-risk profile.

minimization or mitigation of risks, if needed. Therefore, appropriate planning to risk minimization/mitigation allows for products with considerable risk to be approved and maintained into the market. There are several examples of medicinal products, which received marketing authorization or were maintained into the market because of effective risk minimization planning in spite of their high-risk profile (Box 2.2.1 illustrates the example of risk minimization measures for strontium ranelate, indicated for severe osteoporosis).

A modern concept for risk management planning was introduced in 2004 with the guideline "Pharmacovigilance Planning—E2E" developed by the International Conference on Harmonization, which represented the basis for the future guidance both in the United States and the EU (ICH, 2004). In 2005, the US-FDA released guidance for industry on the "Development and Use of Risk Minimization Action Plan (RiskMAPs)" specifically focused for products with borderline benefit-risk balance (FDA, 2005). Later on, the 2007 FDA Amendments Act gave the FDA authority to require postmarketing studies and Risk Evaluation and Mitigation Strategies (REMS) to ensure that benefits of products outweighed their risks. Therefore, REMS replaced RiskMAPs as main US strategy for additional risk minimization. A detailed guidance for industry: "Format and Content of Proposed REMS, REMS Assessments, and Proposed REMS Modifications" was issued in 2009 with further details on distribution requirements and inclusion in REMS being published in 2011 (FDA, 2009, 2011a).

BOX 2.2.1 CARDIOVASCULAR RISK MINIMIZATION MEASURES FOR STRONIUM RANELATE (EMA, 2014C)

In April 2013, the PRAC had recommended restricting the use of strontium ranelate, authorized in the EU to treat severe osteoporosis because of a concern raised during a routine benefit-risk assessment regarding cardiovascular safety beyond the already recognized risk for venous thromboembolism. New risk minimization measures were therefore introduced consisting in contraindications for patients with high risk for ischemic cardiac disorders, recommendation for monitoring the cardiovascular risk factors during the long-term treatment with strontium ranelate, and restrictions of the indication.

Following further in-depth evaluation of the benefits and risks of products containing strontium ranelate, in January 2014 the PRAC recommended the suspension of the marketing authorizations for strontium ranelate, on the basis of serious concerns about whether the contraindications and warnings implemented to mitigate cardiac and thromboembolic risks could have been achievable in clinical practice (considering that strontium ranelate is intended for long-term treatment of a population of elderly patients whose cardiovascular status may deteriorate over time).

The Committee for Medicinal Products for Human Use , which has the final opinion on the benefit-risk assessment of a medicinal product in the EU, considered feasible for practicing physicians to monitor the cardiovascular risk as they mainly rely on accessible information (such as family and patient history, smoking status, body mass index, waist circumference, and blood pressure) and commonly investigated laboratory values (such as blood glucose and lipids) and confirmed the positive benefit-risk balance.

To address the PRAC concern that cardiovascular risk may increase considerably over time in the predominantly elderly target population, the marketing authorization holder proposed regular assessment of the patients' cardiovascular risk and introduced, to support this activity, aRMM, such as a prescribers' checklist and a patient alert card.

In the EU, the first legal requirement for a detailed description of the risk management system, as part of the authorization dossier of innovative drugs, referred to Directive 2001/83/EC and Regulation N. 726/2004 followed up by the release of the "Guideline on Risk Management Systems for Medicinal Products for Human Use" in November 2005 (EMA, 2005). Another key document issued in 2008, the "Guidelines on Pharmacovigilance for Medicinal Products for Human Use (Volume 9A)" was replaced following the revised Pharmacovigilance Legislation implemented in July 2012 by the good pharmacovigilance practices (GVP) guidelines (EC, 2008, 2010). These guidelines are a set of measures drawn up to facilitate the performance of pharmacovigilance in the EU. A focus on risk minimization can be found in the EU GVP Module V and the GVP Module XVI (EMA, 2012a, 2014a).

RISK MINIMIZATION METHODS

The current sets of FDA and European Medicines Agency (EMA) guidance are driven by similar objectives for the identification, monitoring, and minimization of risk to patient safety. They reflect the cultural shift from reactive, process-based risk management to a proactive approach for risk prevention. Rather than waiting for an adverse reaction to occur and then determining a risk minimization, the new approach aims to define strategies to anticipate and detect new adverse reactions as early as possible and identify measures to minimize the possible clinical impact. As a result, risk minimization measures frequently lead to the generation of similar data needs and conceptually similar risk minimization tools in both regions. However, the EU GVP makes the EU RMP mandatory for all newly licensed products, and the different risk minimization tools are classified into routine and additional risk minimization measures (aRMM) (EMA, 2012a), whereas in the United States, the REMS is requested on a case-by-case basis and the principles behind the EU routine risk minimization are not generally applied (Table 2.2.2).

Routine Risk Minimization

Routine risk minimization involves those activities that apply to every medicinal product, including product information, labeling, product pack design and size, and legal status (EMA, 2012a).

A key component in routine risk minimization measures consists of the product information, which describes a medicinal product based on its chemical, pharmaceutical, and pharmacologic properties, defines indications and contraindications, and communicates information about the risks. The product information is an important document at the time of the marketing authorization because it forms the basis for all other communications about the medicinal product. Revisions of the product information can be implemented in the post-authorization phase as a result of new information. Regulatory authorities use different label formats to convey product information. In the United States, the FDA uses the United States Package Insert (USPI) targeted to health-care professionals (HCP) (FDA, 2013a, 2016a), whereas in the EU, the EMA uses the Summary of Product Characteristics (SmPC) targeted to HCP and the patient information leaflet targeted to patients/caregivers (EC, 2009). In the United States, printed patient information such as the Patient Package Insert (PPI) and Medication Guides is not required for all FDA-approved medicinal products; therefore, they are part of REMS and should not be viewed as routine risk minimization measures.

There are some structural differences between the USPI and the SmPC, in particular the order of the information provided and the presentation of the adverse reactions. However, the most relevant safety concerns are communicated in the contraindication section (USPI section 4; SmPC section 4.3) and in the warning and precaution section (USPI section 5; SmPC section 4.4). Warning and precaution section provides information on special patient groups that are at increased risk of experiencing an adverse reaction, any need for specific clinical or laboratory monitoring and any measure to identify patients at risk and prevent the occurrence, or detect the early onset or worsening of adverse reactions, including instructions to manage them. The

Table 2.2.2 The European Medicines Agency (EMA) and FDA Regulatory Tools for Risk Minimization

Risk Minimization Tool	EU-EMA	US-FDA
Routine Risk Minimization		
Product information	• Summary of product characteristics • Patient information leaflet	• United States package insert • Medication guide (targeted to patients)[a] • Patient package insert[a]
Other basic requirements	• Labeling • Pack size • Legal status	• Container label[b] • Carton labeling design[b] • Prescription status[b]
Additional Risk Minimization		
Educational material	• Prescribing/dispensing guides and brochures • Prescriber checklist • Training material • Patient diaries • Patient alert card	• Medication guide[c] • Training material • Reminder system
Communication plan	• Direct health-care professional communication • Other modalities of communication and implementation	• Dear health-care professional letter • Dissemination strategies • Communication tools
Controlled access systems	• Prescriber checklists • Enrollment forms (mandatory) • Patient informed consent • Mandatory screening/monitoring • Controlled dispensing/distribution • Registries • Pregnancy prevention program[d]	• Elements to assure safe use, which may include any or all tools and process intended to mitigate specific serious risks as used in the EU

[a]Not standard measures for all medicinal products and they cannot be considered routine risk minimization tools. A guidance issued in 2011 clarified FDA's authority to require medication guides independent of REMS (FDA, 2011a).
[b]Regulated in FDA guidance on safety consideration to minimize medication errors (FDA, 2013b) and criteria for application of nonprescription (over-the-counter) drugs (FDA, 2002; Brass, 2001). They are considered element to promote safe product dispensing, administration, and use.
[c]Optional requirement for product approved with REMS; can be targeted to both health-care providers and patients and it is provided in addition, to general information sheets for patients.
[d]Combines educational programs with elements of controlled access systems.

therapeutic indication (USPI section 1; SmPC section 4.1) may mitigate the risk by restricting the target population, whereas there are other sections intended to communicate certain types of safety concerns, such as pregnancy issues (USPI section 8.1; SmPC section 4.6) and drug interactions (USPI section 7; SmPC section 4.5). The section pertained to the adverse reactions communicates to HCP, all side effects of the medicinal product, including those considered a lowest priority for risk minimization, so that an informed decision on the treatment can be made.

Labeling and pack design ensure that the critical information necessary for the safe use of a medicine is legible, accessible, and that users of medicines can easily assimilate this information so that any risk of confusion and error is minimized. A relevant example of the importance of appropriate labeling and pack design is provided in the guidance on "Risk Minimization Strategy for High Strength and Fixed Combination Insulin Products" issued by the EMA in 2015 (EMA, 2015a). The guidance was the results of concerns expressed by the Pharmacovigilance Risk Assessment Committee (PRAC) about the potential risk of medication errors associated with the use of high-strength insulins, particularly the mix-up between long-acting (basal) and short-acting (bolus) insulins, and the mix-up between different product strengths. To address these concerns, the following recommendations have been set up in the guidance: (1) the need for a prominent display of the name of the products, active ingredient, and its strength (e.g., sufficient large font, colors chosen to ensure good contrast between the text and the background to ensure maximum legibility, and use of formatting to distinguish products with similar sounding active substance); (2) the need to add and enhance design features to optimally distinguish the new product from others; and (3) the need to use different colors on the labels and also on the devices to clearly distinguish between insulins/strengths and to draw attention to specific information on the label, particularly to enhance recognition of the high strength.

Because every pack size is specifically authorized for a medicinal product, planning the number of dosage units within each pack and the range of pack sizes available can be considered a form of routine risk minimization. Controlling the number of dosage units should also mean that patients will need to see HCP at defined intervals, thus increasing the opportunity for monitoring patient status and compliance to recommended treatments. This measure can be very effective, as demonstrated by the reduction of death due to paracetamol poisoning following the introduction of legislation in England and Wales to restrict pack sizes of products containing paracetamol (Hawton et al., 2013), or the reduction of cases of severe liver injuries following the withdrawal in the EU of all packs containing more than 30 doses of nimesulide products, along with restrictions of the therapeutic indication and limitation of the duration of treatment (EMA, 2012b).

In the EU, the legal status of the medicinal product typically includes information on whether or not the product is subject to medicinal prescription or not. Article 71(1) of EU Directive 2001/83/EC (EC, 2001) states that medicinal products shall be subjected to medical prescription where they (1) are likely to present a danger either directly or indirectly, even when used correctly, if utilized without medical supervision; (2) are frequently and to a very wide extent used incorrectly and as a result are likely to present a direct or indirect danger to human health; (3) contain substances or preparations thereof, the activity and/ or adverse reactions of which require further investigation; or (4) are normally prescribed by a prescriber to be administered parenterally. In the United States, the Durham–Humphrey and Kefauver–Harris Amendments to the Food, Drug, and Cosmetic Act of 1938 define criteria to be used by the FDA in evaluating a new drug application and its classification as prescription only medicine (POM) or over-the-counter (OTC) drug. These amendments require the review of both POM and OTC drugs, thus mandating evidence that an OTC product is safe and effective when used without supervision by HCP (Brass, 2001). Despite these conditions are generally set up during the marketing application, changes might also occur as a result of emerging safety issues. For example, in 2014 the PRAC recommended changes in the use of domperidone-containing products by restricting their use only to relieve symptoms of nausea and vomiting and reducing dose and duration (EMA, 2014b). The review of domperidone was carried out at the request of the Belgian medicines authority over concerns about the product's cardiovascular adverse effects, including QT prolongation and arrhythmias. As a result of this review, several EU countries changed the legal status of domperidone from OTC to POM.

For POM, the EU legislation provides additional conditions that may be imposed by classifying them into those available only on either a restricted medical prescription or a special medical prescription. Medicinal products are subjected to *restricted medical prescription* where they are (1) reserved for treatments that can only be followed in a hospital environment because of its pharmaceutical characteristics or novelty or in the interests of public health; (2) used in the treatment of conditions that must be diagnosed in a hospital environment or in institutions with adequate diagnostic facilities, although administration and follow-up may be carried out elsewhere; or (3) intended for outpatients but its use may produce very serious adverse reactions requiring a prescription drawn up as required by a specialist and special supervision throughout the treatment. On the other hand, medicinal products are subjected to *special medical prescription* where the product (1) contains, in a nonexempt quantity, a substance classified as a narcotic or a psychotropic substance; or (2) is likely, if incorrectly used, to present a substantial risk of medicinal abuse, to lead to addition or be misused for illegal purposes.

Additional Risk Minimization

Safety concerns of a medicinal product are normally adequately addressed by routine risk minimization measures. However, for some drugs, routine measures might not be sufficient and it may be necessary to implement aRMM, such as educational programs for HCP and/or patients, targeted communication, or restrictive systems for drug dispensing/prescribing. These extra measures aim to maintain a positive benefit-risk profile, for example, by early recognition of adverse drug reactions, targeted patient selection or exclusion, and through treatment management (e.g., specific drug preparation and administration, relevant testing, and patient follow-up). These measures are referred to as aRMM in the EU and REMS in the United States (Table 2.2.2).

The decision to implement aRMM/REMS and the choice of appropriate tools are important because additional measures are likely to have major impact on HCP and patients. Successful implementation of aRMM is not always straightforward and requires contributions from all involved stakeholders, including patients, HCP, regulatory authorities, and pharmaceutical companies. Regulatory guidelines do not provide clear criteria or recognized algorithms to establish when additional risk minimization is warranted and what tools are best suited (EMA, 2014a; FDA, 2005, 2009). However, accurate recognition of important risks that need to be minimized is the basic starting point, and prioritization of safety concerns should take into account frequency, seriousness, severity, impact on public health, and preventability. Careful consideration should also be given to whether the goal can be reached with routine minimization activities only, and, if not considered feasible, which additional minimization tools are the most appropriate. Risk minimization tools should be designed to fit within an existing applicable regulatory and legal framework, patient care environment, and health-care system. In addition, the burden of imposing additional risk minimization on stakeholders and the health-care system should be balanced with the expected reduction of the frequency and/or severity of the targeted risks.

Tools for Additional Risk Minimization

There is a wide selection of risk minimization tools that can be chosen to ensure the safe and effective use of a medicinal product beyond routine risk minimization. The GVP Module XVI offers different approaches and several tools can be grouped together as a single aRMM (EMA, 2014a). An REMS submission is generally structured in two parts: a proposed REMS document and REMS supporting documents, which provide additional detailed information (FDA, 2009). Both parts include a medication guide, a communication plan, the elements to assure safe use (ETASU), and an implementation system, with the main difference being the level of details provided in the content. Like in the EU, even REMS programs do not necessarily contain all the possible tools to address a specific safety concern, and a combination of elements is possible. An analysis of the information provided in the FDA website indicates that, by August 2016, of 75 FDA-approved REMS, medication guides were included in 36 cases (48%), communication plan in 26 cases (34.6%), ETASU in 42 cases (56%), and implementation system in 37 cases (49.3%). A combination of the different elements was proposed in 45 cases (60%) (FDA, 2016b).

In spite of the differences between the EU aRMM and the US REMS, there are common features that allow a classification of the risk minimization tools into the following broad categories: educational programs and controlled access systems.

Educational Programs

An educational program is a system consisting of educational materials and targeted communication aimed to provide information that is not sufficiently covered in the product information. They should therefore be developed on the premise that applying this measure is considered essential for minimizing an important risk; they can convey information/recommendations on how to prevent and/or minimize the risk; and risk minimization recommendations are actionable for the targeted stakeholders.

Educational materials can have several different target audiences (e.g., HCP, patients and/or their caregivers, or laboratories) and can address more than one safety concern. In the EU, the need for an educational material, its key elements, and the targeted population is agreed at central level, whereas detailed implementation, including communication and delivery plans, is generally subject to an agreement between the marketing authorization holder and the national competent authority (EMA, 2015b). This is because it is acknowledged there could be relevant differences on how educational tools could be incorporated most easily and effectively into the different health-care systems across the EU. However, there are some situations where some educational tools can be agreed centrally, for example, by engaging the targeted stakeholders (i.e., patients representatives and learned societies) to generate concepts in regard to which tool types pose less potential burden and are more acceptable to use. In the United States, the nearest equivalent of the EU educational materials can be found in the REMS as a part of the Medication Guide and/or PPI and/or ETASU. Examples of relevant materials include HCP training materials, patient educational materials, information on medical monitoring procedures, and data collection forms (FDA, 2009).

The format of a particular tool will depend on the message to be delivered and whether the risk minimization program incorporates a tool to be used before the administration of the medicinal product, such as screening tests or exclusion criteria; or during and/or after the therapy, such as monitoring specific laboratory values or detecting early signs or symptoms of adverse events. For example, *checklists* are increasingly used before the administration of the medicinal product for nonmandatory patient selection, screening procedures, and clinical monitoring as they typically include a sequential list of steps that might be used to identify the eligible patients and to monitor them during the treatment (HPRA, 2016a). Conversely, *brochures and guides* may be more appropriate to provide information on the correct use of a medicinal product, to enhance awareness among the targeted population of specific important risks and possible risk factors, and to instruct on the early recognition and management of adverse reactions during and/or after the therapy (HPRA, 2016b). In case of complex products, brochures and guides may be supplemented with *training materials*, for example, to provide information (with appropriate training programs) on correct storage, preparation, and administration of a particular product generally to reduce the risk of medication errors. Two tools specifically targeted to patients are *patient diaries* and *patient alert cards* (HPRA, 2016c,d). Patient diaries are generally requested to record information on the recommended treatment or particular sign and symptoms that can be discussed with the HCP. Patient alert cards provide concise and focused information about the ongoing treatment with a product and its important risks (e.g., potential life-threatening interactions with other therapies) to ensure that such information reaches the relevant HCP in any circumstances, including patient's incapacity to be communicated, such as in unconsciousness or emergency treatments.

Another part of an educational program is the communication plan, which is a relevant additional risk minimization activity that determines the most appropriate tools and media (e.g., paper, audio, video, web, training programs, and targeted outreach), tailored formats (e.g., to HCP or patients), and dissemination strategies (e.g., direct-to-patients or HCP, through learned societies or patient organizations) to deliver information on the risk of a particular product and to enhance awareness and understanding among the targeted population. In the EU, the objectives and principles on communication of a risk from marketing authorization holders are set up in the GVP Module XV—*Safety Communication* (EMA, 2013). The guideline indicates that key messages for the safety communication (1) should be established at the right time to increase the effectiveness of the risk minimization; (2) should be tailored to the appropriate audience using appropriate language; (3) should be presented in the context of the benefits and include information on seriousness, severity, frequency, risk factors, time to onset, reversibility of potential adverse reactions, and expected time to recovery; and (4) should be presented using appropriate quantitative measures when describing and comparing risks (e.g., absolute risks instead of relative risks). In the United States, strong emphasis is given to communication and the FDA REMS guidance considers the communication plan as a relevant element of REMS if may support its implementation (FDA, 2009). The communication plan may include sending letters to HCP, disseminating information about REMS elements to encourage implementation by HCP or to explain certain safety protocols (e.g., as medical monitoring by periodic laboratory tests), or disseminating information to HCP through learned societies about any serious risks of the drug and any protocol to assure safe use. The FDA has published a guide for communicating benefits and risks, aiming to provide a scientific and structured approach for designing and implementing communication plans (FDA, 2011b).

Communication of important new safety issues is primarily performed by sending paper-based letter to HCP; these are called Direct Healthcare Professional Communication (DHPC) in the EU, or Dear Health Care Professional (DHCP) letter elsewhere. It typically aims to rapidly raise awareness on safety issues and consequent risk minimization actions to be taken. The preparation of the DHPC/DHCP letter requires particular care to convey the right information to HCP; cooperation among the relevant stakeholders might also help to improve the effectiveness of the letter as a risk minimization tool. Current evidence from the EU indicates that DHPC are not always effective in changing HCP behavior. A study was conducted in the Netherlands to systematically assess the effects of 58 safety-related regulatory actions on changes in volume of drug use in ambulatory care, which showed that DHPC lowered drug use in half of the cases in the short term, whereas long-term changes in use were observed for a third of the drugs with a DHPC, resulting in a mean decrease of 26.7% in drug use (Piening et al., 2012a). However, DHPC can be more effective, if safety information is presented in a well-structured way and in case of very serious safety concerns (Reber et al., 2013). Therefore, DHPC/DHCP letter remains a relevant component of the communication plan, but they need to be supported by other tools to increase and maintain long-term effectiveness.

Controlled Access Systems

Controlled access systems are generally requested when other elements of aRMM/REMS, such as the educational programs, are not considered sufficient to mitigate a risk; they are intended to provide safe access for patients to medicinal products with known serious risks that would otherwise be unavailable. Because these measures may be mandatory for HCP and patients, their impact on the use of the medicine (and potential unintended effects) should be carefully evaluated before their introduction. Box 2.2.2 provides the example of a risk minimization program implemented in the United States for preventing fetal exposure to lenalidomide, an immunomodulatory agent.

Examples of requirements that need to be fulfilled before the product is prescribed and/or dispensed and/or used in a controlled access system include

BOX 2.2.2 RISK MINIMIZATION PROGRAM FOR PREVENTING FETAL EXPOSURE TO LENALIDOMIDE (CASTANEDA ET AL., 2008)

Lenalidomide is an immunomodulatory drug and an analogue of thalidomide, a known teratogen. Recent studies have failed to demonstrate malformations in fetuses exposed to lenalidomide. Nonetheless, because of the similarities with thalidomide the drug is only available under a special restricted access program called RevAssist developed by the marketing authorization holder and agreed by the FDA. The principal elements of RevAssist as described in the ETASU section of the REMS program include

- Signatures in the HCP-patient agreement form from both physicians and patients
- Controlled dispensing/distribution through registration of prescribers, patients, and contract pharmacies

- Mandatory educational programs for prescribers, patients, and pharmacists about the risk associated with lenalidomide
- Requirements and counseling for adequate contraceptive measures (at least one highly effective method and one additional effective method) for female patients of childbearing potential and for adult males
- Pregnancy tests before, during, and after treatment among females of childbearing potential
- Monitor and compliance through mandatory prescriber and patient surveys, pharmacy audits, and reporting of abnormal pregnancy test results

screening procedures; enrollment, agreement, and consent forms; controlled dispensing or distribution; and registries. *Screening procedures* are requirements to monitor patients before starting and/or during treatment to ensure compliance with strictly defined clinical criteria, to check for adverse reactions (or early symptoms) and treatment efficacy. Such requirements are also included in the educational programs as checklists, although in controlled access systems they are considered mandatory. For example, in the EU, treatment with abacavir products, indicated to treat HIV infection, should be initiated only after the screening of the HLA-B*5701 allele, which is the only identified pharmacogenetics marker consistently associated with abacavir-related hypersensitivity reactions. *Enrollment, agreement, and consent forms* are intended to document the receipt and understanding of the information provided on the serious risk of the product prior to treatment. For example, the Adempas REMS program requires HCP, the fulfillment of the "Prescriber Enrollment and Agreement Form," where the HCP should acknowledge the teratogenic risk of riociguat (Adempas)—indicated for the treatment of pulmonary hypertension in adults—and the obligation to educate female patients about the REMS program, monitor them appropriately on the risk of serious birth defect and the use of reliable contraception methods, and report any pregnancies to the REMS program. On the other hand, the "Patient Enrollment and Consent Form" requires the acknowledgment that patients have understood that Adempas is available only under the REMS program, that they were counseled by their HCP prior to receiving the treatment, and that they have read the medication guide.

Controlled dispensing and distribution aims to limit access only to appropriate patients. This can be done by ensuring that medicinal products are made available for dispensing only to pharmacies that are registered and approved to dispense the products. The role of the pharmacist is to filling prescription only from certified prescribers or checking that patients meet certain criteria, including the verification of consent forms or laboratory test results. A further level of risk minimization can be achieved by using a set of measures implemented to ensure that the stages of the distribution chain of a medicinal product (i.e., manufacturer, wholesaler, and pharmacist) are tracked up to the prescription and/or pharmacy dispensing the product. These types of actions are mentioned in the description of the controlled distribution system laid down in GVP Module XVI and in the implementation system section of the FDA REMS guidance (EMA, 2014a; FDA, 2009).

Registries are data collection systems that use noninterventional methods to collect uniform data on specified outcomes in a population defined by a particular disease, condition, or exposure. They have valuable role as risk minimization tool only when there is a mandatory requirement for inclusion of patients into the registries to initiate a specific treatment. Otherwise, they can have a relevant role in capturing long-term safety information as a part of an additional pharmacovigilance activity such as PASS (see Chapter 3.3 for more details on registries as data source for PASS). The GVP Module XVI also gives particular emphasis to the so-called *"Pregnancy Prevention Programs (PPP),"* which is a set of interventions aimed to minimize exposure to a medicinal product with known or potential teratogenic effects during pregnancy. Generally, PPP combine several educational tools with elements considered in the controlled access systems. In the United States, the elements of PPP are generally provided within the ETASU in the context of an REMS program.

EFFECTIVENESS OF RISK MINIMIZATION

The effect of risk minimization activities in health-care systems requires assessment to ensure that their objectives are fulfilled and that the measures in place are appropriate, taking into account the benefit-risk profile of the medicinal product and the efforts required to implement them. Such assessment also enables modifications of the initial measures, if warranted, to improve the risk minimization strategy in the context of an iterative process of evaluation, correction, and reaudit integral to the life cycle benefit-risk assessment of the medicinal product (EMA, 2012a). In the EU, monitoring the effectiveness of aRMM is mandatory for both marketing authorization holders and regulatory authorities, although in certain circumstances risk minimization evaluation can be also requested and/or proposed for routine measures, and such effectiveness assessment studies are considered PASS (EC, 2010; EMA, 2014a). In the United

States, an REMS assessment plan needs to be approved in advance of REMS implementation and submitted by 18 months and by 3 years after the REMS is initially approved, and in the 7th year after the REMS is initially approved, with additional dates if more frequent assessments are necessary to ensure that the benefits of the medicinal product continue to outweigh the risks (FDA, 2009).

Models for Risk Minimization Evaluation Post-Authorization Safety Studies

For a comprehensive assessment of the effectiveness of risk minimization measures, several conceptual models have been proposed to date (Prieto et al., 2012; Smith et al., 2013; Zomerdijk et al., 2013). In spite of some differences in the approach, all models recommend the measurement of different metrics and consider process and outcome indicators as common elements for risk minimization evaluation.

Implementation of risk minimization measures (*Process Indicators*) refers to the course of actions taken to put in practice an intervention, which might enable understanding of why an intervention failed to provide the expected outcomes by revealing whether it was inherently ineffective (failure of the intervention concept) or simply poorly implemented. The knowledge gained may be then used to support corrective implementation actions as needed. Depending on the nature of the interventions, one or more process indicators can be identified for the assessment (Table 2.2.3 lists these indicators, for which study design and data collection modalities are described with details later in the chapter).

To correlate the implementation of risk minimization measures with desired health outcomes (e.g., fewer occurrences or less severity of the adverse events),

Table 2.2.3 Process Indicators for Risk Minimization Evaluation

Process Indicator	Purpose
Risk minimization tool coverage, awareness, and usage metrics	To measure to what extent the program has been disseminated, received, and/or used as planned.
Risk knowledge/comprehension metrics	To determine whether the end users have correctly understood the purpose of the risk minimization tools and their key messages.
Behavioral modification	To measure to what extent the behavior of the targeted stakeholders (HCP, patients, or both) has changed because of the recommendation contained in the risk minimization measure (particularly product information and educational materials).

safety outcomes (*Outcome Indicators*) are used to evaluate the effectiveness of risk minimization activities. Outcome indicator's data may be more difficult to obtain but generally define the ultimate success of a risk minimization program. The GVP Module XVI highlights that in some circumstances, when it is fully justified, that the assessment of outcome indicators is unfeasible (e.g., inadequate number of exposed patients, or very rare adverse events), the effectiveness evaluation may be based on the careful interpretation of data from process indicators (EMA, 2014a).

Considering that risk minimization measures vary widely in complexity from a change in routine measure, such as amendments in the product information (e.g., restriction of indication or addition of contraindication), to extensive additional measures, such as PPP, the evaluation strategy should be tailored accordingly. Careful consideration should be also given to the process and outcome measures that can be realistically collected and provide relevant information to avoid generating suboptimal information unable to support regulatory decisions. Designing and conducting a valid and unbiased risk minimization evaluation PASS relies on the common methods employed for epidemiological investigations with their strengths and limitations. However, there are some challenges that are specifically related to these types of evaluations (Banerjee et al., 2014). Careful consideration should be given to the following aspects:

- Lack of comparators: risk minimization measures are generally implemented to the whole targeted population, thus making it difficult to identify a proper control group and to judge the effect of the risk minimization tools. For medicinal products already marketed, process and/or outcome indicators might be estimated in the same study population before and after the introduction of the risk minimization measure, with preintervention information acting as a surrogate control group (i.e., quasiexperimental designs). However, for medicinal products with risk minimization measures required at the time of initial marketing authorization, preintervention information is missing and any effect of the risk minimization measure is difficult to attribute. In absence of preintervention information, the comparison can be made against a predefined reference value taking into account all the possible limitations (e.g., literature review, historical data, expected frequency in general population, or outcome frequency in the pre-authorization clinical trials).
- Lack of measurable outcomes: for complex risk minimization programs, key elements aimed at behavioral changes may not be eligible for analysis because of lack of clear recommended actions (e.g., use the drug with caution, or carefully select patients) (Zomerdijk et al., 2013). The same applies for key elements aimed at knowledge change for which

information can be only collected through rigorous surveys (e.g., information on the most serious adverse reactions of the drug or information on the medical implications of a drug–drug interaction). Therefore, to facilitate rapid risk minimization evaluation, well-defined key elements of the risk minimization strategy should be considered leading to unambiguous actions of the target population.

- Lack of benchmarking and uncertainty about interpretation: it is difficult to predict what acceptable levels of distribution, tool uptake, and impact on knowledge, behaviors, and attitudes, constitute success. Moreover, there is no certainty that process indicators correlate with the safety outcomes. For example, analyses on clinical behavior may demonstrate significant improvements in adherence to risk minimization recommendations, although the frequency or severity of reported adverse drug reactions remains high. Setting standard thresholds for effectiveness assessment is also challenging because the definition of success and failure of the risk minimization may depend on the severity of the adverse events, the preventability of the risk, and the societal perception of the product risks against its benefits.

Risk Minimization Tool Coverage, Awareness, and Usage

Risk minimization tool coverage, awareness, and usage metrics provide relevant information at the basic level of the evaluation strategy on the implementation of the risk minimization measure (Smith et al., 2013). It focuses on whether the material was actually distributed, received, and/or used by the target population. Common process indicators to be considered are proportion of tool distribution or download frequency if electronic tools are provided, and proportion of end users aware of, and using the educational tool.

Risk minimization tool coverage generally does not require properly designed studies on sampled population as the tools are supposed to be distributed to all end users. However, monitoring of tool distribution can be required and estimates of coverage provided on the basis of agreed timeframes. Results of inadequate distribution/coverage should lead to reconsideration of the delivery channels employed or help to determine whether a different tool format is required.

Once risk minimization tools have been distributed, there is no guarantee that targeted stakeholders will use or are aware of them. Indicators, such as HCP requests for refills of consumable risk minimization items, for example, HCP/patient checklist in controlled distribution systems, may also be exploited as proxies of tool utilization. This information may also be gathered through tailored surveys to stakeholders. For example, in a survey of HCP awareness on safety communications, 16% of the HCP were not familiar with DHPC; the majority (58%) also indicated that they read only the DHPC that contained information that was relevant to them (Piening et al., 2012b). Survey PASS results can be analyzed as a whole or stratified to show how specific subgroups are performing, with the aim of highlighting areas where coverage, awareness, and usage is poorer and needs to be improved. In interpreting these results, the structure of the health-care system where the risk minimization measure has been implemented should also be considered, particularly how the system is organized, how the quality of the risk minimization measure is ensured, and how logistics are organized and monitored.

Risk Knowledge/Comprehension

Risk knowledge or comprehension metrics gauge whether target audiences understand both the purpose of the risk minimization tools and their key messages. These messages often relate to the risks, such as important signs and symptoms, or to actions that should or should not be taken, such as performing laboratory tests or not prescribing a drug to specific subpopulations. Common process indicator to be considered is proportion of end users correctly responding to specific questions aimed to measure the understanding of the key messages contained in the risk minimization tool.

Generally, to assess the level of knowledge/comprehension achieved by educational interventions and/or risk communication, rigorous survey methods should be applied. The GVP Module XVI (Appendix I) provides the key elements that should be considered when assessing protocols and results from these survey PASS (EMA, 2014a). However, comprehensive guidelines for survey research can be also retrieved from the published literature (Groves et al., 2004; Aday and Cornelius, 2006; McColl et al., 2001). Overall, the following elements should be considered in the design and implementation of a survey PASS to minimize potential biases and to optimize the generalizability of the results to the intended population: (1) sampling procedures and recruitment strategy; and (2) design and administration of the data collection instruments.

Appropriate sampling procedures should ensure that the sampling frame is not subjected to selection bias leading to a study population that is not similar to, or representative of, the indented population in one or more aspects. Therefore, a randomly selected sampling frame is generally the optimal approach to minimize the risk of selection bias, provided that relevant characteristics of the study population are taken into account in the sampling strategy. In addition, the recruitment strategy of a survey should give careful consideration of the potential recruitment sources, such as HCP lists from learned societies, patients list from local health authorities, web panels, which should be completed and up to date.

The design of the data collection instrument is important to avoid that the proposed questions drive respondents to answer in a particular way that questions do not fully cover all the relevant aspects of the risk minimization tool, or that the instrument is not able to ultimately measure and predict different degrees of knowledge/comprehension. The following are the main principles to follow to ensure that data collection instrument is able to adequately catch the level of risk knowledge of the targeted population:

- *Pretesting and validation:* this involves testing the draft questionnaire on samples of subjects similar to those who will ultimately be studied. Its purpose is to identify questions that are poorly understood, ambiguous, or evoke undesirable responses. Pretests should be carried out using the same procedures that will finally be used in administering the questionnaire.
- *Content validity:* items or variables in the questionnaire should capture all the aspects related to end users knowledge on the risk minimization tool. It is also important that the items or variables included in the questionnaire are clear and unambiguous and that questions pertaining to the implemented regulatory action are avoided (e.g., "do you know that product X is contraindicated for disease Y?").
- *Construct validity:* items or variables in the questionnaire should be developed in a way that they are likely to accurately measure (at different degrees) end-user knowledge/comprehension on the risk minimization tool.

Behavioral Modification

Evaluation of behavioral modification examines the extent of deviations of clinical actions from the recommendations contained in the risk minimization tools. The related process indicators should therefore provide insight into what extent the risk minimization program has been executed as planned by the targeted stakeholders and whether the intended impact on behavior has been observed. Questionnaire-based survey PASS is not well suited to assess behavioral modification because they rely on the respondent self-reporting, thus introducing misclassification of exposure or the Hawthorne effect (e.g., respondents improve or modify an aspect of their behavior in response to their awareness of being observed) (Beiderbeck et al., 2004). Therefore, this evaluation strategy is better addressed with time-trend analyses relying mainly on information from health insurance administrative claims and electronic medical records (EMR). Data from claims and EMR might in fact provide rapid feedback on the effectiveness of risk minimization measures, considering that information on drug exposure and patient characteristics (which might define the adherence to the recommendation contained in product information and/or educational materials) is generally based on secondary data collection. Chapters 3.1 and 3.2 discuss operational details of claims and EMR, respectively. Table 2.2.4 provides a list of relevant criteria to consider in PASS measuring behavioral modification employing claims and EMR.

Table 2.2.4 Criteria to Consider in PASS Measuring Behavioral Modification Employing Claims and EMR Databases

Principle	Criteria for Judgment
Ability of EMR in capturing the prescribed/dispensed medicinal products in a certain population.	• Sales and pharmacy claims data or prescribed drugs in EMR databases are likely to capture most of the information on medicinal products used in primary care. • The validity of the data source should be demonstrated for information on medicinal products restricted to the specialists and for nonreimbursed/over-the-counter drugs.
In multicountry studies, particularly in the EU, differences in drug policies and local clinical practices.	• Differences in drug distribution and reimbursement might result in misleading estimates in drug exposure and HCP behavior across different countries. • Experience from multicountries projects, e.g., EU-ADR, PROTECT, has shown how differences in drug/disease coding, case definitions, and terminologies might affect the ability to compare clinical variables.
Information on dose and duration provides more accurate estimates on drug exposure.	• Sales and pharmacy claims data might be unable to provide information on prescribed daily dose and duration. • Health-care databases are potentially able to provide information on dose and duration, although such information is rarely complete and accurate. • Drug exposure misclassification should always be considered when the recommended daily dose is highly variable (e.g., warfarin) or the drugs are taken sporadically (e.g., NSAIDS).
Operational definitions should always be used for the relevant elements of risk minimization evaluation.	• Operational definitions are algorithms based on the clinical definition of a particular disease, which uses drug/disease coding, text mining, or laboratory and diagnostic procedures to select patients with the disease.
Validity of operational definitions should be demonstrated by their sensitivity and positive predictive values.	• For diseases and conditions with clear-cut diagnosis, e.g., myocardial infarction, simple operational definitions are generally sufficient to demonstrate their validity. • For disease and conditions that are difficult to diagnose, or when diseases, drugs, or procedures are managed outside the primary care setting, complex operational definitions, and tailored validation studies are required.

EU-ADR, exploring and understanding adverse drug reactions project; NSAIDS, nonsteroidal antiinflammatory drugs; PROTECT, pharmacoepidemiological research on outcomes of therapeutics by a European consortium.

Process indicators to consider in time-trend analyses to measure behavioral modifications are changes in drug exposure and changes in HCP behaviors before and after the implementation of the risk minimization measures. Generally, changes in drug exposure are expressed by *drug consumption* (e.g., number of kilograms of a medicinal product sold divided by the average dose, patient-years of use, or defined daily dose/1000 inhabitants day) *and patients prevalence/incidence drug use* (e.g., number of patients exposed with a medicinal product divided by the total study population). On the other hand, changes in HCP behavior are expressed by the proportion of patients exposed to a medicinal product in accordance with the authorized indication; the proportion of contraindicated patients exposed to a medicinal product; or the proportion of patients undergoing recommended diagnostic tests prior, during, or after exposure to a medicinal product.

Time-trend analyses can be designed using the *uncontrolled before–after design,* the *interrupted time series design* in presence of preintervention information, and the *regression discontinuity design* in absence of preintervention information (Briesacher et al., 2013). The uncontrolled before–after design is the simplest as it measures the study endpoints only at two time intervals (Grimshaw et al., 2000). However, it is challenging to attribute the observed changes to the intervention or to the underlying secular trends of the prescribing patterns, and it might potentially overestimate the effects of the intervention. In the case of the interrupted time series design, data are collected at multiple instances over time before and after an intervention (interruption) is introduced. The key assumption of this design is that extrapolating the preintervention level and trend correctly reflects the (counterfactual) outcome that would have occurred without the intervention (Fig. 2.2.1). An advantage of this design is that it allows for the statistical investigation of potential biases in the estimate of the effect of the intervention (e.g., secular trends, seasonal effects, duration, random fluctuations, and autocorrelations). It can be also performed using aggregate-level longitudinal data, although it does require preintervention information (Ramsay et al., 2003).

The regression discontinuity design is most appropriate to assess the impact of regulatory measures that applies to a subgroup of population defined by a continuous measure with a fixed threshold (e.g., contraindication in the elderly) (Fig. 2.2.2). All subjects who score on one side of the cutoff, for example, age ≥ 65 years, are assigned to the intervention group, whereas those scoring on the other side are assigned to a control group. Based on regression equations above or below the assignment threshold, one could predict what the intervention group values would have been if the risk minimization program had no effect. The regression discontinuity design is a reasonably robust quasiexperimental design and may be especially useful when preintervention

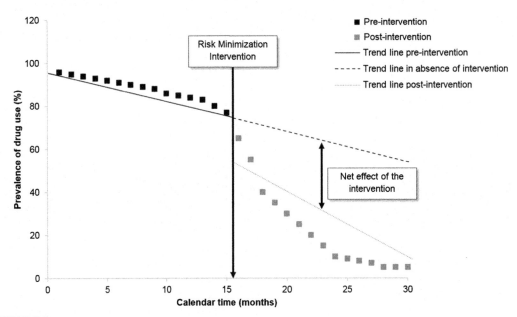

FIGURE 2.2.1
Example of interrupted time series design to evaluate the effectiveness of risk minimization measures.

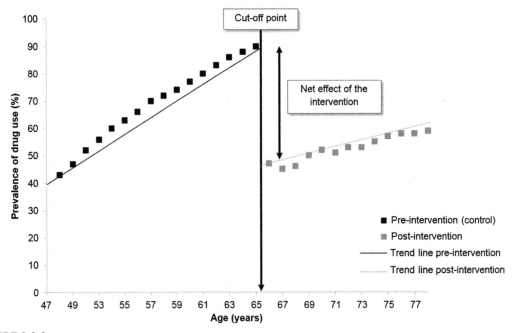

FIGURE 2.2.2
Example of regression discontinuity design to evaluate the effectiveness of risk minimization measures.

data are limited, although it requires individual level data and it is rarely used in medical research (Venkataramani et al., 2016).

Safety Outcomes

The ultimate measures of success of a risk minimization program are the safety outcomes, i.e., the demonstration that the introduction of a risk minimization activity correlates with lower frequency or severity of the adverse events in patients exposed to the medicinal product in routine practice. Outcome indicators to consider are *incidence rate or cumulative incidence* (e.g., number of new adverse reactions in patients exposed to a certain medicinal product divided by the person-time/or size of the exposed population within a specified period) and *reporting rates* (e.g., number of suspected adverse reaction reports attributed to a certain medicinal product over a fixed period). The use of reporting rates should be considered with caution because of the inherent limitations of spontaneous reporting systems, particularly the underreporting and the lack of patient-level linkage between drug exposure and adverse events (Sharrar and Dieck, 2013). The GVP Module XVI outlines that when a direct measure on the risk in the treated population is not feasible (e.g., when the adverse event in the target population is rare), spontaneous reporting data could offer an approximation of the frequency of the adverse reaction in the treated population (EMA, 2014a).

The evaluation of the incidence of the adverse events is often employed through noninterventional PASS using information collected from healthcare databases or registries. A disease registry includes patients based on diagnosis, whereas product registries include patients based on the treatment they receive. The disease registries usually provide more complete information than the product registries because they contain information on patients not exposed to the products under observation. Even in the absence of preintervention information in the exposed population, this might help evaluating the effect of a regulatory measure by providing a background rate of the occurrence of the adverse events in the affected population in the absence of a particular treatment or in association with relevant treatment modalities for comparison. In addition, the information collected in patient registries is less likely to be affected by recall or Hawthorne effect because the investigators are not focused on a specific product.

Compared to claims and EMR databases, registries may be more reliable, particularly when the safety outcome or the target population is likely to be diagnosed/managed in specialist settings, or when accurate detection/measurement of safety outcomes, confounding/risk factors, and characteristics of the target population is requested, such as outcomes like congenital malformations and Stevens–Johnson syndrome.

References

Aday, L.A., Cornelius, L.J., 2006. Designing and Conducting Health Surveys. John Wiley & Sons, Inc., Hoboken (New Jersey).

Banerjee, A.K., Zomerdijk, I.M., Wooder, S., Ingate, S., Mayall, S.J., 2014. Post-approval evaluation of effectiveness of risk minimization: methods, challenges and interpretation. Drug Saf. 37, 33–42.

Beiderbeck, A.B., Sturkenboom, M.C., Coebergh, J.W., Leufkens, H.G., Stricker, B.H., 2004. Misclassification of exposure is high when interview data on drug use are used as a proxy measure of chronic drug use during follow-up. J. Clin. Epidemiol. 57, 973–977.

Brass, E.P., 2001. Changing the status of drugs from prescription to over-the-counter availability. N. Engl. J. Med. 345, 810–816.

Briesacher, B.A., Soumerai, S.B., Zhang, F., Toh, S., Andrade, S.E., Wagner, J.L., Shoaibi, A., Gurwitz, J.H., 2013. A critical review of methods to evaluate the impact of FDA regulatory actions. Pharmacoepidemiol. Drug Saf. 22, 986–994.

Castaneda, C.P., Zeldis, J.B., Freeman, J., Quigley, C., Brandenburg, N.A., Bwire, R., 2008. RevAssist: a comprehensive risk minimization programme for preventing fetal exposure to lenalidomide. Drug Saf. 31, 743–752.

Eichler, H.G., Abadie, E., Breckenridge, A., Flamion, B., Gustafsson, L.L., Leufkens, H., Rowland, M., Schneider, C.K., Bloechl-Daum, B., 2011. Bridging the efficacy-effectiveness gap: a regulator's perspective on addressing variability of drug response. Nat. Rev. Drug Discov. 10, 495–506.

European Commission, 2001. Directive 2001/83/EC of the European Parliament and of the Council of 6 November 2001 on the Community Code Relating to Medicinal Products for Human Use. Available at: http://ec.europa.eu/health/files/eudralex/vol-1/dir_2001_83_cons/dir2001_83_cons_20081230_en.pdf.

European Commission, 2008. Guidelines on Pharmacovigilance for Medicinal Products for Human Use. Available at: http://ec.europa.eu/health/files/eudralex/vol-9/pdf/vol9a_09-2008_en.pdf.

European Commission, 2009. A Guideline on Summary on Product Characteristics. Available at: http://ec.europa.eu/health/files/eudralex/vol-2/c/smpc_guideline_rev2_en.pdf.

European Commission, 2010. Regulation (EU) No 1235/2010 of the European Parliament and of the Council of 15 December 2010 Amending, as Regards Pharmacovigilance of Medicinal Products for Human Use, Regulation (EC) No 726/2004 Laying Down Community Procedures for the Authorisation and Supervision of Medicinal Products for Human and Veterinary Use and Establishing a European Medicines Agency, and Regulation (EC) No 1394/2007 on Advanced Therapy Medicinal Products [online]. Available from: http://eur-lex.europa.eu/LexUriServ/LexUriServ.do?uri=OJ:L:2010:348:0001:0016:EN:PDF.

European Medicines Agency, 2005. Guideline on Risk Management Systems for Medicinal Products for Human Use. Doc. Ref. EMEA/CHMP/96268/2005. Available from: http://www.emwa.org/Documents/Freelancer/riskmanagement/rmp%20guidelines.pdf.

European Medicines Agency, 2012a. Guideline on Good Pharmacovigilance Practices (GVP): Module V – Risk Management Systems. Doc. Ref. EMA/838713/2011. Available from: http://www.ema.europa.eu/docs/en_GB/document_library/Scientific_guideline/2012/06/WC500129134.pdf.

European Medicines Agency, 2012b. Assessment Report for Nimesulide Containing Medicinal Products for Systemic Use. Doc. Ref. EMA/73856/2012. Available from: http://www.ema.europa.eu/docs/en_GB/document_library/Referrals_document/Nimesulide_31/WC500125574.pdf.

European Medicines Agency, 2013. Guideline on Good Pharmacovigilance Practices (GVP): Module XV Safety Communication. Doc. Ref. EMA/118465/2012. Available from: http://www.ema.europa.eu/docs/en_GB/document_library/Scientific_guideline/2013/01/WC500137666.pdf.

European Medicines Agency, 2014a. Guideline on Good Pharmacovigilance Practices (GVP): Module XVI − Risk Minimization Measures: Selection of Tools and Effectiveness Indicators. Doc. Ref. EMA/204715/2012 Rev 1. Available from: http://www.ema.europa.eu/docs/en_GB/document_library/Scientific_guideline/2014/02/WC500162051.pdf.

European Medicines Agency, 2014b. Assessment Report for Domperidone Containing Medicinal Products. Doc. Ref. EMA/152501/2014. Available from: http://www.ema.europa.eu/docs/en_GB/document_library/Referrals_document/Domperidone_31/Recommendation_provided_by_Pharmacovigilance_Risk_Assessment_Committee/WC500168926.pdf.

European Medicines Agency, 2014c. Press Release: European Medicines Agency Recommends that Protelos/Osseor Remain Available but with Further Restrictions. Doc. Ref. EMA/84749/2014. Available from: http://www.ema.europa.eu/docs/en_GB/document_library/Press_release/2014/02/WC500161971.pdf.

European Medicines Agency, 2015a. Risk Minimisation Strategy for High-strength and Fixed Combination Insulin Products. Doc. Ref. EMA/686009/2014. Available from: http://www.ema.europa.eu/docs/en_GB/document_library/Regulatory_and_procedural_guideline/2015/11/WC500196980.pdf.

European Medicines Agency, 2015b. Guideline on Good Pharmacovigilance Practices (GVP): Module XVI Addendum I − Educational Material. Doc. Ref. EMA/61341/2015. Available from: http://www.ema.europa.eu/docs/en_GB/document_library/Regulatory_and_procedural_guideline/2015/12/WC500198761.pdf.

Food and Drug Administration, 2002. Additional criteria and procedures for classifying over-the-counter drugs as generally recognized as safe and effective and not misbranded. Final rule. Fed. Regist. 67, 3060−3076.

Food and Drug Administration, 2005. Guidance for Industry: Development and Use of Risk Minimization Action Plans. Available at: http://www.fda.gov/downloads/RegulatoryInformation/Guidances/UCM126830.pdf.

Food and Drug Administration, 2009. Guidance for Industry. Format and Content of Proposed Risk Evaluation and Mitigation Strategies (REMS), REMS Assessments, and Proposed REMS Modifications. Available from: http://www.fda.gov/downloads/Drugs/GuidanceComplianceRegulatoryInformation/Guidances/UCM184128.pdf.

Food and Drug Administration, 2011a. Guidance for Industry: Medication Guides − Distribution Requirements and Inclusion in Risk Evaluation and Mitigation Strategies (REMS). Available at: http://www.fda.gov/downloads/Drugs/.../Guidances/UCM244570.pdf.

Food and Drug Administration, 2011b. Communicating Risks and Benefits: An Evidence-based User`s Guide. Available at: http://www.fda.gov/downloads/AboutFDA/ReportsManualsForms/Reports/UCM268069.pdf.

Food and Drug Administration, 2013a. Guidance for Industry Labeling for Human Prescription Drug and Biological Products − Implementing the PLR Content and Format Requirements. Available at: http://www.fda.gov/downloads/drugs/guidancecomplianceregulatoryinformation/guidances/ucm075082.pdf.

Food and Drug Administration, 2013b. Guidance for Industry: Safety Considerations for Container Labels and Carton Labeling Design to Minimize Medication Errors. Available at: http://www.fda.gov/downloads/drugs/guidancecomplianceregulatoryinformation/guidances/ucm349009.pdf.

Food and Drug Administration, 2016a. DailyMed. Available at: https://dailymed.nlm.nih.gov/dailymed/.

Food and Drug Administration, 2016b. Approved Risk Evaluation and Mitigation Strategies. Available at: http://www.accessdata.fda.gov/scripts/cder/rems/.

Grimshaw, J., Campbell, M., Eccles, M., Steen, N., 2000. Experimental and quasi-experimental designs for evaluating guideline implementation strategies. Fam. Pract. 17 (Suppl. 1), S11–S16.

Groves, R.M., Fowler, F.J., Couper, M.P., Lepkowski, J.M., Singer, E., et al., 2004. Survey Methodology. John Wiley & Sons, Inc., Hoboken (New Jersey).

Hawton, K., Bergen, H., Simkin, S., Dodd, S., Pocock, P., Bernal, W., Gunnell, D., Kapur, N., 2013. Long term effect of reduced pack sizes of paracetamol on poisoning deaths and liver transplant activity in England and Wales: interrupted time series analyses. BMJ 346, f403.

Health Products Regulatory Authority, Educational Material for Medicine, 2016a. Dianette Prescriber Checklist. Available at: https://www.hpra.ie/docs/default-source/3rd-party-documents/educational-materials/dianette_hcp_checklist-for-prescribers_v1-07-15.pdf?sfvrsn=2.

Health Products Regulatory Authority, Educational Material for Medicine, 2016b. Lixiana Prescriber Guide. Available at: https://www.hpra.ie/docs/default-source/3rd-party-documents/educational-materials/lixiana_hcp_prescriber-guide_v1-09-15.pdf?sfvrsn=2.

Health Products Regulatory Authority, Educational Material for Medicine, 2016c. Rivastigmine Patient Diary. Available at: https://www.hpra.ie/docs/default-source/3rd-party-documents/educational-materials/rivastigmine-sandoz-_patient_patient-diary.pdf?sfvrsn=2.

Health Products Regulatory Authority, Educational Material for Medicine, 2016d. Lixiana Patient Alert Card. Available at: https://www.hpra.ie/docs/default-source/3rd-party-documents/educational-materials/lixiana_hcp_prescriber-guide_v1-09-15.pdf?sfvrsn=2.

International Conference on Harmonisation of Technical Requirements for Registration of Pharmaceuticals for Human Use, 2004. Pharmacovigilance Planning E2E. Available at: http://www.ich.org/fileadmin/Public_Web_Site/ICH_Products/Guidelines/Efficacy/E2E/Step4/E2E_Guideline.pdf.

McColl, E., Jacoby, A., Thomas, L., Soutter, J., Bamford, C., et al., 2001. Design and use of questionnaires: a review of best practice applicable to surveys of health service staff and patients. Health Technol. Assess. 5, 1–256.

Piening, S., Reber, K.C., Wieringa, J.E., Straus, S.M., de Graeff, P.A., Haaijer-Ruskamp, F.M., Mol, P.G., 2012a. Impact of safety-related regulatory action on drug use in ambulatory care in The Netherlands. Clin. Pharmacol. Ther. 91, 838–845.

Piening, S., Haaijer-Ruskamp, F.M., de Graeff, P.A., Straus, S.M., Mol, P.G., 2012b. Healthcare professionals' self-reported experiences and preferences related to direct healthcare professional communications: a survey conducted in The Netherlands. Drug Saf. 35, 1061–1072.

Prieto, L., Spooner, A., Hidalgo-Simon, A., Rubino, A., Kurz, X., Arlett, P., 2012. Evaluation of the effectiveness of risk minimization measures. Pharmacoepidemiol. Drug Saf. 21, 896–899.

Ramsay, C.R., Matowe, L., Grilli, R., Grimshaw, J.M., Thomas, R.E., 2003. Interrupted time series designs in health technology assessment: lessons from two systematic reviews of behavior change strategies. Int. J. Technol. Assess. Health Care 19, 613–623.

Reber, K.C., Piening, S., Wieringa, J.E., Straus, S.M., Raine, J.M., de Graeff, P.A., Haaijer-Ruskamp, F.M., Mol, P.G., 2013. When direct health-care professional communications have an impact on inappropriate and unsafe use of medicines. Clin. Pharmacol. Ther. 93, 360–365.

Sharrar, R.G., Dieck, G.S., 2013. Monitoring product safety in the postmarketing environment. Ther. Adv. Drug Saf. 4, 211–219.

Singh, S., Loke, Y.K., 2012. Drug safety assessment in clinical trials: methodological challenges and opportunities. Trials 13, 138.

Smith, M., Banerjee, A.K., Mayall, S., 2013. Evaluating the effectiveness of risk minimization. In: Bannerjee, A.S., Mayall, S.J. (Eds.), Therapeutic Risk Management of Medicines, first ed. Woodhead Publishing, Cambridge, pp. 241–275.

Vandenbroucke, J.P., Psaty, B.M., 2008. Benefits and risks of drug treatments: how to combine the best evidence on benefits with the best data about adverse effects. J. Am. Med. Assoc. 300, 2417–2419.

Venkataramani, A.S., Bor, J., Jena, A.B., 2016. Regression discontinuity designs in healthcare research. BMJ 352, i1216.

Zomerdijk, I.M., Trifiro, G., Sayed-Tabatabaei, F.A., Sturkenboom, M.C., Straus, S.M., 2013. Additional risk minimization measures in the EU: are they eligible for assessment? Pharmacoepidemiol. Drug Saf. 22, 1046–1053.

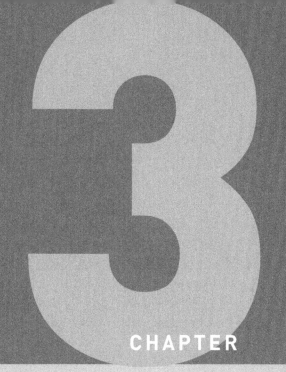

CHAPTER

Data Sources for PASS

3.1 Health Insurance Administrative Claims 49
3.2 Electronic Medical Records 63
3.3 Registries 74
3.4 Big Data 79
3.5 Social Media 92

Health Insurance Administrative Claims

Beth L. Nordstrom, Kathy H. Fraeman, Dimitra Lambrelli

Evidera, Bethesda, MD, United States

INTRODUCTION

Health insurance administrative claims databases provide a convenient source of health-care data on large population of patients exposed to prescription drugs. In the United States and certain other countries, a health insurance claim is generated each time a patient receives a medical or pharmacy service that is covered by the health insurance plan. Claim forms summarize the health-care services rendered and represent bills that are submitted to payers (i.e., health insurers) requesting reimbursement for those services. Although the primary purpose of claims is for billing, they contain a wealth of real-world health-care information that can be valuable for post-authorization safety studies (PASS). Outside of the United States, many countries have administrative databases that are similar to claims databases in their content and data structure; the following chapter relates to those databases and data derived from health insurance claims.

Claims databases are assembled at either the health plan or provider level. Databases containing health plan level information, or closed system databases, include data on all medical services covered by the health plan that are received during a patient enrollment in that health plan. Patients may disenroll from one health plan and move to another, with dates of start and end of enrollment noted in the database. These dates of enrollment provide an important indicator for availability of data for each patient. Closed system databases may include data from a single health plan or combine data from multiple plans.

Open claims databases represent a provider-centered view of patient medical services, rather than a health plan level view. The claims in an open system typically represent not only the claims for members of a particular health plan but also all claims submitted by contributing providers (e.g., hospitals, clinics, and pharmacies). When a database brings together claims from a large number of providers, the resulting patient population can be very large, but the

CONTENTS

Introduction 49

Contents of Claims Databases 50

Strengths and Limitations of Claims Databases 52

Methodological Considerations 55

Claims-Based Post-Authorization Safety Studies 57

References 60

Post-Authorization Safety Studies of Medicinal Products. https://doi.org/10.1016/B978-0-12-809217-0.00003-9

completeness of the data for each included patient cannot be assured. Unlike in the closed system where all covered services within enrollment periods should appear, in an open system there are no dates of enrollment; visits to providers who do not contribute to the system are simply not seen in the data. Most of the claims databases used in drug safety research contain data from the United States, although some use the European administrative databases. PASS requirements for the European Medicines Agency typically stipulate obtaining at least some data from European countries. Still, data from US data sources can often be used to increase sample size, especially for medicinal products that received earlier marketing authorization in the United States than in Europe.

CONTENTS OF CLAIMS DATABASES

The primary content in a claims database consists of procedure codes, diagnosis codes, and prescription drug codes; Fig. 3.1.1 illustrates the general

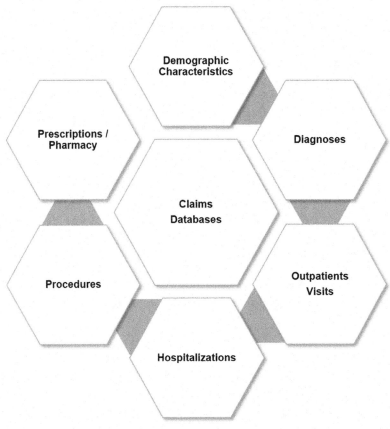

FIGURE 3.1.1
Contents of typical claims databases.

contents of claims data. Each claim includes a date of service representing the date that the patient visits the medical provider or the pharmacy, allowing a longitudinal view of patient medical care over time. All medical claims contain at least one procedure code indicating the service that was provided; visits where no medical procedures are undertaken (including well visits) are indicated by procedure codes for evaluation and management. In the United States, several procedure coding systems are used. Hospitals use International Classification of Diseases (ICD) version 9 or 10 procedure codes (CDC, 1998; WHO, 2016), with ICD-10 having replaced ICD-9 in October 2015 (CMS, 2017a; HHS, 2008). Outpatient clinics, on the other hand, report procedures using Current Procedural Terminology codes (AMA, 2016). Although the specific formatting of the codes differs as does some of the content of these three coding systems, all of these codes can be used within the same analysis for a PASS. Another procedure coding system, Healthcare Common Procedure Coding System (CMS, 2017b), contains codes for medications administered in medical settings, such as injected and infused medicinal products, and nonphysician services, such as ambulance rides and durable medical equipment. In Europe, the procedure coding systems vary by country and data source. Examples include the Office of Population Censuses and Surveys Classification of Interventions and Procedures in the United Kingdom, and the Dutch Classification of Procedures in the Netherlands (WHO, 2016b). The Nordic Medico-Statistical Committee (NOMESCO) introduced the NOMESCO Classification of Surgical Procedures (NCSP) with national versions for Sweden, Norway, Denmark, and Finland; whereas Iceland implemented the Nordic (English language) version of NCSP (NordClass, 2012). In Germany, the Einheitlicher Bewertungsmaßstab system is used for procedures and laboratory tests performed in the outpatient setting (KBV, 2017), whereas inpatient hospital procedures are recorded with the Operationen- und Prozedurenschlüssel coding system (DIMDI, 2017). In Italy, ICD-9 procedure codes are used for hospital procedures (CDC, 1998). Japanese databases use the Japan Classification and Coding for Clinical Laboratory Tests (JLAC10) (Yoshida et al., 2014).

Diagnosis codes are reported as ICD-10 codes in many countries (WHO, 2016a), although older US data and some other countries such as Italy contain ICD-9 codes (CDC, 1998), and some countries use other coding systems, such as Read codes in the United Kingdom (NHS, 2017). These diagnosis codes represent justification for billing for the procedure(s) on the claim. In many cases, they can be used to classify the medical conditions, including indications for medications, comorbidities, and adverse events and other outcomes. Date of onset of a condition is not included in the claims; instead, the date of diagnosis (i.e., the service date on the claim) is used in claims analyses.

Prescribed medications, as noted earlier, can be identified through procedure codes for medications that are administered by health-care providers in a clinic setting. Most medicinal products, however, are found in pharmacy claims. These claims contain records of each dispensing a patient receives, regardless of whether the dispensing represents an initial fill or a refill. Key elements in the pharmacy data include the date of dispensing, number of days of drug supplied, and information that can be used to derive daily dose (including drug strength and quantity dispensed). Unlike in medical claims, the indication for the medication is not included in the pharmacy data; no diagnosis field is present.

In addition to the information on procedures, diagnoses, and medications, most claims databases include some level of detail on patient demographics and—for closed claims systems—enrollment dates. The demographic data available in claims are generally restricted to a small number of variables, including year of birth, gender, and geographic region. Demographic information that may be of strong interest as covariates in some analyses of PASS, but that are not usually available in claims data, include race and ethnicity, educational level, and socioeconomic status. Health plan type (e.g., preferred provider organization vs. health maintenance organization) and start and stop dates of enrollment in the health plan are available for most claims databases. The enrollment start and stop dates define the time period during which the patient can be considered to be under follow-up in the system.

STRENGTHS AND LIMITATIONS OF CLAIMS DATABASES

One of the primary benefits of using claims databases for PASS is the availability of relatively complete health-care information for large populations. Even in the largest claims database, however, newly approved medicinal products may have a lengthy period of gradual uptake, with only small numbers of patients prescribed the product during the early months or years after launch. The products with relatively slow uptake are difficult to study during the first year or two of their availability regardless of the data source. In general, short of constructing a prospective patient registry that attempts to enroll all patients newly prescribed the targeted product, claims databases are likely to allow the largest possible patient population (see Chapter 3.3 for a detailed discussion about registries). If the number of patients is too small to power the analyses soon after launch, additional patients can be accrued into the cohort over time through data updates.

Although most claims databases represent large convenience samples of patients from one or more health plans, they permit selection of an unbiased sample of individuals with the given health insurance type who have been prescribed a medicinal product of interest. This is in sharp contrast with the highly selective process involved in recruiting patients for studies using active follow-up, such as clinical trials or registries. Even other retrospective approaches, such as obtaining medical charts for review through a site-based selection process, may result in a biased sample if clear and systematic selection criteria are not rigorously followed. In general, the representativeness of a patient population identified through claims data can be considered a great strength of these analyses. The national databases such as those from the Nordic countries are of course ideally representative of the population of the country.

Additionally, claims analyses have an advantage over prospective (primary data collection) studies in that the data reveal the real-world patterns of treatment and outcomes with no possibility of intervention. Even in non-interventional studies, when conducted prospectively, the researchers may unwittingly modify the treatment approach, degree and types of monitoring, and other interactions with the patients. Any such modifications may alter the real-world association between treatment and outcome. For a discussion of prospective studies, including interventional and noninterventional designs see Chapter 4.5.

Claims databases containing full pharmacy data for patients provide an excellent source of information on drug exposures. Although unable to pinpoint directly the lack of use of product received, the recording of such refill, with date, quantity, and days of product supplied, permits a relatively accurate assessment of time exposed to a medicinal product. Accuracy is suboptimal, however, with patients who demonstrate poor adherence to the product (i.e., those with a considerably longer interval between refills that indicated by the supply time of the dispensing). In addition, specifying the end date of drug use following a last dispensing can be very imprecise. The patient may have taken only one dose (or even none) from the last dispensing, or continued to take the full supply dispensed as indicated, or taken the full supply with breaks, leading to a later end date than the claims suggest (i.e., the date of last dispensing plus days of drug supplied). Still, the pharmacy data again represent real-world view of prescription drug use that is difficult to obtain through most data sources.

Despite the wealth of medical information available in claims databases, there are a number of limitations that may impact their usefulness for PASS. Missing data on exposures and outcomes can be a serious issue for some analyses. Fig. 3.2.2 in Chapter 3.2 illustrates completeness of data commonly available in health-care databases, including claims. Services that are not covered by health plan will not appear in the data. Most notably, this includes over-the-counter products. An analysis of myocardial infarction as an outcome, for example, would likely benefit from inclusion of aspirin use as a covariate. Although some aspirin use may appear in pharmacy claims data, most is likely to be unreported in claims. Other drug exposure information that is often missed in claims is the use of drug samples. The start date of exposure to a study drug is generally a landmark time point for PASS, as the risk of outcomes associated with the medicinal product begins when the product is initiated and, for many outcomes, declines with continued use of the product. If a patient initiates a product as a sample, with no indication of the sample in the claims, the risk period will be misclassified and the period of highest risk may be missed entirely. Also, products received during an inpatient hospital stay are typically not reported on claims, as their cost is bundled with the other hospital costs.

Missing data related to clinical outcomes can also be problematic. As a rule of thumb, the occurrence of events that do not lead to medical care will not appear in the data. Hence, more minor adverse events, especially at the symptom level (e.g., cough or fever), should be assumed to be largely incomplete in claims. In addition, events that require clinical details such as laboratory tests or pathology results cannot be identified directly in claims, as that information is not available. Proxies for such outcomes through diagnosis codes may suffice in a limited subset of cases (e.g., hypertension identified through a diagnosis code rather than blood pressure measurements will likely identify many but not all cases of new-onset hypertension). Of particular concern for many PASS, most claims databases lack information on death.

As previously mentioned, diagnosis codes in claims are entered for the purpose of justifying the expense of the procedure(s) administered by the medical provider. Although many diagnosis codes appear to reflect accurately the condition of the patient, others are entered to indicate a condition that is being tested by may not be present; such codes are known as "rule-out" codes. For example, a patient being worked up for suspected rheumatoid arthritis, who is found not to have the condition, may still have the diagnosis for rheumatoid arthritis entered on a claim for the laboratory tests relevant to making the diagnosis. It can be difficult to separate rule-out codes from true diagnoses. Still, some measures can be taken to reduce the likelihood of misclassifying disease based on rule-out codes. Some of the approaches that are commonly applied include requirement of multiple claims with the diagnosis of interest separated by some minimum number of days (applicable for chronic conditions) or on an inpatient claims; requirement of a diagnosis plus a related treatment; or restriction to codes on claims for evaluation and management procedures and not codes obtained from claims for laboratory tests, radiology, and other diagnostic procedures (Capkun et al., 2015; Sung et al., 2016). Even aside from rule-out codes, the diagnosis codes entered in claims may be erroneous (e.g., data entry errors). For some outcomes and coding systems, the codes may be too imprecise to pinpoint the outcome. The move from ICD-9 to ICD-10 codes has reduced the latter problem, as ICD-10 codes are more specific than ICD-9 (Ali et al., 2017). For example, Stevens–Johnson syndrome, an event of interest for some PASS, is combined with other skin disorders in ICD-9 codes but has a unique ICD-10 code. Still, all coding systems have their limitations, and not all diagnoses can be identified precisely in any claims database. Even when the coding system allows for precise identification of diagnoses of interest, the codes entered may contain only the higher-level information (i.e., the first several digits or characters of a code) rather than the full, specific code.

In a closed claims system, where start and end dates of enrollment are known, the average duration of enrollment may be relatively brief; for many databases, an average of 2–3 years is seen. If a baseline period of 6–12 months is set, to establish new use of the study drug and examine comorbidities, then the average follow-up duration after the index date (i.e., date of study drug initiation) may be only a year or two. Outcomes that occur quickly after starting a new medicinal product can be studied in this situation, but those that require a lengthy exposure time and/or incubation period (e.g., development of cancer) may not be well-suited for claims database with high membership turnover. Some administrative databases have very low turnover, however, such as those representing national health-care systems (e.g., in the Nordic countries), which typically contain lifetime data for patients unless they emigrate from the country.

Health insurance claims undergo an adjudication process between submission of the claim from the provider and payment being made to the provider for health-care services. This process may be completed very quickly, but in some instances, a claim may not be settled for several months. This delay must be added to the time needed to prepare the claims database for research use, resulting in a lag between the occurrence of medical services and the availability of the claims data on those services that can be any duration from 1 month to over a year (depending on the claims system and their processes for preparing the data for public use). Near real-time analysis of data on newly approved medicinal products is therefore not possible using claims data, as the lag time needs to be accounted for in all analyses.

METHODOLOGICAL CONSIDERATIONS

The enrollment dates that are included in most claims databases define the period when the patient treatment and medical history can be considered to be known. A small number of claims may appear to have service dates outside of the dates of enrollment, although it cannot be assumed that complete information on the patient medical care is available if their enrollment has ended or not yet begun. Accordingly, in a claims analysis it is important to define the baseline and follow-up periods based on periods of continuous enrollment. For same analyses, a 1-month break in enrollment may be permitted while still considering the enrollment period to be continuous, but longer breaks should be excluded from the analyses. The general approach is to censor the data for patients when they disenroll from the health plan, even if one or more additional claims appear after the end of enrollment. It is also typical to require a baseline period prior to the study index date; this baseline period allows a view of the patient preexisting medical conditions and provides reasonable assurance that the study drug was initiated on the index date rather than continuing from earlier use. Fig. 3.1.2 presents a general timeline for cohort definition with baseline and follow-up periods. During the period of continuous enrollment, the assumption is made that all relevant medical care, including treatments, diagnoses, and procedures, are included in the data, and that no relevant medical events occurred without appearing in the data. There is, in essence, no data that can be positively identified as missing; even a complete lack of data during follow-up is interpreted to mean that the patient had no medical visits or drug dispensings during that time.

Another methodological issue that may be important for some analyses relates to the fact that diagnoses are entered as justification for services and do not have dates of onset attached. As a result, it can be difficult to separate a new event of the same type from follow-up care for a prior event. For

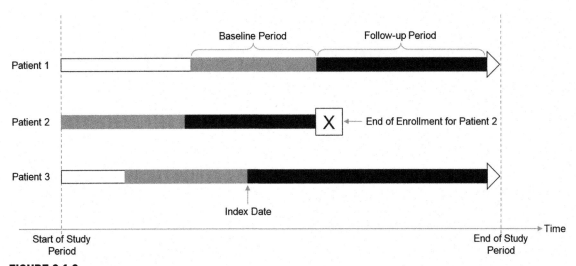

FIGURE 3.1.2
Cohort selection and time periods for claims analysis.

example, a study examining stroke as an outcome may include patients who had a stroke prior to starting the study drug. If the baseline stroke predates a claim for stroke during follow-up by years, it may be safely assumed that the follow-up stroke claim represented a new event. On the other extreme, if a baseline stroke occurred 1 day before the index date, and a follow-up claim with a stroke diagnosis appears on the day after the index date, it is quite likely that the follow-up stroke record is referring to the same event that occurred during baseline. The simplest approach to handle this problem is to exclude the patients with a history during the baseline period of the outcome event. If, however, the inclusion of such patients is an important element of the PASS, it may be possible to construct algorithms to tease apart new from nonnew events during follow-up. Such algorithms may rely on combinations of time between successive claims for the event, start of a new inpatient hospitalization with a primary diagnosis of the event (for events such as stroke that typically result in hospitalization), and treatment (including drugs and procedures) that may indicate a new event. Their validity, however, may be limited (Deshpande et al., 2015; Kumamaru et al., 2014; Wen et al., 2015).

CLAIMS-BASED POST-AUTHORIZATION SAFETY STUDIES

In some limited cases, PASS for regulatory requirements may be conducted using claims data alone; other PASS use claims data as a starting point and link to other sources of health-care information, such as medical charts, to fill gaps in the claims data. The choice of whether a claims database would be an appropriate data source for PASS depends on several factors, as illustrated in Fig. 3.1.3. If the medicinal products of interest, the indication for those products, and the study outcomes all have unique codes in the database coding system, then it might be feasible to conduct a claims PASS. For indications that may appear as rule-out diagnoses or are otherwise questionable in claims, in most cases the presence of a diagnosis code for the indication plus the treatment of interest is sufficient to identify the patient population of interest.

Outcomes, on the other hand, must be identified with good validity in the data if the results are to be meaningful. The existence of a unique diagnosis code for the outcome of interest does not guarantee that all records containing that diagnosis code are truly indicating the event. If studies have previously been conducted in similar databases with linked information that allows confirmation or disconfirmation of the event, such as through a chart review, and an algorithm with high accuracy has been established, then the claims database may be used on its own for PASS, without linking to other types

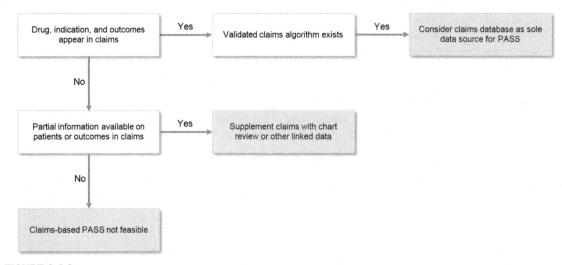

FIGURE 3.1.3
Decision tree for determining whether a claims database is suitable for PASS.

of data. However, if no such validation studies have been published in similar data sources, of if high-performing algorithms were not found, then for a valid PASS, it is necessary to link to another source of data to ensure that the endpoints are correctly identified.

Many drug safety studies, for regulatory and other purposes, have been conducted in claims databases alone, with no other data linked to the claims (Citrome et al., 2013; Correll et al., 2015; Dore et al., 2009; Endres et al., 2016; Liu et al., 2015; McIntyre and Jerrell, 2008; Roughead et al., 2015; Shin et al., 2017; Singh et al., 2016; Tsai et al., 2016; Villines et al., 2015; Wang et al., 2015). Roughead et al. estimated the risk of edema and heart failure associated with the used of thiazolidinediones antidiabetes therapies, taking claims data from six countries: Australia, Canada, Hong Kong, Japan, Korea, and Taiwan (Roughead et al., 2015). In a study using the US claims database, Ingenix Research Data Mart, Dore et al. estimated the relative risk of acute pancreatitis among patients using incretin-based diabetes therapies compared with patients treated with antidiabetes medications with established safety profiles (metformin or glyburide) (Dore et al., 2009). Villines et al. used another US claims database from the US Department of Defense to compare the safety profile of anticoagulant agents with major bleeding as the primary safety outcome (Villines et al., 2015). One component of the latter study assessed the benefit–risk profile observed in routine clinical care compared with that reported in clinical trials. Although all of these studies were published in peer-reviewed journals, given that they were conducted in claims data alone, the validity of the outcomes may be questionable—a fact that was appropriately noted in the paper discussion sections.

Because of the tremendous importance of correctly identifying adverse events in PASS that are intended to address regulatory requirements, most such studies take steps to validate outcomes by linking to another type of data. Even when a validated, high-performing algorithm exists for an outcome, the regulatory agency may stipulate that direct validation of the outcomes in the studies population is needed. There are a number of different types of data that can be linked to claims to fulfill this need. Most commonly, the data linked to claims to validate outcomes are obtained via chart review. With this approach, a screening algorithm is applied to the claims data to identify patients who might have had the outcome of interest. The screening algorithms used are typically designed to cast a wide net in an effort to pull in all true cases even at the expense of reviewing charts for patients who are not found to have the event. In other words, the intent of the screening algorithm is to prioritize sensitivity over specificity. The charts are reviewed and information extracted onto a form designed to summarize all of the information relevant to determining whether the outcome event occurred. The completed forms are typically adjudicated by clinicians who have expertise identifying the outcome. Only cases that are confirmed in the adjudication process are included in the outcome analysis. Examples of studies using claims data with chart reviews to validate outcomes include an assessment of a University of Minnesota claims-based algorithm for detecting severe renal and urinary adverse effects of radiotherapy (Sewell et al., 2013); an examination of hypersensitivity reactions to the HIV drug abacavir in the Ingenix Research Database (Nordstrom et al., 2007); and a study in Medicare claims data on surgical site infections after hip arthroplasty (Calderwood et al., 2013).

To overcome the lack of death data in most claims databases, many drug safety studies link to national or state mortality data. The process generally involves submitting identifying information for all patients who disenroll from the health plan during the risk period for the outcome to a search of the death data. One study linking claims to death data included a third linkage, to electronic medical record (EMR) data, to asses the positive predictive value of opioid overdose and poisoning codes (Green et al., 2017). Chapter 3.2 discusses EMR with details. Other studies link claims with registry data or data from clinical trials; an example of the latter linkage was a study using claims data to follow patients with metastatic prostate cancer who were enrolled in a clinical trial of androgen deprivation therapy; adverse events were identified through Medicare claims (Hershman et al., 2016). Conversely, patients can be identified from claims data and then followed prospectively with clinical assessments or surveys. This approach may be needed for outcomes that are not typically monitored in real-world clinical practice. One study examined self-reported duration of glucocorticoid use and adverse events obtained from a survey of patients identified as glucocorticoid users from a claims database (Curtis et al., 2006).

References

Ali, A.K., Beyrer, J.K., Schroeder, K.M., Wu, J., Haldane, D.C., Mitchell, L., 2017. Case studies on the impact of ICD-9-CM to ICD-10-CM coding transition on studies using real-world data in the United States. Value Health 20 (3), A319.

American Medical Association (AMA). CPT®, 2016. Available from: https://www.ama-assn.org/practice-management/cpt-current-procedural-terminology.

Calderwood, M.S., Kleinman, K., Bratzler, D.W., Ma, A., Bruce, C.B., Kaganov, R.E., et al., 2013. Use of Medicare claims to identify US hospitals with a high rate of surgical site infection after hip arthroplasty. Infect. Control Hosp. Epidemiol. 34, 31−39.

Capkun, G., Lahoz, R., Verdun, E., Song, X., Chen, W., Korn, J.R., et al., 2015. Expanding the use of administrative claims databases in conducting clinical real-world evidence studies in multiple sclerosis. Curr. Med. Res. Opin. 31, 1029−1039.

Citrome, L., Collins, J.M., Nordstrom, B.L., Rosen, E.J., Baker, R., Nadkarni, A., et al., 2013. Incidence of cardiovascular outcomes and diabetes mellitus among users of second-generation antipsychotics. J. Clin. Psychiatr. 74, 1199−1206.

Correll, C.U., Joffe, B.I., Rosen, L.M., Sullivan, T.B., Joffe, R.T., 2015. Cardiovascular and cerebrovascular risk factors and events associated with second-generation antipsychotic compared to antidepressant use in a non-elderly adult sample: results from a claims-based inception cohort study. World Psychiatry 14, 56−63.

Curtis, J.R., Westfall, A.O., Allison, J., Bijlsma, J.W., Freeman, A., George, V., et al., 2006. Population-based assessment of adverse events associated with long-term glucocorticoid use. Arthritis Rheum. 55, 420−426.

Deshpande, A.D., Schootman, M., Mayer, A., 2015. Development of a claims-based algorithm to identify colorectal cancer recurrence. Ann. Epidemiol. 25, 297−300.

Deutsches Institut fur Medizinische Dokumentation und Information (DIMDI), Der Operationen- und Prozedurenschlüssel (OPS), 2017. Available from: http://www.dimdi.de/static/de/klassi/ops/kodesuche/index.htm.

Dore, D.D., Seeger, J.D., Arnold Chan, K., 2009. Use of a claims-based active drug safety surveillance system to assess the risk of acute pancreatitis with exenatide or sitagliptin compared to metformin or glyburide. Curr. Med. Res. Opin. 25, 1019−1027.

Endres, H.G., Kaufmann-Kolle, P., Steeb, V., Bauer, E., Bottner, C., Thurmann, P., 2016. Association between potentially inappropriate medication (PIM) use and risk of hospitalization in older adults: an observational study based on routine data comparing PIM use with use of PIM alternatives. PLoS One 11 e0146811.

Green, C.A., Perrin, N.A., Janoff, S.L., Campbell, C.I., Chilcoat, H.D., Coplan, P.M., 2017. Assessing the accuracy of opioid overdose and poisoning codes in diagnostic information from electronic health records, claims data, and death records. Pharmacoepidemiol. Drug Saf. 26 (5), 509−517.

Hershman, D.L., Unger, J.M., Wright, J.D., Ramsey, S., Till, C., Tangen, C.M., et al., 2016. Adverse health events following intermittent and continuous androgen deprivation in patients with metastatic prostate cancer. JAMA Oncol. 2, 453−461.

Kassenärztliche Bundesvereinigung (KBV), Einheitlicher Bewertungsmaßstab (EBM), 2017. Available from: http://www.kbv.de/html/ebm.php.

Kumamaru, H., Judd, S.E., Curtis, J.R., Ramachandran, R., Hardy, N.C., Rhodes, J.D., et al., 2014. Validity of claims-based stroke algorithms in contemporary Medicare data: reasons for geographic and racial differences in stroke (REGARDS) study linked with medicare claims. Circ. Cardiovasc. Qual. Outcomes 7, 611–619.

Liu, J., Sylwestrzak, G., Ruggieri, A.P., DeVries, A., 2015. Intravenous versus subcutaneous anti-TNF-alpha agents for Crohn's disease: a comparison of effectiveness and safety. J. Manag. Care Spec. Pharm. 21, 559–566.

McIntyre, R.S., Jerrell, J.M., 2008. Metabolic and cardiovascular adverse events associated with anti-psychotic treatment in children and adolescents. Arch. Pediatr. Adolesc. Med. 162, 929–935.

National Health Service (NHS) UK, Read Codes, 2017. Available from: https://digital.nhs.uk/article/1104/Read-Codes.

Nordic Centre for Classifications in Health Care (NordClass), NOMESCO Classification of Surgical Procedures (NCSP), 2012. Available from: http://www.nordclass.se/ncsp_e.htm.

Nordstrom, B.L., Norman, H.S., Dube, T.J., Wilcox, M.A., Walker, A.M., 2007. Identification of abacavir hypersensitivity reaction in health care claims data. Pharmacoepidemiol. Drug Saf. 16, 289–296.

Roughead, E.E., Chan, E.W., Choi, N.K., Kimura, M., Kimura, T., Kubota, K., et al., 2015. Variation in association between thiazolidinediones and heart failure across ethnic groups: retrospective analysis of large healthcare claims databases in six countries. Drug Saf. 38, 823–831.

Sewell, J.M., Rao, A., Elliott, S.P., 2013. Validating a claims-based method for assessing severe rectal and urinary adverse effects of radiotherapy. Urology 82, 335–340.

Shin, J.Y., Song, I., Lee, J.H., Yoon, J.L., Kwon, J.S., Park, B.J., 2017. Differential risk of peptic ulcer among users of antidepressants combined with nonsteroidal anti-inflammatory drugs. J. Clin. Psychopharmacol. 37, 239–245.

Singh, S., Heien, H.C., Sangaralingham, L.R., Schilz, S.R., Kappelman, M.D., Shah, N.D., et al., 2016. Comparative effectiveness and safety of anti-tumor necrosis factor agents in biologic-naive patients with Crohn's disease. Clin. Gastroenterol. Hepatol. 14, 1120–1129.e6.

Sung, S.F., Hsieh, C.Y., Lin, H.J., Chen, Y.W., Yang, Y.H., Li, C.Y., 2016. Validation of algorithms to identify stroke risk factors in patients with acute ischemic stroke, transient ischemic attack, or intracerebral hemorrhage in an administrative claims database. Int. J. Cardiol. 215, 277–282.

Tsai, P.S., Liu, I.C., Chiu, C.H., Huang, C.J., Wang, M.Y., 2016. Effect of valproic acid on dementia onset in patients with bipolar disorder. J. Affect. Disord. 201, 131–136.

US Centers for Disease Control and Prevention (CDC), US National Center for Health Statistics, World Health Organization (WHO), International Classification of Diseases, Ninth Revision (ICD-9), 1998. Available from: https://www.cdc.gov/nchs/icd/icd9cm.htm.

US Centers for Medicare & Medicaid Services (CMS), January 2017a. Physician Quality Reporting System: ICD-10 Section. Available from: https://www.cms.gov/Medicare/Quality-Initiatives-Patient-Assessment-Instruments/PQRS/index.html?redirect=/pqri.

US Centers for Medicare & Medicaid Services (CMS), 2017b. HCPCS—General Information. Available from: https://www.cms.gov/Medicare/Coding/MedHCPCSGenInfo/index.html.

US Department of Health and Human Services (HHS), August 2008. HHS Proposes Adoption of ICD-10 Code Sets and Updated Electronic Transaction Standards: Proposed Changes Would Improve Disease Tracking and Speed Transition to an Electronic Health Care Environment [Press Release]. Available from: http://www.hhs.gov/news/press/2008pres/08/20080815a.html.

Villines, T.C., Schnee, J., Fraeman, K., Siu, K., Reynolds, M.W., Collins, J., et al., 2015. A comparison of the safety and effectiveness of dabigatran and warfarin in non-valvular atrial fibrillation patients in a large healthcare system. Thromb. Haemostasis 114, 1290–1298.

Wang, M.T., Chu, C.L., Yeh, C.B., Chang, L.C., Malone, D.C., Liou, J.T., 2015. Antidepressant use and risk of recurrent stroke: a population-based nested case-control study. J. Clin. Psychiatr. 76, e877–e885.

Wen, J., Barber, G.E., Ananthakrishnan, A.N., 2015. Identification of recurrent *Clostridium difficile* infection using administrative codes: accuracy and implications for surveillance. Infect. Control Hosp. Epidemiol. 36, 893–898.

World Health Organization (WHO), International Classification of Diseases, 10th Revision, 2016a. Available from: http://apps.who.int/classifications/icd10/browse/2016/en.

WHO Collaborating Centre for the Family of International Classifications (FIC) in the Netherlands. CMSV 2.6 (nl), 2016b. Available from: http://www.who-fic.nl/Downloads_en_Links.

Yoshida, Y., Yamakami, H., Hattori, J., Ohe, K., 2014. Development and evaluation of the code finder "J-Lacco" from the JLAC10, the Japan classification and coding for clinical laboratory tests described "Laboratory Test Code Master". Jpn. J. Med. Inform. 34, 129–140.

Electronic Medical Records

Beth L. Nordstrom, Kathy H. Fraeman, Dimitra Lambrelli

Evidera, Bethesda, MD, United States

INTRODUCTION

The use of electronic medical records (EMRs) in clinical practice is expanding, replacing the paper charts that were formally the standard means of tracking health data for patients (King et al., 2012). An EMR contains patient medical information in digital format, allowing for the creation of databases that can be used for research. Drug safety studies in support of regulatory requirements, including post-authorization safety studies (PASS) for European Medicines Agency and postmarketing safety studies for the US FDA, may be conducted using EMR databases with or without additional linked data.

CONTENTS OF ELECTRONIC MEDICAL RECORD DATABASES

EMR databases may contain data for patients from one site or many, or those representing multiple sites; those sites may be using the same EMR system for entering the patient data or using different EMR software. Because these databases represent different collections of sites (i.e., clinical practices or medical facilities) and of EMR software, their contents can differ widely. Many of these databases bring together data from a collection of sites of the same type; for example, there are EMR databases from general practitioners only and others from oncology clinics only. Others provide data from integrated health systems and include a combination of outpatient primary care, outpatient specialty, and inpatient settings. The latter type of databases can allow a complete view of all of the medical care a patient receives within that health system (Fig. 3.2.1).

Information on active diagnoses for patients is an essential part of all EMR databases used for drug safety research. Diagnoses may be entered using a standard coding system, such as ICD-10 (WHO, 2016), or can be entered as free text. The date attached to a diagnosis may represent the date of a visit during which the condition was given consideration by the physician or the original date of diagnosis; some databases provide both of these dates,

CONTENTS

Introduction 63

Contents of Electronic Medical Record Databases 63

Strengths and Limitations of Electronic Medical Record Databases 66

EMR-Based Post-Authorization Safety Studies 68

PASS Using EMR Linked to Other Data 70

References 72

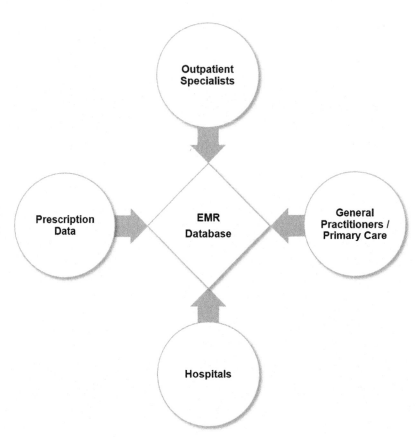

FIGURE 3.2.1
Contents of typical EMR database.

allowing a view of duration of disease and patterns of follow-up care for the disease. Similarly, for any database that might be considered for PASS, some levels of detail are needed on prescription treatments received. Although some EMR databases contain linked pharmacy dispensing data, most include prescriptions only. The database might note, for example, the name of the medicinal product, date prescribed, and dose prescribed; repeat prescriptions would be noted, but the dates on which the patient filled the prescription and any allowed refills would not be available. Supply times allowed in each prescription may or may not be indicated in the data.

One of the hallmarks of most EMR databases is the availability of laboratory results data. Many of these databases contain laboratory test names, either in free text or using a coding system such as Logical Observation Identifiers Names and Codes , along with the results of the test, date of the test, and sometimes the normal range specific to the laboratory that processed the test (LOINC, 2017). The completeness of the laboratory results data depends, in part, on the data entry mechanism used. When the laboratory reports data electronically into the system, completeness is excellent for all laboratory tests measured in that practice. However, when manual entry is required, the results of the tests may not be available consistently. Nonstandard tests that are processed by specialty laboratories are particularly subject to this limitation in many databases; in some cases, the specialty laboratory results appear infrequently if at all.

Although the use of EMR in clinical practice includes an electronic recording of progress notes and other open, free-text information, this component of the record is typically not available in database extracts that can be purchased for analyses by parties other than the data owner. Such open fields may contain patient names and other identifiers; sharing the data would thus violate patient privacy. Some EMR data owners are able to conduct targeted searches of the notes to identify information of interest. The information is placed into separate fields and contains only the data elements of interest. For example, a search of progress notes for any mention of symptoms of psychosis can be used to create new variables indicting the name of the symptom and date recorded. Finding the information within the free-text data is a complex process that requires sophisticated natural language processing to ensure, for example, that a note stating that a patient did not have a given event (e.g., condition or treatment) is not incorrectly coded as the patient having had the event (Xu et al., 2011; Henriksson et al., 2015).

Site-specific EMR databases that reflect, for example, primary care settings only may include some limited information for other settings. Referrals to other specialties, summary information from hospitalizations, and notes of medications that were prescribed elsewhere can appear in some databases. In general, the information that is available on diagnoses and treatments received outside of the EMR system should be used with caution, as it may have a high likelihood of missing or erroneous data. Fig. 3.2.2 presents the relative degree of availability of various types of information in different classes of EMR databases compared with the data available in claims databases (see Chapter 3.1 for detailed discussion about administrative claims databases). Because of the wide variation in EMR databases, however, some specific databases within a given type may differ considerably with respect to availability of one or more data types. A key requirement, prior to embarking on any PASS using an EMR database, is to assess carefully the type and extent of data available in the selected database that is relevant to identifying the study population, predictors, and outcomes.

Variables	Administrative Claims	Electronic Medical Records		
		Primary Care	Specialist Care	Integrated Health System
Diagnosis	●	●	●	●
Demographics	◐	◕	◐	◕
Treatment Prescribed	●	◐	◐	●
Treatment Dispensed	●	○	○	○
Treatment Administered in Hospital	◐	○	◐	●
Comorbidities	●	●	◔	●
Other Concomitant Medication Use	●	◐	◐	◕
Specialist Visits (All Specialties)	●	○	◔	●
Surgical Procedures	●	◔	◐	●
Radiology / Pathology Findings	○	○	◔	◔
Laboratory Tests Performed	●	◐	◔	●
Laboratory Test Results	○	◐	◔	◕
Over-The-Counter Medications	○	○	◔	◔

Data Unavailable ⟵————⟶ Data Available

○   ◔   ◐   ◕   ●

FIGURE 3.2.2

Completeness of data commonly available in claims and EMR databases.

STRENGTHS AND LIMITATIONS OF ELECTRONIC MEDICAL RECORD DATABASES

When the purpose of PASS is to assess major clinical outcomes in a real-world population of patients using the medicinal product of interest, an appropriately selected EMR database may provide the best possible source of data. The population represented in an EMR database is highly generalizable to the types of patients seen in the sites included in the database. Although this population may not be representative of all patients who are prescribed the study drug, it is at least not typically limited by age group or type of health insurance coverage, as is typically the case with a claims database. Patients can be identified for the study based on programming rules that stipulate certain combinations of diagnoses and drugs recorded in the EMR, with far lower opportunity for biased

selection than when enrolling patients by consent or asking physicians to identify suitable patients from their practices.

EMR databases may contain a wealth of clinical detail that can be invaluable
for certain PASS. For example, a study examining the risk of renal outcomes
will benefit from the availability of relevant laboratory measures such as
estimated glomerular filtration rate, in addition to diagnoses of renal disease
and procedures, such as dialysis. These laboratory results may be used not
only to identify the outcomes of interest but also to classify patients with
respect to their renal function at baseline. An important limitation, however,
will arise if the database is site-specific rather than covering all sites of care
(including inpatient, outpatient, and dialysis centers). A database covering
outpatient clinics may have little or no data on hospitalizations; thus, patients
with the most severe outcomes who are hospitalized for the event might have
no indication of the event in the database.

Although the problem of rule-out diagnoses in claims data is well known
(Lawson et al., 2012), researchers may mistakenly assume that any diagnosis
entered into an EMR represents a true diagnosis and not simply a condition
that is being tested but may be found not to be present. Unfortunately,
some of the information entered into an EMR, including diagnoses, may be
used to populate medical claims, and so in general, EMR diagnoses suffer
from the same limitations as in claims. Therefore, care must be taken to avoid
considering a rule-out diagnosis as a true condition. Diagnoses given in
conjunction with a testing procedure, for example, may have a high likelihood of being invalid.

Most EMR databases lack clear information on the time period during which
the patient can be considered under follow-up. Whereas health insurance
plans include dates of start and end of enrollment, and all covered services
can be assumed to be present in the data between those dates; follow-up in
an EMR database often requires creating a proxy for enrollment based on
the earliest and latest visit dates. Any observed gaps in care between those
dates might reflect times when patients received no medical care or when
they received care from outside of the EMR system. Additionally, patients
may receive some care within the EMR system while concurrently receiving
care from a specialist outside of the system. One approach to overcoming
the lack of enrollment data and providing more complete data across all sites
of care is to combine an EMR database with a claims database, using only
subset of patients who appear in both databases. The resulting data set can
provide a powerful tool for assessing drug safety, with the clinical depth in
the EMR data combined with the comprehensive but shallower view of all
health-care services available in claims data. Events and conditions that are
found only in the claims data may be imprecise, without the laboratory results

and other information on clinical findings that are seen in an EMR, but at least no major medical events should be missing from the combined data. The primary, often insurmountable, limitation to these combined databases is that they typically represent a relatively small number of patients (often only 10%−20% of the population in the individual databases). Unless the indication and medicinal product under study are highly common in the population, a combined claims-EMR database is unlikely to provide adequate statistical power.

The prescription drug data available in most EMR databases seem to be relatively complete with respect to the medicinal products prescribed in that setting (i.e., by the providers using the EMR system), but the lack of pharmacy dispensing data adds a level of uncertainty to the dates of exposure to products. A prescription that allows up to a year of refills may have been filled on schedule to the end of the year or may not have been filled at all. On the other hand, some EMR databases contain at least some information on patient's self-reported use of over-the-counter products, which is entirely missing in claims data.

EMR-BASED POST-AUTHORIZATION SAFETY STUDIES

Drug safety studies that have been performed using EMR databases alone, with no other source of linked data, have used a variety of data sources ranging from individual medical center EMR systems to data collected from large, nationwide populations. Several examples of such studies are available (Asche et al., 2008; Hicks et al., 2016; Tatonetti et al., 2011; Nordstrom et al., 2014; Coloma et al., 2011). The outcomes of these studies have also varied widely but in general have focused on events that can be found in the more reliable fields available in EMR data extracts, such as commonly measured laboratory test results and diagnoses identifiable through the EMR diagnosis coding system.

Large EMR databases containing general practitioner or primary care data, with little or no specialist visit data, can offer useful sources of drug safety information if the outcomes of interest are most likely to be treated in the primary care setting. One such study used the General Electric Centricity EMR database to examine the risk of a variety of adverse events among patients with diabetes treated with metformin, a sulfonylurea, or a thiazolidinedione (Asche et al., 2008). The outcomes were identified through combinations of diagnosis codes and laboratory results, as appropriate; they included diarrhea, nausea, vomiting, abdominal pain, dyspepsia, dizziness, headache, weight gain, hypoglycemia, edema, lactic acidosis, heart failure, and liver enzyme elevations. Although the most severe outcomes that resulted in hospitalization and the mildest outcomes, for which the patient did not seek medical care, were likely to have been absent from the data, this data source provided a good source of information for the study outcomes, given that most of these events would typically be treated—at least in part—in the primary care setting.

Another primary care database that is frequently used for PASS is the Clinical Practice Research Datalink (CPRD) from the United Kingdom. A study used this database to investigate the risk of breast cancer among patients with diabetes who were prescribed incretin enhancer antidiabetes medications (Hicks et al., 2016). Although breast cancer is not typically treated by general practitioners, the authors cited evidence that the cancer diagnosis found in CPRD demonstrates good concordance with the diagnosis in the country's National Cancer Data Repository. Studies of cancer as an outcome require lengthy follow-up to allow development and diagnosis of the malignancy. The CPRD offers long-term follow-up data for most patients, although any PASS of a newly authorized medicinal product will necessarily include only a limited follow-up duration for the first year after marketing authorization.

EMR databases that include data from a single medical practice are likely to be too small for PASS, but combining several such databases may result in adequate statistical power for some studies. One study used data from three academic medical centers to investigate changes in blood glucose levels among patients treated concurrently with pravastatin lipid-lowering therapy and paroxetine antidepressant therapy (Tatonetti et al., 2011). Analyses were conducted in the separate databases and in a combined cohort. When combining multiple EMR databases, it is important to examine the results in each database separately to determine whether the results are too heterogeneous to allow valid combining. Of course, the desired approach is to combine the databases to maximize power, but if one or more databases produce markedly different findings than the others, the combined data should include only the databases with relatively homogeneous patterns of results. Standard statistical methods for assessment of heterogeneity used in metaanalyses can be performed to evaluate this issue (Higgins et al., 2003).

Databases containing EMR data from specialist practices may be used for certain PASS, for events that are expected to be seen primarily in the specialty clinic. Adverse events that are likely to be treated in other settings such as primary care or hospitals would be poor candidates for specialist-only databases. As with other types of EMR databases, specialist databases may be combined to increase statistical power. A study in two outpatient oncology clinic databases maintained by Varian Medical Systems and Elekta/Impac Medical Systems examined the risk of several hematologic and other laboratory-based adverse events associated with use of bendamustine chemo-therapy (Nordstrom et al., 2014). Other events that cannot be identified through laboratory tests, such as fatigue and alopecia, were also assessed but reflect only those events that were noted by the provider. Assessments of laboratory-based events such as anemia or neutropenia may be more valid than non−laboratory-based outcomes because the laboratory results show normal and abnormal findings. Diagnostic data typically have no negative findings; the assumption is that the absence of a diagnosis means that the diagnosis was not present.

In the present era of overexpanding databases for health-care research, very large combined EMR databases are being created that contain data on huge populations. The Exploring and Understanding Adverse Drug Reactions project has used a distributed data network to link patient data from eight databases in four countries: Denmark, Italy, the Netherlands, and the United Kingdom. A study of the incidence of upper gastrointestinal bleeding associated with use of nonsteroidal antiinflammatory drugs (NSAIDs) was performed in this data network (Coloma et al., 2011). Nearly 20 million patients were included in the analysis, a sample size that would provide ample power for analyses of far more rare events than their selected outcome. Rather than collecting raw data extracts from each database, the distributed data network approach allows the original data to remain behind the data owner firewalls. Data extracts are converted into common data model, and the same programming is applied to the converted data from each data source separately. Only then the results are brought together in aggregate form. Such an approach alleviates concerns regarding the privacy of patient's health-care data and allows the data owners, who have the deepest understanding of their data, to perform the data manipulation as appropriate to the health-care and recording practices used within their system. More discussion on big data and analytic platforms, including common data models is presented in Chapters 3.4 and 5.4.

PASS USING EMR LINKED TO OTHER DATA

Linkage of EMR data to other types of data can be accomplished for specific study objectives, although more and more linked data sources are becoming available. For example, the CPRD contains EMR data from general practitioners with an established link to other data sources such as the Hospital Episode Statistics (HES) and national mortality data. A study assessing the risk of venous thromboembolism with testosterone treatment used this linked data set (Martinez et al., 2016). The availability of hospital data and cause of death information allowed a far more valid identification of the outcome than would the general practitioner data alone. In addition, comorbidities that may be treated in the hospital rather than by the general practitioner were assessed with greater completeness using the linked HES data. Although the HES database contains diagnostic and procedure information that would be relevant to this study, it lacks laboratory results data. Thus, outcomes that rely on inpatient laboratory data would require a different data source.

In the United States, linked EMR and claims databases may provide the most complete retrospective/secondary use of data available. The Geisinger Health System EMR database, for example, can be accessed in conjunction with full medical and pharmacy claims data for the patients who are also enrolled in the Geisinger health plan; the resulting subset represents $\sim 30\%$ of all patients in the EMR database. If the reduced sample size is still sufficient to power the analyses, PASS can be greatly strengthened by adding the relatively complete (i.e., across sites of care) data from claims to the deeper clinical detail provided in an EMR. A study in this database examined the risk of chemotherapy-induced febrile neutropenia (Weycker et al., 2013). The identification of the outcome in claims data, without the inclusion of laboratory results, was only partially successful. Still, the addition of full inpatient and outpatient claims may indicate outcomes that are not included in an EMR database, such as when a patient receives care for an event outside of the health system represented in the EMR.

A similar database to CPRD, The Health Improvement Network (THIN) database, also contains general practitioner data from the United Kingdom. One study in this database compared the risk of upper gastrointestinal bleeding among patients treated with conventional NSAIDs with those receiving COX-II inhibitors (Toh et al., 2011). Although the outcome was identified through diagnosis codes entered in the diagnostic data, they were also validated through a manual review of anonymized free-text notes, which do not form part of a standard extract of the THIN data. This important validation step reduced the number of bleeding cases from 468 to 183. Clearly, the event rate would have been greatly overestimated if only the diagnostic data had been used. The manual review of notes provided an essential source of linked data, although the time needed for this process is substantially longer than use of automated data alone. Manual chart review and other methods of data collection, including both secondary and primary data collection, may lead to highly robust identification of study outcomes. If an outcome event is not typically reported in medical records in usual practice (e.g., if the outcome requires measurement of a diagnostic test that is not commonly performed), then prospective/primary data collection is needed to ascertain the outcome. However, most drug safety outcomes investigated in PASS are expected to appear in some form in retrospective/secondary use of data. Some studies use a combination of EMR database only for some outcomes and linked data for others. For example, a study using a distributed data network in three databases: the Altos outpatient oncology clinic database; the US Department of Veterans Affairs EMR database; and the PHARMO database from the Netherlands used laboratory results from these EMR databases to identify liver enzyme elevations (Shantakumar et al., 2016). The study also examined the risk of drug-induced liver injury, an outcome that requires a hybrid of laboratory results, diagnostic data, and evaluation from an experienced hepatologist to determine with any validity. Hence, manual chart review and case adjudication by an expert clinical panel was performed to validate the drug-induced liver injury outcome. For more discussion on enriched/hybrid study designs, please see Chapter 4.4.

References

Asche, C.V., McAdam-Marx, C., Shane-McWhorter, L., Sheng, X., Plauschinat, C.A., 2008. Association between oral antidiabetic use, adverse events and outcomes in patients with type 2 diabetes. Diabetes Obes. Metab. 10 (8), 638–645.

Coloma, P.M., Schuemie, M.J., Trifiro, G., et al., 2011. Combining electronic healthcare databases in Europe to allow for large-scale drug safety monitoring: the EU-ADR Project. Pharmacoepidemiol. Drug Saf. 20 (1), 1–11.

Henriksson, A., Kvist, M., Dalianis, H., Duneld, M., 2015. Identifying adverse drug event information in clinical notes with distributional semantic representations of context. J. Biomed. Inf. 57, 333–349.

Hicks, B.M., Yin, H., Yu, O.H., Pollak, M.N., Platt, R.W., Azoulay, L., 2016. Glucagon-like peptide-1 analogues and risk of breast cancer in women with type 2 diabetes: population based cohort study using the UK Clinical Practice Research Datalink. BMJ 355, i5340.

Higgins, J.P., Thompson, S.G., Deeks, J.J., Altman, D.G., 2003. Measuring inconsistency in meta-analyses. BMJ 327 (7414), 557–560.

King, J., Patel, V., Furukawa, M.F., December 2012. Physician Adoption of Electronic Health Record Technology to Meet Meaningful Use Objectives: 2009–2012. ONC Data Brief, No. 7. Office of the National Coordinator for Health Information Technology, Washington, DC.

Lawson, E.H., Louie, R., Zingmond, D.S., et al., 2012. A comparison of clinical registry versus administrative claims data for reporting of 30-day surgical complications. Ann. Surg. 256 (6), 973–981.

Logical Observation Identifiers Names and Codes (LOINC), 2017. Available from: https://loinc.org/.

Martinez, C., Suissa, S., Rietbrock, S., et al., 2016. Testosterone treatment and risk of venous thromboembolism: population based case-control study. BMJ 355, i5968.

Nordstrom, B.L., Knopf, K.B., Teltsch, D.Y., Engle, R., Beygi, H., Sterchele, J.A., 2014. The safety of bendamustine in patients with chronic lymphocytic leukemia or non-Hodgkin lymphoma and concomitant renal impairment: a retrospective electronic medical record database analysis. Leuk. Lymphoma 55 (6), 1266–1273.

Shantakumar, S., Nordstrom, B.L., Djousse, L., et al., 2016. Occurrence of hepatotoxicity with pazopanib and other anti-VEGF treatments for renal cell carcinoma: an observational study utilizing a distributed database network. Cancer Chemother. Pharmacol. 78 (3), 559–566.

Tatonetti, N.P., Denny, J.C., Murphy, S.N., et al., 2011. Detecting drug interactions from adverse-event reports: interaction between paroxetine and pravastatin increases blood glucose levels. Clin. Pharmacol. Ther. 90 (1), 133–142.

Toh, S., Garcia Rodriguez, L.A., Hernan, M.A., 2011. Confounding adjustment via a semi-automated high-dimensional propensity score algorithm: an application to electronic medical records. Pharmacoepidemiol. Drug Saf. 20 (8), 849–857.

Weycker, D., Sofrygin, O., Seefeld, K., Deeter, R.G., Legg, J., Edelsberg, J., 2013. Technical evaluation of methods for identifying chemotherapy-induced febrile neutropenia in healthcare claims databases. BMC Health Serv. Res. 13, 60.

World Health Organization (WHO), International Classification of Diseases, 10th Revision, 2016. Available from: http://apps.who.int/classifications/icd10/browse/2016/en.

Xu, H., Jiang, M., Oetjens, M., et al., 2011. Facilitating pharmacogenetic studies using electronic health records and natural-language processing: a case study of warfarin. J. Am. Med. Inf. Assoc. 18 (4), 387–391.

Registries

Stella Blackburn
IQVIA, Durham, NC, United States

CONTENTS

Introduction 74

European
Registries 75

Registry-Based
Post-Authorization
Safety Studies 76

References 78

INTRODUCTION

Registries have the potential to be a powerful tool for post-authorization safety studies (PASS) and for post-authorization efficacy study (PAES). However, the word "registry" has different meaning to different people, ranging from a single excel spread sheet with sparse details on a few patients seen by one physician to a multicenter fully functional database covering a range of diseases. The European Union good pharmacovigilance practices defines a registry as an organized system that uses noninterventional methods to collect uniform data on specified outcomes in a population defined by a particular disease, condition, or exposure (EMA, 2017). In the United States, the Agency for Healthcare Research and Quality defines a patient registry as an organized system that uses noninterventional study methods to collect uniform data to evaluate specified outcomes for a population defined by a particular disease, condition, or exposure and serves one or more predetermined scientific, clinical, or policy purposes (Gliklich et al., 2007).

The most suitable type of registry for PASS will depend on the questions that led to the registry being set up. The two most common types of registries that are used for PASS are product registries and disease registries, but there are also registries that cover a range of products (e.g., biological registries) and registries that cover conditions (e.g., pregnancy registries) or procedures (e.g., the European Bone Marrow Transplant registry) (Watson et al., 2005; APR, 2012; EBMT, 2016). Approximately 9% of the medicinal products authorized by the European Medicines Agency (EMA) via the centralized procedure between 2005 and 2013 were required to have a registry (Bouvy et al., 2017). Of those, 35% were disease registries compared with 65% product registries. For disease registries, 55% of these were new, whereas 90% of product registries were new. The majority (67%) of the requested registries concerned new products treating rare diseases.

As the name suggests, product registries relating to (usually) a single medicinal product, which are established to answer-specific questions relating to that product. They are frequently set up by pharmaceutical companies at the request of regulatory agencies. The most common reason is to answer a safety question, but there may also be questions relating to the duration of effectiveness or the heterogeneity of effect. Registries are frequently requested for orphan medicinal products because the number of patients exposed in pivotal clinical trials is often small, and so the safety profile of the products is not well established at the time of authorization. Because the exposure is rare, a product registry can often be the most efficient method to follow patients treated with a particular product over a longer period.

One of the main flaws with product registries is that patients may switch between treatments and so be lost to follow-up once they are no longer taking the product of interest. In addition, unless the product registry has a control group, it is often difficult to determine whether adverse outcomes are due to the disease or the product of interest. For these reasons, disease registries are usually preferable to product registries. Disease registries can also provide much needed information on the natural history of the disease, and if started early enough, can be used to identify patients for clinical trials and providing a valuable post-authorization research tool. For example, Action Duchenne has a registry of Duchenne and Becker muscular dystrophy patients with details of the precise genetic mutation in the dystrophin gene, which has led to the disease (Action Duchenne, 2016). The stated purpose of their registry is a good example of the main uses for a disease registry, which is to (1) develop and encourage the development of more research into Duchenne and Becker muscular dystrophy; (2) facilitate research by collecting relevant data and making it available for specified research projects; (3) use the information to understand the disease better; (4) establish contact between clinicians, other health-care professionals, researchers, and registry participants; and (5) enhance clinicians and other health-care professionals ability to deliver treatments for this disease.

For those diseases where there are multiple therapeutic options, disease registries can help develop optimal treatment regimens for treating the disease by looking at outcomes of different combinations of therapies delivered at different times. For those diseases where there are no disease specific drug treatments, the effect of different supporting treatments (e.g., corticosteroids, physiotherapy, or ventilation) on relieving symptoms and reducing progression can be tackled in a disease registry and can also be valuable in establishing best practices.

EUROPEAN REGISTRIES

The Nordic countries (Denmark, Finland, Iceland, Norway, and Sweden) have all established population-wide registries that can be linked using the personal identity numbers given to each citizen. Of these, the Danish, Norwegian, and Swedish registries are most used for PASS. Most of the Nordic countries have registries on births, deaths, cancer, prescriptions, and hospital treatment—though the extent of hospital treatment and prescription coverage differs between countries (Ludvigsson et al., 2015). Although individually, the registries would not be considered as fitting the registry definition given earlier because they can be linked and so can provide longitudinal data on specified outcomes, they are often considered as such. All research using these databases must be approved by an ethical committee and all impose stringent conditions on access to protect sensitive patient data (Bouvy et al., 2017). Chapter 4.4 provides an overview of approaches for linking primary and secondary data sources for efficient PASS.

In Europe, there have been several initiatives designed to promote the development of European Registries. Some have been funded under the Seventh Framework Program for Research (EC, 2016). Initiatives vary from funding to setting up individual registries, to integrated platforms designed to connect registries, biobanks, and clinical bioinformatics for rare disease research (TREAT-NMD, 2016; RD Connect, 2016). Orphanet has collected information on registries associated with rare diseases (Orphanet, 2017). As of 2017, a total of 703 registries are available, of which, 69 regional, 496 national, 61 European, and 77 global. Four countries (France, Germany, Italy, and the United Kingdom) host 60% of the total number. Although 83% of the total are designated as public registries, this most likely refers to the affiliation of the organization hosting them—frequently academic and does not imply access. Another European initiative was the PARENT joint action initiative, which supports member states in developing comparable and interoperable patient registries in fields of importance (PARENT, 2016). Its two main deliverables were a fledgling registry of registries and methodological guidelines and recommendations for efficient and rational governance of patient registries. Recognizing the need for registries collecting data important for regulatory decision-making, the EMA established an initiative for patient registries in 2015 (EMA, 2015). The prime aims are to facilitate both use of existing patient registries and to establish new ones if there is a need. As part of this initiative, two workshops have been held during 2017 looking at multiple sclerosis and cystic fibrosis registries.

REGISTRY-BASED POST-AUTHORIZATION SAFETY STUDIES

The decision to use a registry for PASS is governed by a number of factors. The most important factor is the questions needing to be answered by the PASS. Long-term follow-up of a rare exposure is a prime example when a registry could be useful. As mentioned in previous chapters, the rarity of the exposure means that alternative methods, such as EMR, may not contain enough patients to get meaningful results. The next step is to see whether there are existing registries, which could be utilized for the PASS. This step is often harder than it sounds as although the resources mentioned earlier provide some information on existing registries, these are not exhaustive.

If existing registries have been found, the next step is to get details of the information held and the ability to access the data. The key criteria are whether the registry contains information on the medicinal product of interest, outcomes, and other important variables to answer the research question and whether the data are of sufficient quality to be useful. As registries are noninterventional/observational, it is not realistic to expect dual entry source verified data as found in many clinical trial data sets. What matters is whether it is of sufficient quality to answer the questions. If an important variable is missing from the data, it may be possible to add collection of this data to the registry if this is acceptable to both the registry owners and the patients.

The inclusion and exclusion criteria for the registry are important as although the data may be theoretically present in the registry; these can affect what questions can be answered. For example, some registries may confine entry to authorized indications. As such, this would not be useful for looking at drug utilization because any off-label use will not be included. Disease registries will only include information on the specific disease, so if studying medicinal products with multiple indications (e.g., immunomodulating biologics), data from different registries may need to be combined or more likely analyzed separately.

If there are no existing registries suitable for the proposed PASS, it may be necessary to develop a new registry. For the reasons stated above, disease registries are usually preferable to product registries but are likely to be more expensive. However, as in the case of the antiretroviral pregnancy registry, costs can be mitigated by marketing authorization holders of the different products creating a joint registry. An example in the United States is the medullary thyroid carcinoma (MTC) registry, which is a multisponsor disease registry established in 2010 and funded by pharmaceutical companies with marketed long-acting glucagon-like peptide-1 receptor agonists to evaluate the potential association between these antidiabetes medications and the occurrence of MTC (Koro et al., 2016).

Registries are a powerful tool for both PASS and PAES and can help provide important information on both safety and effectiveness over a period. Their usefulness will be determined by the research questions being asked and the proposed study design. With the increasing emphasis on personalized medicine and rare diseases, it is likely that registries will be of increasing importance because patient populations will be relatively small in number and an international registry may be the only way to get sufficient power to answer important safety and effectiveness questions.

References

Action Duchenne, The Action Duchenne Registry. Available from: http://www.actionduchenne.org/registry/the-uk-duchenne-muscular-dystrophy-registry/.

Antiretroviral Pregnancy Registry (APR), 2012. Available from: http://www.apregistry.com/HCP.aspx.

Bouvy, J.C., Blake, K., Slattery, J., De Bruin, M.L., Arlett, P., Kurz, X., 2017. Registries in European post-marketing surveillance: a retrospective analysis of centrally approved products, 2005–2013. Pharmacoepidemiol. Drug Saf. 26, 1442–1450.

European Society for Blood and Marrow Transplantation (EBMT), Annual Report, 2016. Available from: https://www.ebmt.org/Contents/Resources/Library/Annualreport/Documents/EBMT_AnnualRep_2016.pdf.

European Commission (EC), The 7th Framework Programme, 2016. Available from: https://ec.europa.eu/research/fp7/index_en.cfm.

European Medicines Agency (EMA), Initiative for Patient Registries, September 2015. EMA/176050/2014. Available from: http://www.ema.europa.eu/docs/en_GB/document_library/Other/2015/10/WC500195576.pdf.

European Medicines Agency (EMA), October 2017. Guideline on Good Pharmacovigilance Practices (GVP) Annex I—Definitions (Rev 4). EMA/876333/2011 Rev 4. Available from: http://www.ema.europa.eu/docs/en_GB/document_library/Scientific_guideline/2013/05/WC500143294.pdf.

Gliklich, R., Dreyer, N., Leavy, M. (Eds.), April 2007. Registries for Evaluating Patient Outcomes: A User's Guide, third ed. Available from: https://effectivehealthcare.ahrq.gov/sites/default/files/pdf/registries-guide_research.pdf

Koro, C.E., Hale, P.M., Ali, A.K., Qiao, Q., Tuttle, R.M., 2016. The rationale, objectives, design and status of the medullary thyroid carcinoma (MTC) surveillance study: a case-series registry. Thyroid 26 (S1). A-125.

Ludvigsson, J.F., Håberg, S.E., Knudsen, G.P., Lafolie, P., Zoega, H., Sarkkola, C., von Kraemer, S., Weiderpass, E., Nørgaard, M., 2015. Ethical aspects of registry-based research in the Nordic countries. Clin. Epidemiol. 7, 491–508.

Orphanet, May 2017. Orphanet Report Series: Rare Disease Registries in Europe. Available from: http://www.orpha.net/orphacom/cahiers/docs/GB/Registries.pdf.

PARENT, 2016. Available from: http://patientregistries.eu/general-objectives.

RD Connect, 2016. Available from: http://rd-connect.eu/.

TREAT-NMD, 2016. Available from: http://www.treat-nmd.eu/.

Watson, K., Symmons, D., Griffiths, I., Silman, A., 2005. The British Society for Rheumatology biologics register. Ann. Rheum. Dis. 64, iv42–iv43.

Big Data

Jeremy Rassen[1], Sebastian Schneeweiss[1,2]

[1]*Aetion, Inc., New York, NY, United States;* [2]*Brigham and Women's Hospital and Harvard Medical School, Boston, MA, United States*

INTRODUCTION

The use of large databases has become widespread and of critical importance to the evaluation of the safety of medicinal products in the Phase IV post-authorization setting. Increasing regulators and other bodies are looking to databases of drug use in the real-world (large databases covering millions of patient lives) to inform regulatory decision-making about the safety and effectiveness of medicinal produces (Berger et al., 2017; Wang et al., 2017).

Although many studies could benefit from large databases, this chapter will focus on the case of post-authorization safety studies (PASS) unique requirements. In particular, PASS often require large data sets to obtain the precision necessary to verify a safety signal for a rare outcome or to detect frequent outcomes earlier. Confounding adjustment is often required to counter the effect of channeling bias. More generally, PASS has complexity that goes beyond general research, with the absolute requirement for comprehensive documentation, audit support, and other research governance.

CONTENTS

Introduction 79

Big Data for Post-Authorization Safety Studies 79

Creation of "Bigness" 81

Methodological Considerations 85

Modern Methods for Post-Authorization Safety Studies Employing Big Data 87

References 88

BIG DATA FOR POST-AUTHORIZATION SAFETY STUDIES

In the context of PASS, the terms "big data" and "real-world data" are closely linked. Here, big data generally refers to large, multimillion patient data sets, as opposed to other big data in medicine (e.g., radiology data, genetic data, or data from wearable devices), which creates extremely large data but on relatively few patients. Large, multimillion patient databases are almost exclusively created from the observation of patient's routine, real-world interactions with the health-care system. In the United States, these databases are held by government agencies such as the Centers for Medicare and Medicaid Services or licensed commercially by contract research companies. In Europe and Asia, true "big data" usable for PASS purposes, such as the national health-care databases of countries such as France or Japan, are almost exclusively held by government agencies and made available to researchers via academic

Table 3.4.1 Selected Sources of Big Data Usable for Post-Authorization Safety Studies Purposes

Region	Data Source Example	Patient Lives (Millions)
United States and Canada	Truven Health MarketScan	110
	Optum Clinformatics	60
	Medicaid Analytic eXtract[a]	60
	Medicare Claims[a]	40
	Canadian Provincial Databases[a]	1–10
Europe	French Système national d'information interrégimes de l'Assurance Maladie[a]	65
	Spanish Regional Databases[a]	1–10
Asia	South Korean Health Insurance Review and Assessment	50
	Japanese Medical Data Vision	8

[a]Available primarily or exclusively to academic institutions.

institutions on a case-by-case basis. Table 3.4.1 lists selected data sources for PASS; far more sources are available worldwide. Chapter 5.5 provides examples where big data are employed in proactive safety surveillance of medicinal products and also discusses opportunities and challenges to conducting surveillance using big data.

These administrative databases cover a large number of patient lives and have broad scope but do not have the clinical details that would be found in smaller databases such as electronic medical record (EMR) or registries (which on the downside may be longitudinally less complete). Databases will record a unique patient identifier (often decoupled from patients actual national identifiers) and, to varying degrees, the inpatient stays, outpatient visits, and prescription drug dispensings the patient experiences, along with some clinical information such as diagnosis codes, procedure codes, and medication details. However, physician observations, images, laboratory results, or other more detailed clinical information are not recorded. As such, and as mentioned in Chapter 3.1, administrative databases are ideal for PASS where the exposures are recorded clearly in such administrative data, and the outcomes are discernible from diagnosis and procedure codes but do not require detailed clinical information.

In commonly available sources of big data, exposures such as oral prescription medicinal products (Wang et al., 2005; Fralick et al., 2017), infused or injected therapies (Schneeweiss et al., 2008), or specific medical procedures are measureable (Chen et al., 2015; Schneeweiss et al., 2012). Less measurable are over-the-counter products, complex treatment pathways, or inclusion criteria or exposures defined in some way by laboratory results (e.g., diabetes as defined by a specific glycosylated hemoglobin—HbA1c threshold). In these commonly available sources, clearly defined outcomes such as myocardial infarction, hemorrhages requiring transfusion, and acute kidney or liver failures are easily measured. On the other hand, subtle complications, changes in laboratory values, or factors that are generally patient reported are less measurable. Death is an outcome that requires special consideration with respect to data sources. Although most major data sources list death as an outcome, they may not be sensitive to all mortality. For example, in US claims data sources, inpatient or hospice deaths are well recorded but out of hospital or even ambulance deaths may not be. Linking such claims data to government records can improve sensitivity, but these data must be taken in context. For example, linkage to the US Social Security Master File can improve sensitivity, but there may be incomplete reporting such as in cases where on partner of a married couple dies but the living partner continues to draw social security benefits. In the end, precise death data can be expensive; in the United States, complete capture of death is available in the National Death Index, but their per-record pricing can become cost-prohibitive for large data sets.

CREATION OF "BIGNESS"

Big data can also be created from the actual or virtual pooling or linkage of smaller databases, via two primary methods. The first, so-called *"horizontal pooling,"* which creates a larger data set by increasing patient count: data from multiple databases, each containing records on a different population of patients, are brought together into a single analysis (Friedenreich, 1993; Kim et al., 2017). An example of horizontal pooling is the federated data model used by safety surveillance systems, where a single analysis draws from data that is stored across multiple administrative claims or EMR systems but is analyzed as a pooled group (Toh et al., 2012). Horizontal pooling creates our traditional idea of "big data" in the PASS context, where data sets increase in rows (number of patients) but column size (amount of information per patient) stays the same.

The other, *"vertical linkage,"* creates a larger data set by augmenting patient records with additional information about those patients from additional sources. Unlike horizontal pooling, vertical linkage does not create additional patients (does not increase patient pool, adding new rows), but rather adds data to each patient record (links new data, adding new columns). Vertical linkage is not the usual notion of "big data," at least in the context of PASS but can create large-sized data sets through, for example, the addition of genetic or biomarker data or through bringing in unstructured information (e.g., natural language processing for text data). It can also substantially increase the richness of data sets (Lin and Schneeweiss, 2016).

An important distinction between horizontal pooling and vertical linkage is the methods needed to coalesce the data and the statistical analyses required. Horizontal pooling fixes the number of columns, so for each patient, there is a defined (and sometimes limited) amount of information. Each patient in the analysis will have, at a minimum, a patient ID and a data source ID. For the PASS application, other columns will necessarily include exposure status, outcome status, covariates, subgroup indicators, and other factors needed to conduct a safety study. It is most straightforward, though not required, that each data set reports a substantially similar portion of the information on each patient. That is, each data source would ideally record all data elements for all patients, with no data source omitting single variables (e.g., blood pressure or other clinical parameters) across the board. If this is not the case, methods for analysis with substantial missing data will be required (Franklin et al., 2015). Assuming complete data across all data sources in a horizontally linked data set, a cohort of patients may then look like the example in Table 3.4.2. Vertically linked data may resemble the data structure in Table 3.4.3.

Table 3.4.2 Example of Horizontally Pooled Data Set

Data Source ID	Patient ID	Exposure Status	Outcome Status	Age	Gender	Covariates 1 to n
1	1	Yes	No	58	Female	Value 1 to n
1	2	Yes	Yes	65	Female	Value 1 to n
1	3	No	Yes	71	Male	Value 1 to n
2	1	Yes	No	62	Male	Value 1 to n
2	2	No	Yes	53	Female	Value 1 to n

Table 3.4.3 Example of Vertically Linked Data Set

Columns in Data Source 1 (Administrative Claims)	Columns in Data Source 2 (Electronic Medical Record)	Columns in Data Source 3 (Cancer Registry)
Patient ID	Patient ID	Patient ID
Age	Systolic blood pressure	Tumor site
Sex	Diastolic blood pressure	Tumor stage
State	Height	Tumor recurrence
Inpatient events	Weight	Treatment type

Clearly, for most applications—especially PASS, where outcome event counts tend to be low, it is best to have the largest data set with the information needed to identify exposures and outcome and to measure relevant confounders. This will yield both the highest statistical confidence in any result (highest precision), along with the best confounding adjustment available (highest validity). With that said, it is often not possible to fully link or pool data sets. Key barriers include

- *Governance:* Many organizations will not allow their data to be sent to other parties, for reasons of governance, proprietary information, or information security (Platt et al., 2012).
- *Privacy:* Linking databases can lead to identifiability of patients, especially through vertical linkage where the addition of data elements may uniquely identify patients. For example, if one database contains information on the zip code and age of a patient and another contains diagnostic information for a rare cancer, the combination of the two databases could lead to the patient being made identifiable.
- *Lack of reliable unique identifier:* Many databases do not have reliable identifiers that can lead to two issues. For vertical linkage, it may be possible to precisely match one patient to another but could require the use of probabilistic matching techniques (Victor and Mera, 2001). For horizontal pooling, it may be difficult to distinguish the same patient appearing in two data sets, which can lead to an overestimate of the precision of any result because a repeated patient is not an independent observation (Stang et al., 2010).

In many cases, governance can be overcome through metaanalysis. A horizontally pooled data set used to identify or confirm safety signals can be broken into its component parts (in the example in Table 3.4.2, by Data Source ID) and analyzed individually. An identical estimate can be obtained by analyzing each part singly and obtaining a combined result through metaanalytic techniques (Rassen et al., 2009). This has a practical utility in that no data need to be physically combined; rather, an analysis can occur locally and then a combined estimate obtained through a simple combination of the local results. This is illustrated in Table 3.4.4, where the result obtained through metaanalysis is equivalent to that obtained through combination of data sets and stratification. The data in the table were drawn from a published study and were reanalyzed using the R "meta" analysis software package (Kim et al., 2017). Locally created results can of course take advantage of any available confounding adjustment technique, such as multivariate regression or propensity score matching (analytical approaches to minimize bias in PASS are discussed in Chapters 5.1–5.3).

Table 3.4.4 Example of Combination of Data Sources Through Metaanalysis

| Data Analysis Source | Exposure | | Comparator | | Rate Ratio (95% CI) |
	No. of Events	Person-Years	No. of Events	Person-Years	
Data Source 1 (Medicare)	17	1841	50	3954	0.73 (0.42–1.27)
Data Source 2 (Pharmetrics)	10	2061	20	4465	1.08 (0.51–2.31)
Data Source 3 (MarketScan)	9	2999	19	6726	1.06 (0.48–2.35)
Combined data set stratified by data source	36	6901	89	15,145	0.88 (0.60–1.29)
Inverse variance weighted, fixed-effects metaanalysis	–	–	–	–	0.88 (0.60–1.29)
Random-effects metaanalysis	–	–	–	–	0.89 (0.60–1.31)

Privacy is most challenging and will often require a head-on tackling of the issue with the involved parties. In the United States, this will often require that organizations enter into business associates agreements or other contracts and use the resulting combined data set in strict accordance with privacy regulations. Privacy-preserving methods for multivariate analysis have been developed for horizontally partitioned data (Rassen et al., 2010a,b) and vertically partitioned data (Bohn et al., 2017). Another barrier in creating big data sets is lack of unique identifiers. In the case that it is hard to link data about a single patient across multiple databases, probabilistic techniques will need to be used in many cases. In the case that there is possible unknown repetition of patients, the confidence interval of results can be adjusted through an estimation of the amount of repetition of patients (Dom, 2014; Munder et al., 2013).

Traditional claims and EMR data are the standard for safety studies depending on large databases. With that said, there is increasing availability of data from sources that today would be considered novel or nontraditional, especially in the context of PASS. This includes health data from wearable and mobile devices, stationary devices with telemetry, and other feeds of information that come at a volume and frequency far beyond that of medical records or administrative claims. These devices may continuously transmit key clinical values such as pulse or blood pressure. Genomic data, consumer data, and geolocation data are all potential sources for big data usable in PASS.

No matter what the source of data is, however, key pharmacoepidemiological principles must always apply. In particular, *time* is critical and we must always take the basic study timeline into account. Considering the typical cohort study design (Schneeweiss, 2010a) (Chapter 4.3), there will be an "index date," generally the date on which the patient enters the study and the exposure status is determined. Baseline characteristics must be measured before the index date lest they become intermediates on the causal pathway (Weinberg, 1993). Outcomes must be measured after this index date, or else outcomes will allow to occur before exposure. Follow-up must begin at the same time in each exposure group or else immortal person-time might be introduced (Suissa, 2008). Finally, and as mentioned in earlier chapters, a plan for handling missing data must be established, especially if working with laboratory data or EMR, in which missing data are frequent (Schneeweiss et al., 2012).

A newer but also important issue is that as values are measured more frequently, the researcher must decide how to treat values that are measured multiple times. For example, in a PASS of the safety of antihypertensive medications, a key clinical value at baseline would be blood pressure. Wearables and other devices may offer frequent blood pressure readings. As such, an investigator would need to design the study carefully to assess, for each patient, what the baseline blood pressure is in the context of the study; it could be the highest value, the value most proximal to exposure, the lowest value, a moving average, or another value derived from the data. The "correct" value in a given study will be circumstance-driven; for example, if blood pressure drives an immediate treatment decision, then the measurement directly before exposure may be most useful (Franklin et al., 2017).

METHODOLOGICAL CONSIDERATIONS

Large databases are ideal for raising potential safety signals and for validating or refining them. Traditionally, a variety of common signal detection algorithms have been used, such as group monitoring methods, the maximum sequential probability ratio test, statistical process control rules, and disproportionality analyses (Gagne et al., 2012). Newer tree-based scan and time-sequential screening methods are seen as helpful in identifying signals that cluster in time or cluster in specific disease codes or code hierarchies (Kulldorff et al., 2013). However, alerts from these algorithms are simply suggestions of safety issues and must thus be viewed as hypotheses to test rather than confirmed safety issues, a distinction that principally arises from the lack of causality in signal detection.

More generally, relying on P-values in big data is problematic; in almost any reasonably sized data set, it will be possible to obtain a P-value $<.05$. For this reason, among many others, a focus on validity is key. A large database will usually yield a precise result, but without careful consideration of study design and execution may well not yield a valid result. A focus on *P*-values and other naïve methods can lead to very poor results; in particular, frequent false positives can lead to cases where decision-making is stymied by a lack of trusted information. Good decision-making relies on good information (especially in high-stake decisions, such as whether to inform health-care professionals and patients that a medicinal product may have safety issues). In turn, good information must come from robust methodologies and trusted execution. Lacking good information, a decision maker may choose to make no decision at all, which is an important decision in and of itself.

For this reason, a focus on signal strengthening or confirmation is more fruitful for decision-making. Signal confirmation arises when the investigator has identified a hypothesis through one or more channels and has concluded the appropriate study to examine that hypothesis. That study will follow accepted design principles (Schneeweiss, 2010b); will be constructed as to avoid key biases; and will take place only in circumstances where the data will be able to support the measurement of exposure, outcome, and key confounders. Big data is frequently used in signal confirmation PASS, which often use the large commercial databases that are available and/or a specialized data set. Chapters 4.1 through 4.5 describe common PASS designs.

Indeed, the combination of large databases with techniques such as high-dimensional propensity scoring (hd-PS) can be practically effective (Schneeweiss et al., 2009; Rassen et al., 2011). The hd-PS technique uses available data to empirically identify several hundred confounders or proxies for confounders, measures those variables, and constructs a propensity score to use the information in those variables to adjust for confounding, and thus reduce bias. This method derives a portion of its power from the bigness of data sets; usually the incremental information that can be gleaned as data sets grow, there is even greater opportunity to identify potential confounding factors. However, in data sets of any size, the hd-PS technique can strongly increase validity of PASS by removing biases that may have eluded an investigator and producing an estimate of treatment effect that is much more strongly confirmatory than a *P*-value, or even a traditionally designed, fully investigator-driven safety study. Chapter 5.1 provides an overview of exposure propensity scores in pharmacoepidemiologic research.

No matter the database or the analytic method—or even the database size, good pharmacoepidemiologic methods must be applied (FDA, 2009; EMA, 2017). Study design is paramount: in the common sources of big data for PASS, an active comparator will often outperform a nonexposed group. A new-user design will allow for an "apple to apple" comparison of patients at like points in their treatment regime (Ray, 2003). Exposure must be characterized properly and outcomes duly assessed, with an eye toward an appropriate balance of sensitivity and specificity (Rothman et al., 2008). Covariates must be measured at the correct time relative to exposure to avoid potentially adjusting for intermediates on the causal pathway or introducing immortal person-time (Weinberg, 1993; Suissa, 2008). Appropriate confounding adjustment techniques must be applied, and the resulting point estimates must be interpreted carefully (Austin, 2007). Chapters 5.1 through 5.3 cover common analytical approaches to account for bias and confounding in PASS.

In studies that consider multiple, horizontally pooled data sets, the potential for treatment effect heterogeneity must be considered (Rassen et al., 2009). In particular, two cases are important: true treatment effect heterogeneity because of differences in how the treatment performs in various populations versus more "artificial" treatment effect heterogeneity that results from more versus less complete confounding adjustment in various populations. The former case can arise from differences in each data set population, differences in how health care is delivered in each population, or other factors; but it is required in all circumstances to assess whether a pooled point estimate should be reported or whether individual point estimates are more appropriate. The latter case often arises from data sets that measure key confounders at varying levels of completeness or quality and requires careful thought about how to achieve better confounding adjustment in all data sets, or whether to consider study design to focus the analysis on data sets that can provide all necessary confounding information.

MODERN METHODS FOR POST-AUTHORIZATION SAFETY STUDIES EMPLOYING BIG DATA

The field of pharmacoepidemiology has often taken a one-off, study-by-study approach to evaluating the safety of medicinal products. After the formulation of a protocol, line programming in Statistical Analysis System (SAS) or other statistical analysis environments is undertaken to implement the study as designed. However, these approaches are becoming less prevalent as analytical platforms are in many instances replacing traditional methods. The reason for the shift from line programming is rooted in the parallel initiatives around the field to increase transparency and replicability (Berger et al., 2017; Wang et al., 2017). As evaluation of real-world evidence becomes an ever-increasing part of the routine, evaluation of safety and effectiveness of medicinal products and decision-making is increasingly focused on real-world data, new methods are required to maintain quality, transparency, and collaboration among stakeholders (e.g., pharmaceutical companies, payers, and regulators).

The methods we have relied on in the past can often fail us. As compared with analytical platforms, line programming is slow, error-prone, and nontransparent. It can also be slow: line programming often requires detailed implementation and testing, whereas platforms are designed to streamline the process from study concept to final output; differences in time required can vary by an order of magnitude or more. With respect to errors and nontransparency, even with the same protocol, two experienced programmers working on SAS will frequently attain different results; this is most often not due to errors in coding but rather misunderstanding of the protocol at hand. Further error is introduced by usual sources: coding bugs, table transcription, and other such items. On the other hand, an analytic platform that simultaneously maintains control of input, measurement, analysis, and output and supports the user by ensuring correct study implementation and full documentation, virtually eliminates such sources of error. Such platforms use natural language interfaces to describe studies (including all assumptions made, all analytic choices taken, and references to the scientific literature) and have full transparency/auditability. This makes analytic platforms able to be validated against standards or quasistandards such as the FDA Sentinel modules (Wang et al., 2016). Moreover, platforms enforce a standard of quality in study design, e.g., known time-related biases are readily avoided. Chapter 5.4 provides a discussion on data analytic platforms and common data models, and Chapter 8 introduces transparency for PASS in the context of the European public register of PASS protocols and final study reports.

Pharmacoepidemiology has firmly entered the era of big data and will further expand in that direction by adding new data sources from within the healthcare system and beyond, representing both increasing numbers of patients and increasing clinical detail and lifestyle parameters. This new information will offer the chance to improve the validity and precision of PASS but will not alter the need for consistent application of fundamental principles of good pharmacoepidemiologic design and analysis. Use of such information in critical, causally focused decision-making highlights the need for rapid response with consistently high-quality implementation. Modern analytic platforms bring together the strong design, analysis, speed, and quality needed to support effective decision-making using big, real-world data.

References

Austin, P.C., 2007. The performance of different propensity score methods for estimating marginal odds ratios. Stat. Med. 26 (16), 3078–3094. https://doi.org/10.1002/sim.2781.

Berger, M.L., Sox, H., Willke, R.J., et al., 2017. Good practices for real-world data studies of treatment and/or comparative effectiveness: recommendations from the joint ISPOR-ISPE special task force on real-world evidence in health care decision making. Value Health 20 (8), 1003–1008. https://doi.org/10.1016/j.jval.2017.08.3019.

Bohn, J., Eddings, W., Schneeweiss, S., 2017. Conducting privacy-preserving multivariable propensity score analysis when patient covariate information is stored in separate locations. Am. J. Epidemiol. 185 (6), 501–510. https://doi.org/10.1093/aje/kww155.

Chen, C.-Y., Stevenson, L.W., Stewart, G.C., et al., 2015. Real world effectiveness of primary implantable cardioverter defibrillators implanted during hospital admissions for exacerbation of heart failure or other acute co-morbidities: cohort study of older patients with heart failure. BMJ 351, h3529.

Dom, P.R.D., 2014. Sample Overlap in Meta-analysis, pp. 1–18. http://metaanalysis2014.econ.uoa.gr/fileadmin/metaanalysis2014.econ.uoa.gr/uploads/Bom_Pedro.pdf.

European Medicines Agency (EMA), 2017. The European Network of Centres for Pharmacoepidemiology and Pharmacovigilance (ENCePP) Guide on Methodological Standards in Pharmacoepidemiology (Revision 6), pp. 1–93. http://www.encepp.eu/standards_and_guidances/documents/ENCePPGuideofMethStandardsinPE_Rev6.pdf.

Food and Drug Administration (FDA), 2009. Guidance for Industry and FDA Staff, pp. 1–16. https://www.fda.gov/downloads/MedicalDevices/DeviceRegulationandGuidance/GuidanceDocuments/ucm071013.pdf.

Fralick, M., Schneeweiss, S., Patorno, E., 2017. Risk of diabetic ketoacidosis after initiation of an SGLT2 inhibitor. N. Engl. J. Med. 376 (23), 2300–2302. https://doi.org/10.1056/NEJMc1701990.

Franklin, J.M., Eddings, W., Schneeweiss, S., Rassen, J.A., May 2015. Incorporating linked healthcare claims to improve confounding control in a study of in-hospital medication use. Drug Saf. 1–12. https://doi.org/10.1007/s40264-015-0292-x.

Franklin, J.M., Schneeweiss, S., Solomon, D.H., 2017. Assessment of confounders in comparative effectiveness studies from secondary databases. Am. J. Epidemiol. 185 (6), 474–478. https://doi.org/10.1093/aje/kww136.

Friedenreich, C.M., 1993. Methods for pooled analyses of epidemiologic studies. Epidemiology 4 (4), 295–302. https://doi.org/10.1097/00001648-199307000-00004.

Gagne, J.J., Rassen, J.A., Walker, A.M., Glynn, R.J., Schneeweiss, S., 2012. Active safety monitoring of new medical products using electronic healthcare data. Epidemiology 23 (2), 238–246. https://doi.org/10.1097/EDE.0b013e3182459d7d.

Kim, S.C., Solomon, D.H., Rogers, J.R., et al., February 2017. Cardiovascular safety of tocilizumab versus tumor necrosis factor inhibitors in patients with rheumatoid arthritis - a multi-database cohort study. Arthritis Rheumatol. https://doi.org/10.1002/art.40084.

Kulldorff, M., Dashevsky, I., Avery, T.R., Chan, A.K., Davis, R.L., Graham, D., Platt, R., et al., 2013. Drug safety data mining with a tree-based scan statistic. Pharmacoepidemiol. Drug Saf. 22 (5), 517–523. https://doi.org/10.1002/pds.3423.

Lin, K.J., Schneeweiss, S., 2016. Considerations for the analysis of longitudinal electronic health records linked to claims data to study the effectiveness and safety of drugs. Clin. Pharmacol. Ther. 100 (2), 147–159. https://doi.org/10.1002/cpt.359.

Liu, J., Sylwestrzak, G., Ruggieri, A.P., DeVries, A., 2015. Intravenous versus subcutaneous anti-TNF-alpha agents for Crohn's disease: a comparison of effectiveness and safety. J. Manag. Care Spec. Pharm. 21, 559–566.

Munder, T., Brütsch, O., Leonhart, R., Gerger, H., Barth, J., 2013. Researcher allegiance in psychotherapy outcome research: an overview of reviews. Clin. Psychol. Rev. 33 (4), 501–511. https://doi.org/10.1016/j.cpr.2013.02.002.

Platt, R., Carnahan, R.M., Brown, J.S., et al., 2012. The U.S. Food and Drug Administration's Mini-Sentinel program: status and direction. In: Platt, R., Carnahan, R. (Eds.), Pharmacoepidem Drug Safe, vol. 21 (Suppl. 1), pp. 1–8. https://doi.org/10.1002/pds.2343.

Rassen, J.A., Choudhry, N.K., Avorn, J., Schneeweiss, S., 2009. Cardiovascular outcomes and mortality in patients using clopidogrel with proton pump inhibitors after percutaneous coronary intervention or acute coronary syndrome. Circulation 120 (23), 2322–2329. https://doi.org/10.1161/CIRCULATIONAHA.109.873497.

Rassen, J.A., Avorn, J., Schneeweiss, S., 2010a. Multivariate-adjusted pharmacoepidemiologic analyses of confidential information pooled from multiple health care utilization databases. Pharmacoepidemiol. Drug Saf. 19 (8), 848–857. https://doi.org/10.1002/pds.1867.

Rassen, J.A., Solomon, D.H., Curtis, J.R., Herrinton, L., Schneeweiss, S., 2010b. Privacy-maintaining propensity score-based pooling of multiple databases applied to a study of biologics. Med. Care 48 (6 Suppl.), S83–S89. https://doi.org/10.1097/MLR.0b013e3181d59541.

Rassen, J.A., Glynn, R.J., Brookhart, M.A., Schneeweiss, S., 2011. Covariate selection in high-dimensional propensity score analyses of treatment effects in small samples. Am. J. Epidemiol. 173 (12), 1404–1413. https://doi.org/10.1093/aje/kwr001.

Ray, W.A., 2003. Evaluating medication effects outside of clinical trials: new-user designs. Am. J. Epidemiol. 158 (9), 915–920. https://doi.org/10.1093/aje/kwg231.

Rothman, K.J., Greenland, S., Lash, T.L., 2008. Modern Epidemiology. Wolters Kluwer Health/Lippincott Williams & Wilkins, Philadelphia.

Schneeweiss, S., 2010a. A basic study design for expedited safety signal evaluation based on electronic healthcare data. Pharmacoepidemiol. Drug Saf. 19 (8), 858–868. https://doi.org/10.1002/pds.1926.

Schneeweiss, S., 2010b. A basic study design for expedited safety signal evaluation based on electronic healthcare data. Pharmacoepidemiol. Drug Saf. 19 (8), 858–868. https://doi.org/10.1002/pds.1926.

Schneeweiss, S., Seeger, J.D., Landon, J., Walker, A.M., 2008. Aprotinin during coronary-artery bypass grafting and risk of death. N. Engl. J. Med. 358 (8), 771–783. https://doi.org/10.1056/NEJMoa0707571.

Schneeweiss, S., Rassen, J.A., Glynn, R.J., Avorn, J., Mogun, H., Brookhart, M.A., 2009. High-dimensional propensity score adjustment in studies of treatment effects using health care claims data. Epidemiology 20 (4), 512–522. https://doi.org/10.1097/EDE.0b013e3181a663cc.

Schneeweiss, S., Rassen, J.A., Glynn, R.J., et al., 2012. Supplementing claims data with outpatient laboratory test results to improve confounding adjustment in effectiveness studies of lipid-lowering treatments. BMC Med. Res. Methodol. 12 (1), 323. https://doi.org/10.1186/1471-2288-12-180.

Stang, P.E., Ryan, P.B., Racoosin, J.A., et al., 2010. Advancing the science for active surveillance: rationale and design for the observational medical outcomes partnership. Ann. Intern. Med. 153 (9), 600–606. https://doi.org/10.7326/0003-4819-153-9-201011020-00010.

Suissa, S., 2008. Immortal time bias in pharmacoepidemiology. Am. J. Epidemiol. 167 (4), 492–499. https://doi.org/10.1093/aje/kwm324.

Toh, S., Reichman, M.E., Houstoun, M., et al., 2012. Comparative risk for angioedema associated with the use of drugs that target the renin-angiotensin-aldosterone system. Arch. Intern. Med. 172 (20), 1582. https://doi.org/10.1001/2013.jamainternmed.34.

Victor, T.W., Mera, R.M., 2001. Record linkage of health care insurance claims. J. Am. Med. Inf. Assoc. 8 (3), 281–288.

Wang, P.S., Schneeweiss, S., Avorn, J., et al., 2005. Risk of death in elderly users of conventional vs. atypical antipsychotic medications. N. Engl. J. Med. 353 (22), 2335–2341. https://doi.org/10.1056/NEJMoa052827.

Wang, S.V., Verpillat, P., Rassen, J.A., Patrick, A., Garry, E.M., Bartels, D.B., 2016. Transparency and reproducibility of observational cohort studies using large healthcare databases. Clin. Pharmacol. Ther. 99 (3), 325–332. https://doi.org/10.1002/cpt.329.

Wang, S.V., Schneeweiss, S., Berger, M.L., et al., 2017. Reporting to improve reproducibility and facilitate validity assessment for healthcare database studies V1.0. Value Health 20 (8), 1009–1022. https://doi.org/10.1016/j.jval.2017.08.3018.

Weinberg, C.R., 1993. Toward a clearer definition of confounding. Am. J. Epidemiol. 137 (1), 1–8. https://doi.org/10.1093/oxfordjournals.aje.a116591.

Social Media

Andrew Paul Cox, Evie Merinopoulou

Evidera, Bethesda, MD, United States

CONTENTS

Introduction 92

Social Media
Sources 93

Social Media and
Pharmacovi
gilance 94

Challenges With
Social Media
Listening 95

Methodological
Considerations 98

Ethical
Considerations 99

References 102

INTRODUCTION

The first social media site, "six degrees," was created in 1997, and the first blogging site appeared in 1999. Between 2000 and 2006, many of the most popular social media sites, such as LinkedIn, Facebook, and Twitter, were created. Since then, social media has grown and diversified exponentially. Its popularity is in no small part because of the fact that it facilitates the basic human need to communicate and exchange information; it also helps humans to have an innate interest in the conversations of others. Social media manages to remove the geographical barriers to communication, connecting people across the world. As time passes, each of these social media sites holds a historical record of conversations across time. At the time sites have been diversified, for almost any topic, there is likely to be a specialized social media site connecting people with similar interests. Social media can be broadly divided into two types: large, generic platforms that most people will be familiar with (e.g., Google+, Facebook, Twitter, etc.) and smaller platforms that are devoted to specific topics and interests. However, this is not a completely clear divide, as the generic platforms also allow specialist communities to create special interest groups.

Among the "specific" social media platforms or forums are a large number of health care—related sites, which span almost every condition and disease. Some are set up and managed by patients and some by charitable organizations such as MacMillan Center Support or the American Cancer Society (MacMillan, 2015; ACS, 2017). It is impossible to measure the number of health care—related conversations recorded across all these websites and available through the internet. One start-up company that regularly monitors data from health-related social media reports accessing more than 2.5 billion patient posts from 50 million health care users, but this is still likely to be a small portion of available information (dMetrics, 2017). Each website can hold historical conversations dating back several years. For example, there are more than 333,747 breast cancer—related posts spanning 17 years in the Cancer Survivors Network forum of the American Cancer Society, a number that increases daily (ACS, 2016). A large US study estimated that looking for health information is the third most popular online activity, with 80% of internet users looking online for health information (Fox, 2011). The same study reported that as 25% of the US population does not go online, the results of this survey suggest that 59% of the entire US adult population seeks health information online (i.e., 80% of the 75% that go online). Surveys suggest that patients are in favor of social media posts being used in research if it benefits the patients and advances treatment. The results of a survey of more than 3000 social media users showed that ~70% of patients with a medical condition believed that information they posted could be used to discriminate against them (Grajales et al., 2014). Conversely, in spite of this strong reservation, more than 90% were willing to share their health data to help improve care or help research. Approximately 80% would share information with pharmaceutical companies to help make safer medicinal products or learn more about their diseases.

Social media is an increasingly important feature of the modern health-care landscape. It allows patients—and their families and friends—to communicate and find information and support when geographic isolation would otherwise make this type of communication impossible. Patients use social media for a number of reasons, and the purpose varies depending on the condition. Patients use these forums to exchange information about their treatments, and attempt to understand and make sense of the large amount of information a patient needs to become familiar with to receive treatment for their condition. This frequently involves forum users sharing their condition-specific history or treatments and adverse events, experiences, and other important information regarding the condition. The forums are also used to discuss how to manage the side effects of treatment and can highlight misuse of products by patients and others.

SOCIAL MEDIA SOURCES

There is diversity among social media types; however, there are generic social media sites and applications characterized by the fact they are not topic-specific, although they may have topic-specific pages or groups of users. Twitter has ~342 million active users generating 58 million "tweets" per day; Facebook has 1,721,000,000 monthly active users and 74,200,000 pages (Statistic Brain Research Institute, 2016). Although the imposing scale of these sites makes them an attractive target for drug safety surveillance, they have several drawbacks. Their large scale and lack of specificity makes searching for safety events difficult. In this case, the ratio of noise to information is high. Secondly, many of the larger generic sites are very prescriptive about how content is accessed. Twitter provides a free service to access tweets, which are generally rate-limited. However, it is restrictive in other ways, such as larger samples of live tweets being allowed only through expensive subscription services, and in what types of organizations may subscribe. Historical tweets are available through third-party organization for a fee (Twitter, 2017). Facebook is also very prescriptive about use of its content. It is possible to analyze Facebook pages inside your own network, but using data outside your network is restricted. By contrast, specialist social media sites contain more focused content with a lower noise-to-information ratio. Most sites are public facing; however, permission to access and use content is often unclear and, in general, has neither been fully permitted nor restricted. Some sites, such as Smart Patients (www.smartpatients.com), adopt a policy of working with authentic researchers.

SOCIAL MEDIA AND PHARMACOVIGILANCE

Given the vast number of recorded discussions across these forums and how frequently patients discuss the occurrence and management of the side effects of their treatments, it would appear that social media is a large source of "raw" information for those concerned and tasked with monitoring drug safety. Social media in pharmacovigilance is a relatively new phenomenon; in our experience, it tends to polarize opinion. Many pharmaceutical companies have created applications and platforms that monitor adverse events, and they appear to push a plethora of information and material that promises a revolution in monitoring drug safety. In addition, there have been a number of initiatives—with varying degrees of success—to develop effective surveillance systems using social media (Trend Miner, 2011; IMI, 2014; Desai, 2015; Tozzi and Bass, 2015; MedWatcher, 2017). Presently, the value of social media to pharmacovigilance and PASS is not *"if it should be used"* but *"how can it be used effectively?"* and *"how should it be integrated into pharmacovigilance activities and PASS"*. While there is little doubt social media is of value, the technology to provide useful information is still in development. It is a field where it is necessary to exercise a sensible degree of caution, as there is a great deal of overexaggerated claims and hyperbole.

The use of social media in pharmacovigilance falls into three broad areas: (1) websites and platforms owned and maintained by pharmaceutical companies; (2) the use of social media by pharmaceutical companies for marketing and exchanging information with consumers; and (3) the monitoring of social media and other online sources for adverse event signals.

Pharmaceutical companies may create social media platforms to interact with their product users, to allow participants of clinical trials to communicate with each other and the company, as a service to patients with a specific condition, or specifically to allow the reporting of adverse events for their products.

In addition to the usual regulatory framework surrounding pharmacovigilance activities and responsibilities, guidance related to this type of social media activity exists (CIOMS, 2001; EMA, 2017; FDA, 2011, 2014a,b,c; PMCPA, 2017). For example, the good pharmacovigilance practices Module VI states that marketing authorization holders should regularly screen the internet and/or digital media under their purview for potential reports of suspected adverse reactions (EMA, 2017). Additionally, pharmaceutical companies may interact with patients through established social media frameworks that are not under their control or ownership; an example of this may be interactions through Twitter or Facebook. Increasingly, major pharmaceutical companies are engaging with patients in this way.

There is a dearth of guidance or recommendations in regard to the monitoring of social media for adverse event signals. The Council for International Organizations of Medical Sciences did not believe it was necessary for regulators or companies routinely to "surf" the internet beyond their own sites for individual spontaneous adverse event reports (CIOMS, 2001). However, surveillance or studies focusing on social media data sources for intelligence may prove useful as part of an overall pharmacovigilance strategy. Social media has a number of important advantages over traditional spontaneous adverse event reporting channels—it is much closer to real time (occurring in close proximity to the event) and potentially much richer in content. Although social media would never replace these channels of routine pharmacovigilance activities, it could augment existing pharmacovigilance strategies. Just like spontaneous reporting systems, analysis of social media should only be suitable for signal detection and hypothesis generation rather than signal evaluation and risk assessment purposes.

CHALLENGES WITH SOCIAL MEDIA LISTENING

It is believed that much of the reluctance of many pharmaceutical companies to incorporate social media listening into their routine pharmacovigilance activities that will open the floodgate to an unmanageable level of potential adverse event reports that will need to be followed-up and qualified. Undoubtedly, pharmaceutical companies have been held back from the full range of social listening activities prevalent in other industries because of the current lack of clarity and guidance on their regulatory obligations. The FDA defined four criteria for an adverse event to be reported (FDA, 2001):

- *An identifiable patient:* the online post contains sufficient information to lead the reviewer to believe that a patient is involved.
- *An identifiable reporter:* the post contains sufficient contact information to allow follow-up by the reviewer, including an e-mail address, telephone number, or mailing address.

- *A specific medication:* the post must mention a specific medicinal product by brand name or the chemical name of a product if the compound is unique to one specific pharmaceutical brand.
- *An adverse event:* the post describes a reaction that a "reasonable person" would consider to be an adverse event, such as death, hospitalization, vomiting, swelling, or any side effect that is either unknown or expected with the medication.

A study sought to quantify the frequency that messages in social media content met all the above criteria (Maher, 2015). It found that less than 1% of posts/ messages met all four criteria and concluded that the volume of adverse events in social media would not exceed what can be managed by existing reporting channels established for offline reporting methods. However, even this small number of potentially reportable adverse events is likely to be subject to further significant attrition when other issues are considered (e.g., the report may not be current—may be several years old). Another complication is how to contact the medication user who experienced the event, if the only way is through posting follow-up messages on the social media boards, this would require registering to the site, which may be regarded as ethically questionable. Although this is a subject of further discussion for regulatory authorities, it is impractical—if not impossible—for any pharmaceutical company to monitor all social media channels for potential adverse event reports.

When patients discuss their treatment experience and their condition, they tend to talk about symptoms rather than using technical medical and clinical terminology. As in the example of peripheral neuropathy, patients would tend to talk about tingling, numbness, dizziness, throbbing, stabbing, falling, and/or weakness. They would rarely mention peripheral neuropathy unless they had been given this diagnosis by health-care professionals or had researched the causes of possible symptoms. Because of this use of symptom-oriented language, identification of signals requires construction and use of specialized ontologies that can map symptoms to potential clinical terms.

One reservation frequently raised in the context of social media when it is used for research purposes is that of bias. The common perception is that data derived from social media forums are somehow biased and unrepresentative. A common critique is that the mean age of users must be generally younger because older people tend not to use the internet. This may be true to a certain extent, but there is an increasing trend of older users or "silver surfers" engaging in online activities. Historically, older adults have lagged behind younger adults in their adoption, but now a clear majority (58%) of senior citizens use the internet (Perrin and Duggan, 2015). In addition, it is very common for caregivers, family members, and friends to participate in social media on behalf of those patients less able to use this form of communication themselves. We recently found that among posts from the four most popular renal cell carcinoma forums, among users reporting advanced metastatic staging, nearly 40% of the forum users are family, friends, or caregivers posting on behalf of a patient. A second frequent criticism is that how do we know that a patient posting on social media is genuine. This may be true in isolated cases; however, common sense dictates that it is highly unlikely that users pretending to be patients are common and will be present in enough numbers to influence results or produce false safety signals.

Although posts are comprehensible to humans, manually reading through them to analyze the content is not practical. To process large volumes of posts, it is necessary to automate analyses; however, for machines, written language can be inscrutable. This is particularly true for social media, where the language is much more diverse than standardized, corrected, and copye-dited textual content encountered in books, publications, and web pages. The difficulty is that for machines, social media dialog as a data source is inherently "fuzzy" and ambiguous. Concepts and meanings are vague, imprecise, and lacking a fixed schema that allows accurate interpretation. Table 3.5.1 demonstrates some of the issues with classifying social media posts. All of the 11 variants shown are referring to treatment with docetaxel chemotherapy and peripheral neuropathy adverse event. Issues can include typos (variant 1); abbreviations (variants 2, 3, 9, 10, and 11); name variation (variants 5 and 6); misspelling (variants 3 and 5); referring to possible incidents in the past (variant 2); the subject is another person (variant 11);

Table 3.5.1 Example of Lexical Diversity of Social Media Posts

Variant	Post
1	I am on docetaxel and have peripheral neuropathy as a result.
2	I was on tax 6 years ago, they told me I could get peripheral neuropathy.
3	I hear docy can give you peripheral neuropathy
4	I did not get peripheral neuropathy when I was taking docetaxel.
5	Did you get p-n when you took docetaxel?
6	I am on Taxotere, I never heard of peripheral neuropathy
7	I am on my first course of tax;I have some tingling in my hands and feet
8	I am on my first course of tax; I thought I had some tingling in feet but my shoes were too tight.
9	Watch out for feeling nauseous when you are on x.
10	When I was undergoing chemo my life was outside life was on hold, I was paralyzed, I did not even manage to do my self-assessment tax return in time.
11	If you have been on x you might be experiencing a side effect called peripheral neuropathy
12	Oh yeah sure, as soon as I start tax I always get PN, every time!!

symptoms rather than clinical terminology (variants 7, 8, and 9); subject is not treatment- or side-effect related (variant 10); negation (variant 4); humor (variant 8); sarcasm (variant 12); multiple word meanings (variants 7 and 12); and reporting knowledge (variants 2 and 3). Only the first example in this list appears to be less ambiguous, yet even here, it is not clear if the patient has already had this diagnosis identified and reported. When searching hundreds of thousands or possibly millions of postings for adverse events, this lingual diversity creates difficulties, including lexical and meaning-related diversity.

METHODOLOGICAL CONSIDERATIONS

To utilize social media pharmacovigilance purposes—potentially, including post-authorization safety studies (PASS), a number of specialist skills are required, the most important of which are natural language processing (NLP), machine learning, and programming skills in an environment such as Python or the R statistical language. Although NLP is possible in other programming environments, these two are the most commonly used. A corpora of posts need to be obtained first; this can be achieved through a "web scraping" exercise where the elements of interests from websites are transferred from the World Wide Web to a file that can be manipulated for analyses. Alternatively, such information can be obtained from third-party organizations on a commercial basis.

There are two general approaches to identifying posts containing potential adverse event reports: *lexical approach* and *machine learning* (or pattern recognition) approach. Lexical approaches attempt to use dictionaries and ontologies to map the diversity of words relating to a standardized medicinal product name or adverse event. Such approaches need to account for the lexical diversity in social media. In the earlier example, an entry in the dictionary for every variation, abbreviation, and typo used in the online patient community to refer to docetaxel would be needed. This dictionary would effectively relate all the variations back to the standardized term and possibly to a formal coding system. Although this approach can be successful, there are a number of difficulties. Most posts that mention a medicinal product and a potential adverse event are not actually reports for that product. Secondly and perhaps the more difficult task is the diversity of possible words and phrases used in common language to describe adverse events and the entanglement of those words with other irrelevant phrases and synonyms. An example of this might be the words "pain" and "painful"; incorporating these words into your dictionary could lead to a large number of false-positive results (e.g., "it was a real pain" vs. "it was a pain in the neck"). Decisions also need to be made on including similar words, such as "hurt/hurting." There are many other examples of these types of decisions—for rash, which itself has a double meaning ("I had a rash" vs. "he was very rash"), the terms "redness," "red patch," and "spots" might all be used to describe a real side effect of treatment or something completely unrelated. Careful thought needs to be made before including words in the dictionaries to avoid false-positive results.

In addition, it is desirable for the method used to be able to have some ability to interpret meaning and context from surrounding words. Single posts of more than 1000 words are not uncommon and can mention multiple potential adverse events and treatments; thus, it is challenging to correctly interpret if the adverse event mentioned and the treatment are associated. *Association rule mining* is a technique that has been used to establish the relationship between entities (e.g., product–event pairs), in which, a set of labeled examples of text where the adverse event does and does not refer to the medicinal product are provided. A supervised machine learning is then used to learn the patterns that predict when the adverse event and the medicinal product are associated. For social media applications, the high lexical diversity means that large training data sets are required for this to be accurate.

Similar to association rule mining, *pattern matching* approach also uses supervised machine learning. A set of prelabeled posts (positive and negative product–event pairs) are provided to learn the pattern that indicates posts that are potential or protoadverse event reports. The machine learning algorithm is then used on new posts to highlight which posts are protoadverse event reports. The drawback with this method is the large volume of training data that needs to be supplied to the machine learning algorithm to facilitate accurate learning and prediction. If the target of the study is multiple treatments with multiple adverse events, the amount of training data required increases. These training data need to be labeled manually, which can involve a considerable human input. Such algorithms also need to be updated to account for new products and adverse events, and an evolving vocabulary. The fact that actual adverse event reports are rare creates a problem of class imbalance for machine learning techniques, learning or predicting potentially rare events can be challenging for machine learning approaches. For the future, as both these approaches have different strengths and weaknesses, it is likely that they will continue to be incorporated into a single unified approach.

ETHICAL CONSIDERATIONS

Social media in real-world data and analytics is a new frontier, with important implications for patient safety and understanding of the patient perspective. Currently, there is little thought given to the ethical and legal issues surrounding use of what is highly personal and potentially sensitive information. Health-related social media has become an increasingly frequent target for research, with a review having found 284 publications on this topic since 2000 (Hamm et al., 2013). A number of companies are continually collecting billions of patient posts and are commercially marketing proprietary software and services based on the ability to interpret them (dMetric, 2017; Treato, 2017). The "web crawlers" of such companies constantly revisit and update information from social media sites. All of this is done on the basis that the information is in the public domain with little or no consideration of permissions, ethics, or site terms and conditions. A further concern is potential violation of permissions set out in terms and conditions by website proprietors. Website owners clearly have an important stake in their site content being used for research purposes. Web crawlers and scraping software used by researchers to obtain posted information can cause a site to crash if they are not professionally and responsibly programmed. Many website proprietors also own the copyright of the material within the site, so there are multiple stakeholders.

All websites and social media sources have terms and conditions, and their complexity and coverage vary widely. Typically, such terms and conditions contain a restriction of use for personal and noncommercial use of the site and contents. Most contain some statements of copyright ownership and that permission should be sought before use. Occasionally, terms and conditions will prohibit access or scraping of the website by crawlers or software. Sometimes, terms imply permission to use the information, if used in a synthesized form. Overwhelmingly, it is unclear how these terms and conditions apply in regard to use for research, including pharmacovigilance activities. Copyright law applies to material available on the World Wide Web; wholesale copying and reuse of material is a breach of copyright. However, for research purposes, this can be avoided by not reproducing text verbatim (directly copying) and presenting only a summary-level synthesis of the material.

Another concern is the identification of individuals. Scattered over multiple postings, social media users give away a staggering amount of personal data that could be used to identify the individuals. The concern is that identification could lead to discrimination, such as denial of health-care benefits or job opportunities, or for marketing of products or services. In fact, outside of the health-care field, social media has been used to identify and criminally prosecute individuals (CBC News, 2011; NHTSA, 2012).

Different perspectives are available for framing ethical considerations of the use of social media. Patients with rare diseases may be more likely to risk (inadvertently) identification. However, that situation could be different to those with chronic diseases. Because there are large volumes of posts from multiple sites, risk of identification may be less of a concern. Some conditions, though, may carry social stigma. Patients with HIV infection or with mental health conditions may be averse to the potential risk of being identified. Stakeholders are likely to have differing views on the ethical and legal issues involved.

Presently, there are no clear guidelines or legislation that addresses the use of social media in research. Many view this type of posted text as an immensely rich and important source, open and free for use. In contrast, social media posts may also be highly personal and contain sensitive information that should be treated with the goal of preserving personal privacy. There is therefore a strong need for industry guidance or a concise guide to professional best practices. Creation of guidelines involves input from a range of interested parties. Potential best practice starting points may be

- Report-synthesized or summary-level data from forums, posts, or parts of posts. Do not repeat or show directly copied text. This minimizes the possibility of identifying individuals and guards against copyright infringement.
- Do not access or use material present on sites that require registration and/or passwords. Deal only with material that is in the public domain, unless explicit permission has been granted to use the protected material.
- Collect data from websites in a responsible manner and build safeguards into crawling and scraping programs to avoid overloading or crashing websites.
- When publishing research results using social media data, include a statement describing the ethical and legal policy safeguards used. Journals should require demonstration of ethical conduct from authors.
- When publishing research results, posts or social media content should never be reproduced verbatim. It should not be possible to rediscover the source post using the presented information and a search engine.
- The intended research should demonstrate intent that it is being conducted for the benefit of the patient.

An important point that is often overlooked regarding ethical considerations is that, analysis of social media posts can adopt the same conventions as studies that deal with similarly sensitive electronic health records. The FDA collaborated with a health informatics company to develop the digital data-mining platform (MedWatcher Social), which deals with large amount of data from social media sites that are stripped of identifying information before being used for data analysis (FDA, 2015; MedWatcher, 2017).

Presently, most of the major pharmaceutical companies engage with their consumers, key opinion leaders, stakeholders, and wider audiences through social media channels, but compared with the patient and clinical communities, the engagement is small. Adoption of this form of interaction is likely to grow as the industry "catches up" with the trend (Ogilvy Commonhealth Worldwide, 2015). There is a growing interest and debate around the use of social media alongside all stages of clinical trials (The Lancet Oncology, 2014). There is an opportunity for social media–based safety studies to augment pharmacovigilance activities, especially as regulatory agencies have incorporated this type of data sources in their guidelines. The tools to carry out these types of studies are available, but the legislative framework is still uncertain and it is unlikely to be completely specified. At present, the main use of social media in pharmacovigilance is for the detection of potential signals and for product misuse. Any PASS employing social media should be construed as hypothesis-generation studies, which detect signals that can be followed-up by more targeted and formalized investigations.

References

American Cancer Society (ACS), Cancer Survivors Network Discussion Boards, 2016. Available from: https://csn.cancer.org/forum.

American Cancer Society (ACS), Homepage, 2017. Available from: https://www.cancer.org/.

CBC News, Police Overwhelmed by Social Media Evidence, 2011. Available from: http://www.cbc.ca/news/canada/british-columbia/vancouver-police-shift-blame-for-riot-1.995380.

Council for International Organizations of Medical Sciences (CIOMS). Current Challenges in Pharmacovigilance: Pragmatic Approaches. Report of CIOMS Working Group V. 2001. Available from: https://cioms.ch/wp-content/uploads/2017/01/Group5_Pharmacovigilance.pdf.

Desai, S., December 2015. Unleashing the Potential of Social Media in Drug Safety: Exploring the Increasing Use of Diginal Forums in Pharmcaovigilance. Global Forum. Available from: https://www.sciformix.com/wp-content/uploads/GF-Dec2015-SDesai-Social-Media-in-PV.pdf.

dMetrics. Homepage, 2017. Available from: https://dmetrics.com/.

European Medicines Agency (EMA), July 2017. Guideline on Good Pharmacovigilance Practices (GVP). Module VI-Collection, Management and Submission of Reports of Suspected Adverse Reactions to Medicinal Products (Rev 2). EMA/873138/2011 Rev 2. Available from: http://www.ema.europa.eu/docs/en_GB/document_library/Regulatory_and_procedural_guideline/2017/08/WC500232767.pdf.

Food and Drug Administration (FDA), 2001. Guidance for Industry: Postmarketing Safety Reporting for Human Drug and Biological Products Including Vaccines. Available from: https://www.fda.gov/downloads/BiologicsBloodVaccines/GuidanceComplianceRegulatoryInformation/Guidances/Vaccines/ucm092257.pdf.

Food and Drug Administration (FDA), December 2011. Guidance for Industry: Responding to Unsolicited Requests for Off-Label Information about Prescription Drugs and Medical Devices. Draft Guidance. Available from: https://www.fda.gov/downloads/drugs/guidances/ucm285145.pdf.

Food and Drug Administration (FDA), 2014a. Guidance for Industry: Fulfilling Regulatory Requirements for Postmarketing Submissions of Interactive Promotional Media for Prescription Human and Animal Drugs and Biologics. Draft Guidance. Available from: https://www.fda.gov/downloads/drugs/guidances/ucm381352.pdf.

Food and Drug Administration (FDA), 2014b. Guidance for Industry: Internet/Social Media Platforms with Character Space Limitations—Presenting Risk and Benefit Information for Prescription Drugs and Medical Devices. Draft Guidance. Available from: https://www.fda.gov/downloads/drugs/guidances/ucm401087.pdf.

Food and Drug Administration (FDA), 2014c. Guidance for Industry: Internet/Social Media Platforms: Correcting Independent Third-Party Misinformation about Prescription Drugs and Medical Devices. Draft Guidance. Available from: https://www.fda.gov/downloads/drugs/guidances/ucm401079.pdf.

Food and Drug Administration (FDA), 2015. Mining Social Media for Adverse Event Surveillance. Available from: https://www.fda.gov/ScienceResearch/SpecialTopics/RegulatoryScience/ucm455305.htm.

Fox, S., 2011. Pew Research Center. Health Topics. Available from: http://pewinternet.org/Reports/2011/HealthTopics.aspx.

Grajales, F., Clifford, D., Loupos, P., et al., 2014. Social Networking Sites and the Continuously Learning Health System: A Survey. Available from: https://nam.edu/perspectives-2014-social-networking-sites-and-the-continuously-learning-health-system-a-survey/.

Hamm, M.P., Chisholm, A., Shulhan, J., et al., May 09, 2013. Social media use among patients and caregivers: a scoping review. BMJ Open 3 (5).

Innovative Medicines Initiative (IMI), 2014. WEB-RADR: Recognising Adverse Drug Reactions. Available from: https://www.imi.europa.eu/content/web-radr.

MacMillan Cancer Support (MacMillan), 2015. Online Community. Availale from: https://community.macmillan.org.uk/.

Maher, A., 2015. Adverse Event Reporting and Social Medial. Available from: http://www.fdanews.com/ext/resources/files/Conference2/SM15Presentations/Maher-Adverse-Event-Reporting-and-Social-Media.pdf.

MedWatcher, Boston Children's Hospital, Harvard Medical School, Homepage, 2017. Available from: https://medwatcher.org/.

Michigan Office of Highway Safety Planning (NHTSA), 2012. 2012 Annual Evaluation Report, p. 21. Available from: https://www.nhtsa.gov/sites/nhtsa.dot.gov/files/mi_fy12annualreport.pdf.

Ogilvy Commonhealth Worldwide, 2015. Connecting the Dots: Which Pharma Companies are Succeeding in the Social Media Space? Available from: https://www.slideshare.net/OgilvyCommonHealth/connecting-the-dots-47203629.

Perrin, A., Duggan, M., June 26, 2015. Americans' Internet Access: 2000–2015. Pew Research Report. Available at: http://www.pewinternet.org/2015/06/26/americans-internet-access-2000-2015/.

Prescription Medicines Code of Practice Authority (PMCPA), 2017. Digital Communications. Available from: http://www.pmcpa.org.uk/advice/digital%20communications/Pages/default.aspx#.

Statistic Brain Research Institute, 2016. Twitter Statistics. Available from: http://www.statisticbrain.com/twitter-statistics/.

The Lancet Oncology, May 2014. #trial: clinical research in the age of social media. Lancet Oncol. 15 (6), 539.

Tozzi, J., Bass, D., 2015. For Bloomberg. Your Google Searches Could Help the FDA Find Drug Slie Effects. Available from: https://www.bloomberg.com/news/articles/2015-07-15/your-google-searches-could-help-the-fda-find-drug-side-effects.

Treato, Homepage, 2017. Available from: http://treato.com.

European Commission, Homepage, 2011. Available from: http://www.trendminer-project.eu/.

Twitter, 2017. Twitter Developer Documentation. Available from: https://dev.twitter.com/rest/public.

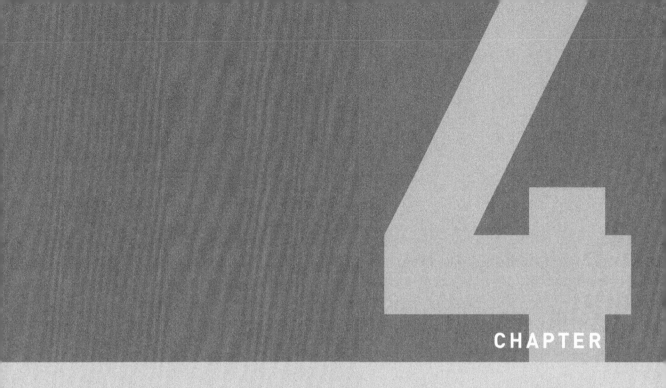

CHAPTER

4

Study Designs for PASS

4.1 Drug Utilization and Prescription-Event Monitoring Studies 107
4.2 Self-Controlled Studies 120
4.3 Cohort and Nested Case-Control Studies 139
4.4 Enriched Studies 150
4.5 Prospective Studies 158

Drug Utilization and Prescription-Event Monitoring Studies

Massoud Toussi[1], Deborah Layton[2]
[1]*IQVIA, Cedex, France;* [2]*IQVIA, London, United Kingdom*

INTRODUCTION

Drug utilization studies (DUS) were defined by the World Health Organization as studying the marketing, distribution, prescription, and use of medicinal products in a society, with special emphasis on the resulting medical and socioeconomic consequences (WHO, 2003). This definition focuses on the marketing of the medicinal products that has been amended and further expanded to other uses of products over time to include the reasons for medication use, the profile of prescribers and patients, and notions such as adherence to mediation (Elseviers et al., 2016). An alternative definition of DUS is the electronic collection of descriptive and analytical methods for the quantification, understanding, and evaluation of the processes of prescribing, dispensing, and consumption of medicinal products and for the testing of interventions to enhance the quality of these processes (Hartzema et al., 2008). In the context of post-authorization safety studies (PASS), DUS may be conducted for a variety of reasons, including understanding of drug exposure, consumption, off-label use, misuse, medication errors, and treatment dynamics. Additionally, DUS can be used to assess the effectiveness of risk minimization measures.

Knowledge about the exposure to medicinal products is of utmost importance. By quantifying the number of patients who are exposed—or will be exposed—to a product, the impact of its potential adverse events can be measured, including off-label use, misuse, or medication errors. For example, drug exposure (measured in person-years) is used as a denominator for normalizing the number of spontaneously reported adverse events for the product in the periodic safety update reports submitted by the marketing authorization holder. The extent of exposure is usually reported by country and period,

CONTENTS

Introduction 107

Methodological Considerations .. 108

Data Source for Drug Utilization Studies 110

Prescription-Event Monitoring Studies 111

Modified Prescription-Event Monitoring Studies 114

Specialist Cohort-Event Monitoring Studies 116

References 117

Post-Authorization Safety Studies of Medicinal Products. https://doi.org/10.1016/B978-0-12-809217-0.00004-0

which often needs to be extrapolated at country level. When exposure in terms of patient-years is difficult to determine, the understanding of its consumption in terms of units of product sold can provide useful insights. A common research question in DUS is whether the variation of the consumption across geographic regions and time is correlated with the extent of its reported adverse events. This approach is especially useful for the study of rare safety outcomes that are associated with commonly used products, e.g., liver transplant and paracetamol overdose (Gulmez et al., 2015).

DUS can provide direct insights on how a product is used in real-world conditions, including product withdrawals related to safety concerns, switches to another better tolerated product, or the study of adherence to treatments. Evaluation of the extent of off-label use, misuse, or medication errors is generally conducted through DUS. For example, to determine whether the product is prescribed to the right patient with the right dosage and route of administration. Based on the context of product use and its conditions of appropriate prescribing, a variety of designs and data sources can be considered (see Prescription-event monitoring studies).

When there is reasonable likelihood that a medicinal product is used inappropriately, a number of additional actions on top of routine risk minimization activities are proposed to mitigate risks associated with the product. According to the good pharmacovigilance practices, the effectiveness of these additional risk minimization measures should be evaluated. At process implementation level, DUS are commonly used to evaluate the impact of these measures, for example, by determining whether the off-label use rate in specific populations falls after the implementation of the additional risk minimization program (Mazzaglia et al., 2017). More detail on risk minimization measures and effectiveness assessment PASS is presented in Chapter 2.2.

METHODOLOGICAL CONSIDERATIONS

Commonly, a DUS is descriptive as its main purpose is to determine how the product is used in real-world settings. However, it can also be conducted as an analytic study, e.g., for determining the drivers of appropriate product use or the study of the effect of off-label or poor adherence with the frequency of adverse reactions. Similarly, the conditions of use are generally evaluated for a given point in time, e.g., at the time of prescription issuance. One's natural tendency is to consider the DUS design as longitudinal as soon as the conditions are checked in the patient history. However, it is sometimes useful to consider the patient history as an attribute of patient at the time of prescription. For example, consider sodium valproate, which is avoided in pregnant women unless no other antiepileptic agent is available. At clinical practice, the verification shall be conducted at the time of prescribing. If this study is conducted through electronic medical records (EMR), the information about pregnancy shall be sought from the patient history in the past. However, it is useful to consider collecting this information from patient history and create an attribute (pregnant, yes/no) at the moment of prescription, which will make it a cross-sectional DUS. In other cases, longitudinal designs are more appropriate, e.g., when evaluating whether the off-label rate gets better over time or the appropriateness of treatment duration.

In the context of PASS, most DUS are single arm in design as they are conducted to determine the conditions of use for a specific medicinal product. However, sometimes it makes sense to conduct comparative studies, e.g., when the extent of off-label use of a product is compared to a comparator or its pharmacologic class. Evaluation of the variation of the conditions of use of a product over time can be useful, especially in the context of risk minimization measures or other interventions. In such context, metrics of medication errors or appropriate prescribing can be compared before and after the interventions (pre–post design) (Bo et al., 2007). If the measurements can be done in several points of time, the interrupted time series analysis provide insights about the trends (Anand et al., 2017). See Fig. 2.2.1 for an example in the context of assessing the effectiveness of risk minimization activities.

The scope of DUS as a commitment for European regulatory requirements is generally over the European population to which the medicinal product was marketed. It is not necessary to include all European countries in the study, but it is generally expected that the population of the study represents the target population treated with the product of interest. For example, in case the product is authorized in entire Europe, it is expected that the sample of participating countries in the study covers different country profiles with different prescribing and health-care cultures. Consequently, it is wise to include Nordic and Eastern European countries as well as Central, Western, and Southern countries while paying attention to include a mix of small, medium, and large countries within each region. In practice, it is difficult to build a sample of individuals from different countries to represent their real distribution in the population. Therefore, it is important to conduct sample weighting, in which the proportions and measurements obtained for the different strata of the sample are adjusted to take into account the real distribution of the strata in the target population. Sometimes, e.g., exposure measurement, it is also important to extrapolate the information from the sample to obtain the real number of patients exposed to a product (this is of less importance though when proportions are the metrics of interest, e.g., proportion of off-label use).

DATA SOURCE FOR DRUG UTILIZATION STUDIES

In line with the variety of research questions and designs available for DUS, various data collection methods are available for such studies, including primary data collection and secondary use of data. One of the caveats of primary data collection for DUS is the fact that, in many cases, the data collected specifically for a given research question are prone to information bias, whereas routinely collected secondary data generally provide the actual use of a medicinal product in real-world settings.

Primary data collection sources for DUS include surveys, data extraction and abstraction from patient records and chart review, and prospective observational cohorts and registries. Data collected through questionnaires administered among health-care professionals or patients can be valuable in providing information about drug consumption. Surveys among the households and health people are sometimes the only way to collect information about drug misuse or abuse (Matheson et al., 1990; Perry et al., 2005; Bertoldi et al., 2008). When data are available in patient records in forms that are not accessible electronically, extraction from patient records using a questionnaire can be an option. This is especially useful for hospitalized patients where observations related to patients are recorded (Elseviers et al., 2010).

Collection of data from a cohort of patients over time and in periodic ways is very common and is one of the data sources for drug use. When combined with data from health-care professionals, patient logs and diaries can provide insights about how the medicinal product is actually used by the patients. Prospective cohorts collect data for specific study and research questions, whereas registries collect data for a broader scope and usually intended to be used for future studies. When used for a new study, established registries are considered as secondary source of data, e.g., the Nordic drug and patient registries (Wettermark et al., 2007; Furu et al., 2010). Chapter 3.3 discusses registries as one of the data sources for PASS, and Chapter 4.5 introduces prospective PASS designs.

On the other hand, secondary data sources include drug sales data, pharmacy records, administrative claims, EMR, social media, wearables and electronic devices, and prescription-event monitoring. In general, it is preferred to use secondary data whenever they are available and fit for purpose, as they allow collection of information with minimal clinical intervention. Information about product sales provides insights about the extent of sales of a product in the market for a given country. As mentioned before, these are specifically useful in providing the context of exposure to a product for ecological studies. Pharmacy dispensations of products are electronically registered in most industrialized countries and provide a very useful source of information about patterns of drug use (Richter et al., 2015; Skelly et al., 2017). Claims and EMR are invaluable sources of information about drug use. They allow verification of drug prescriptions or reimbursements and provide useful information about patient profile, e.g., diagnoses, comorbidities, and comedications. They are an excellent data source for the evaluation of off-label use, especially when the conditions to check are complex and involve some algorithms for measurement (Bücheler et al., 2002; Murray et al., 2004). Electronic devices collecting information about medication use such as mobile applications of patient diaries provide data valuable for DUS; similarly, social media can provide some information about the use of dynamics of medication use, including switches, discontinuations, and off-label use. Detailed discussions on claims, EMR, and social media data are presented in Chapters 3.1, 3.2, and 3.5, respectively.

The prescription-event monitoring is a specific scheme available in a number of countries, including the United Kingdom, Australia, and Japan. Details about this approach are provided below.

PRESCRIPTION-EVENT MONITORING STUDIES

In the United Kingdom, it was acknowledged that the spontaneous reporting system was best placed to detect dramatic and very rare adverse events (<0.01%), which is contrasted with the ability of clinical trials to detect common adverse events (1%−10%). However, there were calls for a system to bridge the gap between these extremes, detecting adverse drug events that occurred uncommonly (0.1%−1%). Several systems were proposed with limited success or were considered too expensive, including "registered release" of new medicinal products, where marketing authorization holders should provide evidence of use of the product with freedom from toxicity in a restricted group of patients (between 5000 and 10,000 for a commonly prescribed product) (Dollery and Rawlins, 1977); "recorded release," which required prescribers to complete a special prescription form that would be sent for registration to a central agency and follow-up would include completion of a questionnaire by the prescriber to report adverse events (Wilson, 1977); and "monitored release," in which the dispensing pharmacist would transcribe information onto a registration form that would be submitted to a central agency and follow-up would be directly undertaken with the prescribing physician (Lawson and Henry, 1977).

A scheme described as the "retrospective assessment of drug safety" was suggested with the intent to generate safety signals, but the proposal was hindered because of economic difficulties (Inman and Dollery, 1981). In 1980, the

Prescription-Event Monitoring Studies (PEMS) design was proposed to provide an improved method for early detection of potential drug hazards, not only for new products but also for established medicines according the criteria in Box 4.1.1 (GMSC, 1980). The PEMS scheme was at inception and remains the only national scheme in England available to all primary care general practitioners, in addition to the Yellow Card Scheme, used to monitor the safety of recently authorized medicinal products, under real-world conditions of general practice. A summary of study design and data collection process for PEMS in England is presented in Table 4.1.1. Unlike other countries, such as Japan and New Zealand, the unique structure of National Health Service in the United Kingdom has a central processing system for prescriptions and requires the general population to register with general practitioners; this permits creation of longitudinal medical records that hold all health-care consultations and interventions that occurred during the life of each patient. In addition to providing drug utilization information, the PEMS provide estimates of incidence rates for events reported in the exposed cohort and also provide the opportunity for further clinical evaluation of selected events of interest using bespoke follow-up questionnaires.

The PEMS methodology relies on the identification of a single inception cohort (new user design) assembled on the basis of a common exposure (i.e., the medicinal product under surveillance). More detail on cohort designs

BOX 4.1.1 ESSENTIAL CRITERIA FOR PRESCRIPTION-EVENT MONITORING STUDIES (INMAN AND DOLLERY, 1981)

- Should measure the relative incidence of adverse events in populations of patients treated with various drugs. To achieve this it will be necessary to obtain both the numerator (the adverse event) and the denominator (the number of patients treated).
- Events rather than adverse drug reactions should be recorded, irrespective of whether or not they are related to treatment. This has several advantages, including no need for medical opinion about the probability of a causal relationship between drug and event.
- Conducted retrospectively and should be clearly distinguished from postmarketing (Phase IV) clinical trials in which participants are recruited in advance. There should be no preselection of patients, and the study should not in any way

interfere with normal prescribing or record keeping.
- Should provide for long-term follow-up. It should be appreciated that, at present, it is very unlikely that a doubling or even greater increase in the incidence of cancer or other serious disease caused by a drug would be detected.
- Would in no way affect freedom to prescribe.
- Because prescribers would not be reporting opinions about the cause of adverse events occurring during treatment, the medicolegal risk of participation should be considerably less than that associated with other currently available methods of drug safety monitoring.
- Collaboration would be voluntary.
- Methods of recording information should be simple and not time-consuming.
- Should be inexpensive

Table 4.1.1 Operational Characteristics of Prescription-Event Monitoring Studies in England

Characteristic	Description
Selection of medicines	According to defined criteria independent of regulator
Comparator	No internal comparator
Setting	Primary care
Route of establishing cohort	Dispensed prescriptions via national prescription remuneration scheme
Special conditions	New users (inception cohort)
Start of observation	Market launch
Period of follow-up	Patients censored at 6–12 months
Prescribers surveyed	General practitioners
Survey frequency	Single time
Desired sample size	10,000 patients
Primary outcome and exposure data source	Drug utilization, events, and selected risk factors from secondary use of prescriber-held patient medical records
Additional data source	None
Signal generation	Assessment of event risk and rate differences between periods
Ethics and consent	Ethics waiver, consent not required

for PASS is presented in Chapter 4.3. Each study is national in scale and attempts to sample for all general practitioners in England. It is possible that the cohort may be subject to selection bias, arising from phenomena such as channeling or switching, which may affect the generalizability of study results. Channeling occurs prescribers preferentially prescribe the product to subsets of patients defined by a specific characteristic, such as having a condition resistant to previous therapy, or preexisting risk factor may be a precaution for use or contraindication to certain treatments. Switching could be attributed by past experience with an alternative medicinal product that modifies the risk of adverse events associated with the current use of the product of interest under study.

Furthermore, selection bias may be introduced through nonresponse, which becomes important if the characteristics of the study cohort are systematically different in nonresponders. For example, there may be depletion of susceptibles bias if general practitioners selectively respond for those patients who tolerate and continue to use the product of interest. The reverse is also possible whereby prescribers may be more likely to respond if patients have experienced adverse events with a new product. Another limitation of standard PEMS is the paucity of information on baseline characteristics for the whole cohort such as medical history, comorbidities, and treatment patterns.

In the context of PASS, PEMS can be classified into modified PEMS (M-PEMS) and specialist cohort-event monitoring studies (SCEMS) (Layton and Shakir, 2014, 2015). Collectively, the methodology is noninterventional, retrospective in nature, based on secondary use of data from existing medical records and regarded as a surveillance methodology employed to bridge the gap in generating safety signals of uncommon or rare outcomes that could be missed in clinical trials because of size or missed in spontaneous reporting systems because of underreporting and background noise.

MODIFIED PRESCRIPTION-EVENT MONITORING STUDIES

The first M-PEMS design was introduced in 1998, whereby the "green form" questionnaire was updated to identify subsets of patients with important cardiovascular risk factors for sildenafil, an erectile dysfunction treatment (Shakir et al., 2001; Boshier et al., 2004). This modification was in response to the emergence of the requirements for risk management of medicinal products (EC, 2008) and in parallel with pharmacoepidemiological developments in general (Epstein, 2005; ENCePP, 2013). A number of further enhancements have since been made to the PEMS to facilitate more targeted safety surveillance of safety concerns, enhance data quality, and provide increased scope for more robust data analysis in terms of signal generation and hypothesis strengthening.

The M-PEMS approach was evolved in attempt to overcome some of the limitations of the standard PEMS through innovation in design, application of new analytical methods, and remuneration to prescribers. M-PEMS retain the advantages of the original method but with enhancements that permit specific questions to be addressed in accordance with the needs of the pharmacovigilance plan, including additional pharmacovigilance activities such as PASS.

In both standard PEMS and M-PEMS, dispensed prescription data sources and EMR are used to provide data for eligible patients. Exposure data are derived from dispensed prescriptions issued by general practitioners, and study outcomes and other data are derived from the EMR at the general practitioner level. Data collection begins immediately after market launch of the product of interest until the targeted sample size has been reached. There are no specific exclusion criteria; however, one key difference between the two approaches relates to the per protocol sample size. For the M-PEMS, the study is powered to achieve sufficient numbers of patients to provide a reliable estimate of the primary objective—that being the key risk of concern, which generally requires fewer patients than other safety surveillance studies. For

Table 4.1.2 Comparison Between Standard Prescription-Event Monitoring Studies (PEMS) and Modified PEMS (M-PEMS)

Characteristic	Standard PEMS	M-PEMS
Sample size	≥10,000	Bespoke to targeted event
Follow-up period	6–12 months	3–12 months and longer
Survey intervals	One	Multiple
Questionnaire format	Short, single page "green form"	Long, multiple pages
Drug utilization	All populations	Targeted subgroups at risk
Risk factors	Event specific	Selected factors for all patients
Outcome surveillance	General	General and targeted
Analysis	Measures of frequency and impact	Regression models
Prescriber remuneration	No	Yes
Considered as PASS	No	Yes
Registration in EU PAS Register	Not required	Required

EU PAS, *The European Union electronic register of post-authorization studies;* PASS, *post-authorization safety studies*

example, the median cohort size of 19 standard PEMS for psychotropic products was 11,735, whereas those of six M-PEMS were 3586. This might be due to the difference in principal study objectives. Standard PEMS are intended for general surveillance with a target size of a minimum of 10,000 patients to allow for the detection of rare events occurring with a frequency of at least one in 2000 patients (assuming the background rate is zero) with 85% power (Machin et al., 1997). Table 4.1.2 describes the differences between standard PEMS and M-PEMS. In general, M-PEMS are frequently used as PASS and therefore, they are required to be registered in the European Union electronic Register of post-authorization studies (see Chapter 8 for more details on transparency of PASS).

In terms of duration of observation, for both approaches a minimum of 3 months lag is required to allow information to be shared between patients and prescribers after the date of each first prescription issued to the patient. Thereafter, relevant outcome data can be collected from study questionnaires sent to each prescriber at predefined periods (a standard 6-month observation period for PEMS). In M-PEMS, the duration of follow-up is driven by the expected pattern of risk for events identified within the study primary objectives. The M-PEMS permit data collection in multiple waves for both short- and long-term risk surveillance patterns, e.g., 3–12 months. This permits stratification of data collection to focus on collecting more detailed information on early onset (acute) risks, treatment details at initiation, selected risk factors and medical history, concomitant medications, changes in morbidity and product posology over time, and selected prescriber or patient behaviors close to the index date of starting the medicinal product of interest. Additionally, events of interest may be followed up for purposes of further evaluation. In recognition of the additional work effort, remuneration is offered to general practices for each completed M-PEMS questionnaire returned. For each returned questionnaire/patient data, trained coding staff prepares a computerized, longitudinal record of demographic, exposure, and outcome data, including additional follow-ups when needed.

SPECIALIST COHORT-EVENT MONITORING STUDIES

In 2008, an additional adaptation to the PEMS methodology was introduced that addressed an existing need for safety surveillance of new medicinal products initiated in secondary care settings, e.g., hospitals (Layton and Kimber, 2014). In the United Kingdom, secondary care data, particularly around prescribing, are not well captured in EMR databases, such as the Clinical Practice Research Datalink (CPRD). The SCEMS application was developed in the recognition that PASS conducted exclusively in the primary care settings may be at risk of biased conclusions about the frequency of adverse events and prevalence of the types of patients prescribed new products because of the potential for exclusion of patients who are managed predominately within hospitals. These patients, who may be started their treatment under the care of a specialist health-care professional, may have different characteristics and health experiences than those treated—for similar indications—by general practitioners in the primary care settings. There is a need for data capture across both health-care settings to ensure all relevant exposure populations are characterized and monitored. The SCEMS approach of PEMS enables cohorts of patients who were prescribed a new product in hospitals to be monitored.

The principal differences between M-PEMS and SCEMS relate to the route of identification of patients and requirements for consent and ethics approval. Patients are identified through networks of specialists that are established by the National Institute of Health Research Clinical Research Network. Similar to M-PEMS, SCEMS are powered to examine the principal safety issue of concern; and all specialist consultations, exposure data, and outcome data that have been recorded in the patients medical records are derived from the questionnaire sent to the specialist treating the patient at predefined periods after the date of each first prescription issued.

In general, M-PEMS and SCEMS provide a method to systematically monitor the safety of medicinal products following introduction into clinical practice. They are considered hypothesis-generating designs permitting the examination of the characteristics of prescribers and populations of new product users and contribute to the accumulation of safety data through the conduct of both quantitative and qualitative data analyses. Qualitative analysis of PEMS provides insights on drug utilization factors, prescribing decisions, and use in vulnerable populations for whom off-label prescribing has occurred. Quantitative analyses also underpin the main approach to signal detection, e.g., crude event rates (usually incidence densities for a fixed period expressed in units of first event reported per 1000 patient-months) are calculated to give estimates of real-world frequency. Calculation of incidence density differences between periods of observation is an effective approach for signal detection. The enhancements to PEMS allow to investigate safety signals due to additional information, including demographics and other confounding factors, which can be accomplished by the application of survival analysis methods and estimation of incidence densities within and between special populations of interest (Layton and Kimber, 2014).

References

Anand, K., Sketris, I., Zhang, Y., Levy, A., Gamble, J.-M., December 2017. The impact of US FDA and health Canada warnings related to the safety of high-dose simvastatin. Drugs Real World Outcomes 4 (4), 215–223.

Bertoldi, A.D., Barros, A.J., Wagner, A., Ross-Degnan, D., Hallal, P.C., 2008. A descriptive review of the methodologies used in household surveys on medicine utilization. BMC Health Serv. Res. 8 (1), 222.

Bo, S., Valpreda, S., Scaglione, L., Boscolo, D., Piobbici, M., Bo, M., Ciccone, G., 2007. Implementing hospital guidelines improves warfarin use in non-valvular atrial fibrillation: a before-after study. BMC Publ. Health 7, 203.

Boshier, A., Wilton, L.V., Shakir, S.A., 2004. Evaluation of the safety of sildenafil for male erectile dysfunction: experience gained in general practice use in England in 1999. BJU Int. 93 (6), 796–801.

Bücheler, R., Schwab, M., Mörike, K., Kalchthaler, B., Mohr, H., Schröder, H., et al., June 1, 2002. Off label prescribing to children in primary care in Germany: retrospective cohort study. BMJ 324 (7349), 1311–1312.

Dollery, C.T., Rawlins, M.D., 1977. Monitoring adverse reactions to drugs. Br. Med. J. 1 (6053), 96–97.

Elseviers, M.M., Vander Stichele, R.R., Van Bortel, L., October 1, 2010. Drug utilization in Belgian nursing homes: impact of residents' and institutional characteristics. Pharmacoepidemiol. Drug Saf. 19 (10), 1041–1048.

Elseviers, M., Wettermark, B., Almarsdottir, A.B., Andersen, M., Benko, R., Bennie, M., Eriksson, I., Godman, B., Krska, J., Poluzzi, E., Taxis, K., Vlahovic-Palcevski, V., Stichele, R.V. (Eds.), 2016. Drug Utilization Research: Methods and Applications.

Epstein, M., 2005. Guidelines for good pharmacoepidemiology practices (GPP). Pharmacoepidemiol. Drug Saf. 14 (8), 589–595.

European Commission (EC), September 2008. Volume 9A - Pharmacovigilance for Medicinal Products for Human Use. Available at: http://ec.europa.eu/enterprise/pharmaceuticals/eudralex/vol-9/pdf/vol9a_09-2008.pdf.

European Network of Centres of Excellence for Pharmacoepidemiology, Pharmacovigilance (ENCePP), June 18, 2013. Guide on Methodological Standards in Pharmacoepidemiology (Revision 2). EMA/95098/2010 Rev.2. Available at: http://www.ema.europa.eu/docs/en_GB/document_library/Scientific_guideline/2014/09/WC500172402.pdf.

Furu, K., Wettermark, B., Andersen, M., Martikainen, J.E., Almarsdottir, A.B., Sørensen, H.T., February 1, 2010. The Nordic countries as a cohort for pharmacoepidemiological research. Basic Clin. Pharmacol. Toxicol. 106 (2), 86—94.

GMSC, 1980. Prescription-event monitoring: pilot study approved. Br. Med. J. 281 (6254), 1579—1584.

Gulmez, S.E., Larrey, D., Pageaux, G.-P., Bernuau, J., Bissoli, F., Horsmans, Y., et al., September 2015. Liver transplant associated with paracetamol overdose: results from the seven-country SALT study. Br. J. Clin. Pharmacol. 80 (3), 599—606.

Hartzema, A.G., Tilson, H.H., Chan, K.A. (Eds.), 2008. Pharmacoepidemiology and Therapeutic Risk Management, first ed.

Inman, W., Dollery, C., 1981. Post-marketing drug surveillance. In: Cavalla, J. (Ed.), Risk-benefit Analysis in Drug Research: Proceedings of an International Symposium Held at the University of Kent at Canterbury, England, 27 March 1980. Springer Netherlands, New York, pp. 141—161.

Lawson, D.H., Henry, D.A., 1977. Monitoring adverse reactions to new drugs: "restricted release" or "monitored release"? Br. Med. J. 1 (6062), 691—692.

Layton, D., Shakir, S.A.W., 2014. Prescription-event monitoring (PEM): the evolution to the new modified PEM and its support of risk management. In: Mann, R.D., Andrews, E.B. (Eds.), Pharmacovigilance, 3 ed. Wiley Blackwell, Chichester, UK, pp. 359—384.

Layton, D., Kimber, A., 2014. Feasibility of adjusted parametric methods to model survival data as a tool for signal strengthening: an example in modified prescription-event monitoring (M-PEM). Pharmacoepidemiol. Drug Saf. (S1), 1—497.

Layton, D., Shakir, S.A., 2015. Specialist cohort event monitoring studies: a new study method for risk management in pharmacovigilance. Drug Saf. 38 (2), 153—163.

Machin, D., Campbell, M., Fayers, P., et al., 1997. Sample Size Tables for Clinical Studies. Table 7.1. Blackwell Science Ltd, Oxford, UK.

Matheson, I., Kristensen, K., Lunde, P.K.M., May 1, 1990. Drug utilization in breast-feeding women. A survey in Oslo. Eur. J. Clin. Pharmacol. 38 (5), 453—459.

Mazzaglia, G., Straus, S.M.J., Arlett, P., da Silva, D., Janssen, H., Raine, J., Alteri, E., November 9, 2017. Study design and evaluation of risk minimization measures: a review of studies submitted to the European medicines agency for cardiovascular, endocrinology, and metabolic drugs. Drug Saf. https://doi.org/10.1007/s40264-017-0604-4 (Epub ahead of print).

Murray, M.L., de Vries, C.S., Wong, I.C.K., December 1, 2004. A drug utilisation study of antidepressants in children and adolescents using the General Practice Research Database. Arch. Dis. Child. 89 (12), 1098—1102.

Perry, P.J., Lund, B.C., Deninger, M.J., Kutscher, E.C., Schneider, J., September 2005. Anabolic steroid use in weightlifters and bodybuilders: an internet survey of drug utilization. Clin. J. Sport Med. 15 (5), 326.

Shakir, S.A., Wilton, L.V., Boshier, A., Layton, D., Heeley, E., 2001. Cardiovascular events in users of sildenafil: results from first phase of prescription event monitoring in England. BMJ 322 (7287), 651—652.

Richter, H., Dombrowski, S., Hamer, H., Hadji, P., Kostev, K., 2015. Use of a German longitudinal prescription database (LRx) in pharmacoepidemiology. Ger. Med. Sci. 13. Doc14.

Skelly, A., Carius, H.J., Bezlyak, V., Chen, F.K., 2017. Dispensing patterns of ranibizumab and aflibercept for the treatment of neovascular age-related macular degeneration: a retrospective cohort study. Adv. Ther. 34 (12), 2585—2600.

Wettermark, B., Hammar, N., MichaelFored, C., Leimanis, A., Otterblad Olausson, P., Bergman, U., et al., July 1, 2007. The new Swedish Prescribed Drug Register—opportunities for pharmacoepidemiological research and experience from the first six months. Pharmacoepidemiol. Drug Saf. 16 (7), 726—735.

Wilson, A.B., 1977. Post-marketing surveillance of adverse reactions to new medicines. Br. Med. J. 2 (6093), 1001—1003.

World Health Organization (WHO), 2003. Introduction to Drug Utilization Research. WHO, Oslo, Norway.

Self-Controlled Studies

Shirley V. Wang[1], Ayad K. Ali[2]

[1]*Division of Pharmacoepidemiology and Pharmacoeconomics, Department of Medicine, Brigham and Women's Hospital and Harvard Medical School, Boston, MA, United States;* [2]*Eli Lilly and Company, Indianapolis, IN, United States*

CONTENTS

Introduction 120

Assumptions and Data Requirements 121
Across Approaches ... 121
Approaches Using Person-Time Before the Outcome 123
Approaches Using Person-Time After the Outcome 124

Types of Self-Controlled Designs 125
Case-Crossover 126
Self-Controlled Risk Interval 129
Sequence Symmetry Analysis 130
Self-Controlled Case-Series 131

Methodological Considerations .. 132
Population Trends in Exposure Over Time . 132
Healthy-User/Sick-Quitter Effects 134
Event-Dependent Exposures 136

References 137

INTRODUCTION

There are many designs in analytic choices available for post-authorization safety studies (PASS). In an effort to increase transparency, to facilitate appropriate design and analytic choices, and to reduce false-positive and false-negative signals due to bias, the FDA Sentinel Program created a structured taxonomy with decision tables (Gagne et al., 2012). Self-controlled designs are one arm of this taxonomy. The primary appeal and benefit of self-controlled designs are the use of within-person comparisons. This comparison means that all characteristics that do not vary with time, including factors that are often unrecorded in large health-care databases, cannot bias the analysis (Maclure, 1991; Farrington, 1995; Fireman et al., 2009; Madigan et al., 2011; Maclure et al., 2012). In addition to characteristics that do not vary with time, long-term health habits or health events that occurred in the distant past do not confound within-person comparisons that sample more proximal person-time (Madigan et al., 2011). Like other designs, self-controlled methods require additional adjustment to account for time-varying confounders whose status changes across the within-person time sampled for comparison (Suissa, 1995; Farrington et al., 2009; Wang et al., 2011a). For example, proximal changes in health-care utilization, exercise, smoking, or alcohol consumption behaviors are related to exposures and outcomes.

Self-controlled PASS designs are best suited for evaluating intermittent exposure in relation to abrupt onset outcomes in situations where there is little misclassification of timing of exposure and outcome as well as negligible time-varying confounding. The Sentinel Taxonomy recommends use of self-controlled designs for signal refinement when key assumptions are fulfilled; however, in situations where one or more assumptions are not met, cohort type approaches are preferred (see Chapter 4.3) (TPW, 2010). It is important to keep in mind that conceptually, cohort and self-controlled studies address different questions (Maclure, 2007). The former asks the question "why me?—is it because I am a user of product X?" In contrast, the latter asks the question "why now?—is it because today is one of the days that I used product X?"

There are many variations of self-controlled designs, each of which use different strategies for sampling within-person comparison time. However, at the heart of each approach is the comparison of the observed rate of events during a postulated at-risk window following exposure to the expected or "usual" rate of events during unexposed time within an individual. Depending on how within-person time is sampled to estimate the expected rate of events, different challenges have been identified. These include bias because of population-level time trends in exposure or outcome (Suissa, 1995; Fireman et al., 2009), protopathic bias (Wang, 2013), bias due to mixing of intermittent and persistent users (Hallas et al., 2016), or outcomes influencing future exposure within the patient (Farrington et al., 2009).

ASSUMPTIONS AND DATA REQUIREMENTS

There are several assumptions and conditions that must be met for unbiased estimation with self-controlled PASS conducted using large health-care databases. Some are common across approaches, others are relevant for designs that only use person-time prior to the outcome, and others are relevant for approaches that include person-time after the outcome. Selection of a self-controlled design and within-person sampling strategy for PASS should be based on consideration of many factors, including the strength of the potential bias due to violation of assumptions.

Across Approaches

Across approaches, the outcome under investigation should be one with an abrupt onset whose timing can be identified clearly from the available data (TPW, 2010). The timing of diagnoses and procedures related to health-care encounters is accurately and prospectively recorded in large health-care data sources (see Chapter 3.1 for claims and Chapter 3.2 for EMR data sources). Regardless of study design, outcomes that do not generate a health-care encounter or that are difficult to identify with reasonable sensitivity and specificity are difficult to study. For self-controlled designs, there is added importance to ascertain timing of health-care encounter versus timing of actual outcome. Misclassification of the timing of the outcome can result in incorrect attribution of outcomes to risk window or reference window (Greenland, 1996). Furthermore, there is risk of findings due to reverse causality from exposures that occur after the outcome but prior to detection. Therefore, it is ideal to study outcomes that are serious, can be identified well using large health-care databases, and have abrupt onset (necessitating immediate health-care contact) when using a self-controlled study design.

Another assumption is the exposure of interest is intermittent (i.e., transient), meaning it varies within person. For case-crossover and self-controlled risk-interval approaches, the exposure or exposure effect should be brief (Maclure, 1991); however, longer exposure duration can be used with self-controlled case-series approach (Whitaker et al., 2009). The timing of exposure effect should be ascertainable with the data available. As stated in previous chapters, large health-care databases, e.g., administrative claims, have excellent prospective recording of timing of dispensations of prescribed medicinal products, whereas EMR can accurately capture timing of issued prescriptions. However, the timing of actual exposure may not correspond directly with a prescription or dispensation. Whether and when a patient is exposed depends on first obtaining a prescription, then filling it, and then taking the medication. Prescription records do not capture whether or when a patient fills their prescription and will misclassify exposure due to nonadherence, whether primary (patient never fills the first prescription) or secondary (patient does not fill as prescribed). Even if a prescription is dispensed, dispensation claims cannot capture whether or when a patient actually consumed the prescribed treatment. Misclassification of the timing of exposure effect (i.e., the risk window) can result in incorrect attribution of outcomes to exposure status within individuals.

The ability of large databases to capture timing of actual exposure may vary according to data type and the clinical question (see Chapter 3.4 for a discussion about big data). For example, prescriptions of a short intended duration for a symptomatic condition versus an indefinite prescription for long-term prevention of an asymptomatic condition. Defining timing of exposure can be complicated when the intended course of treatment is long or indefinite. Patients may stockpile products and refill at irregular intervals, resulting in apparent transitions in exposure that change depending on the algorithms for defining exposure. The sensitivity of self-controlled designs to misclassification of timing of exposure and the necessity of transitions in exposure within individual to contribute to safety evaluations make them best suited for PASS of point exposures (e.g., vaccines) or exposures of intended short duration (e.g., antimicrobials) as opposed to exposures of intended longer duration (e.g., antihypertensives).

The induction period, duration of treatment, and pharmacokinetics and pharmacodynamics of the medicinal product should be considered when operationalizing the definition of timing of exposure effect. Operational decisions should be based on subject matter knowledge (i.e., clinical expertise) and consider data availability and limitations. Timing of vaccinations in a clinic can be identified easily; however, timing of the effect of exposure will vary depending on vaccination and outcome (Chapter 7.3 discusses PASS options for vaccines) (Yih et al., 2011). Drug exposures can be defined based on pre-scription dates or dispensation dates, with or without inclusion of data on days supply, use of stockpiling algorithms, inclusion of exposure extension windows, or bridging of adjacent exposure episodes.

Moreover, immeasurable time can bias self-controlled designs. When using large health-care databases to conduct self-controlled analyses for PASS, it is important to evaluate whether exposure and outcome can be ascertained over the compared within-person time windows based on enrollment in data source and the coverage of that data source. For claims data, exposure and outcome status cannot be captured outside of patient's enrollment period. In addition, many US claims databases have outpatient dispensations but are not linked to inpatient dispensations. This means that exposure during hospi-talization time cannot be determined. For EMR data, it is often difficult to tell whether a patient is receiving care outside of the practice or health-care system. Any exposure or outcome that is prescribed or treated outside of the EMR source is not measurable.

Approaches Using Person-Time Before the Outcome

Some self-controlled designs, such as the unidirectional case-crossover design, only sample person-time prior to the outcome (Maclure, 1991). The observed probability of exposure during time just prior to the case-defining event is compared to the expected probability of exposure estimated in person-time further back in the patient history. A benefit of only sampling person-time prior to the outcome is that bias due to changes in probability of exposure caused by the outcome are averted. However, when there is a trend in probability of exposure over time before the outcome, this can result in inaccurate estimation of the usual or expected frequency of exposure (Suissa, 1995; Wang et al., 2011a, 2013). Therefore, stable probability of exposure in these approaches is an additional assumption to consider.

PASS may encounter situation with exposure time trends. For example, when a medicinal product enters the market, there may be rapid uptake, resulting in the probability of exposure in the population being systematically higher at later dates (Fig. 4.2.1). For case-crossover PASS conducted during this period of calendar time, the probability of exposure during historically sampled person-time would be an underestimate of the expected probability of exposure at the time of the case-defining event and result in measures of asso-ciation that are biased up (Wang et al., 2014). The bias from population-level trends in exposure probability would continue until the population reaches a steady state of starting and stopping the medicinal product of interest. This

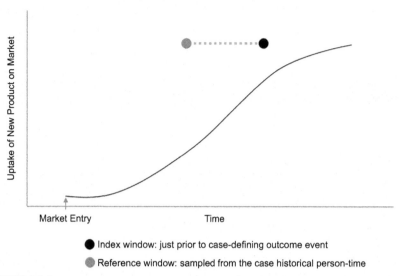

FIGURE 4.2.1
Population-level trends in exposure in case-crossover designs.

bias may also be seen during periods when the market share of a product declines sharply around the time of changes in drug insurance policies or formularies or other sources of ecological shifts in exposure probability over time (Madigan et al., 2011).

Another example of a situation when there may be changes in the probability of exposure over time is when prodromal signs and symptoms related to the case-defining event lead to health-care seeing behavior, resulting in proto-pathic bias (Horwitz and Feinstein, 1980; Ali, 2015). When this occurs, patients experience more health-care encounters and may be exposed to more medical interventions just prior to the case-defining event than usual (Wang et al., 2013). Because the impending outcome promoted exposure to medical interventions, any observed association would be due to reverse causality. Similarly, knowledge of impending health events (e.g., death) may lead some health-care professionals or patients to discontinue exposure to long-term preventive medications (e.g., antihypertensives) whose benefits are unlikely to be realized (Glynn et al., 2001; Wang et al., 2013). This discontinuation can lead to observed crossover in exposure status just prior to a case-defining event.

Approaches Using Person-Time After the Outcome

Some self-controlled designs such as the self-controlled case-series approach include sampling of person-time that occurred after the occurrence of a case-defining event (Farrington et al., 1995). These designs assume that events within individuals occur as part of a nonhomogeneous Poisson process, in which the observed rate of outcomes during exposed time is compared with the usual or expected rate of outcomes when not exposed. These methods perform best when the case-defining event is rare or recurrent case-defining events are independent (Whitaker et al., 2006). In practice, if events are not independent (e.g., the first occurrence increases the probability of another occurrence), this can be handled analytically by grouping clusters of outcomes into distinct episodes and analyzing the episodes as independent outcomes (Farrington et al., 1995), or if the outcome is rare, one can keep only the first occurrence in the analysis (Whitaker et al., 2006). Thus, rare or independent recurrent events should be considered as an assumption in these approaches.

Another critical assumption that must be met for unbiased treatment effect estimation when including within-person time sampled after the case-defining event is that the outcome does neither influence subsequent probability of exposure nor does it censor the observation period (i.e., no event-dependent exposure) (Whitaker et al., 2006, 2009). To illustrate why this is important, if the occurrence of an outcome results in a reduced probability of treatment for a limited period(e.g., vaccination delayed following a seizure) and the probability of another outcome during the delay is temporarily lowered before returning to baseline, this will inflate the relative incidence for exposed compared with unexposed person-time. Occurrence of an outcome can result in more extreme interference with exposure probability if it results in a permanent contraindication to exposure, and the patient remains under observation, or if occurrence of an outcome censors the observation window. The latter can happen if occurrence of the outcome increases the short-term rate of death. Death censors observation for the patient, making the probability of future exposure zero.

TYPES OF SELF-CONTROLLED DESIGNS

The many variants of self-controlled designs may be broadly categorized as those that sample only person-time before the outcome, those that sample only person-time after the outcome, and those that include person-time both before and after the outcome of interest. They can be further divided into "exposure-indexed" or "outcome-indexed" designs (Table 4.2.1). Exposure-indexed approaches start by defining the risk window from exposure and sampling the reference person-time not in the risk window. In contrast, outcome-indexed approaches start by defining the window prior to the outcome during which exposure could have had an effect on outcome and sampling reference person-time outside of the window. We note that, while

Table 4.2.1 Types of Self-Controlled Designs for Post-Authorization Safety Studies

Design	When is Person-Time Sampled Within Individuals in Relation to the Outcome?		
	Before	After	Before and After
Outcome-indexed	Case-crossover[a]		
Exposure-indexed		Self-controlled risk interval[a]	Self-controlled case-series Sequence symmetry

[a]*Could be bidirectional, sampling person-time before and after the outcome.*

variants in implementation of the case-crossover and self-controlled risk interval can be bidirectional (Wang et al., 2011b), sampling person-time from both before and after the outcome, those approaches are not typically used in pharmacoepidemiology. Furthermore, the implementation and assumptions become virtually identical to the self-controlled case-series.

In all types of self-controlled designs, the use of within-person comparison means that only individuals who have crossover in exposure and the outcome contribute analytically to the estimated effect of treatment. This can make the construction of analytic data sets from longitudinal streams of health-care data simpler, as only individuals with the event of interest who also have exposure at some point in their recorded history must be identified.

Case-Crossover

The case-crossover design is an outcome-indexed self-controlled approach that can be applied to evaluate transient effects of exposure as a trigger for abrupt onset outcomes (Maclure, 1991). PASS typically apply unidirectional case-crossover designs, where within-person comparisons are based on person-time prior to the case-defining event (Consiglio et al., 2013). These involve comparison of the observed probability of exposure just prior to the outcome to the expected probability of exposure estimated in historical person-time within the same individual.

When designing case-crossover PASS, researchers must consider how to parameterize index and reference windows (Fig. 4.2.1). The index window includes person-time prior to the case-defining event when exposure could potentially have an effect on the outcome. The reference window includes person-time prior to the case-defining event when exposure could not have had an effect on the outcome. Multiple reference windows may be sampled within individual to increase power. Including washout periods between windows of person-time allows potential carryover effects of exposure to subside.

As an illustrative example, Fig. 4.2.2 depicts 20 days of time within the lives of five patients. The exposed time is represented by black blocks, the unexposed

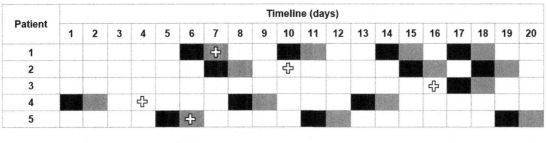

FIGURE 4.2.2
Illustration of timeline of exposure and outcome for patients.

time by white blocks, and case-defining outcome events by white cross. Because of a brief induction period and short half-life, the hypothesized effect of exposure on the outcome occurs 1 day after exposure begins and continues until 1 day after exposure ends (gray blocks). Because the case-crossover design is outcome-indexed, we align the outcomes for each patient at time 0 (Fig. 4.2.3A). We operationalize the within-person comparison as a comparison between an index window (person-time during which exposure could have an effect on outcome) and the reference window (person-time during which exposure is not expected to be able to have an effect on outcome). Given our assumptions about the exposure effect period, for each case, we define the index window as the day prior to the outcome and the reference window as 3 days prior to the outcome. This allows a washout of 1 day in between the reference and index windows to allow potential carryover effects of exposure to subside.

Because of the within-person comparison, only cases that have crossover in exposure within the compared windows can contribute to the effect estimate. In our example, patient 3 does not have crossover in exposure during the within-person time sampled for comparison; therefore, this patient does not contribute to the effect estimate. The observed probability of exposure during the index window is compared with the expected probability of exposure at that time if there were no effect of exposure on outcome. The latter is estimated by the probability of exposure observed in the reference window. In the simplest setting, with one historical reference window of the same length as the index window sampled for each case, the odds ratio (OR) can be estimated as a ratio of discordant pairs (i.e., ratio of cases who crossed from unexposed to exposed to cases who crossed from exposed to unexposed) (Maclure, 1991).

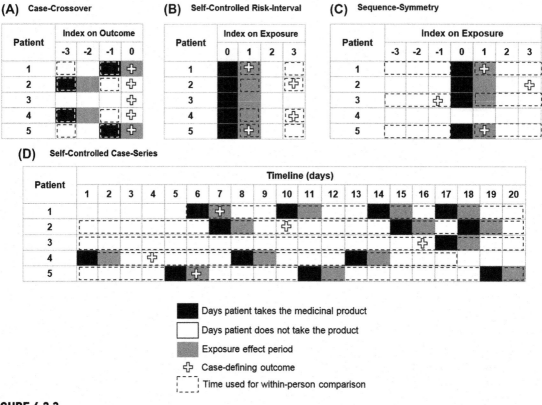

(A) Case-Crossover

Patient	Index on Outcome			
	-3	-2	-1	0
1			■	✚
2	■			✚
3				✚
4	■			✚
5			■	✚

(B) Self-Controlled Risk-Interval

Patient	Index on Exposure			
	0	1	2	3
1	■	✚		
2	■			✚
3	■			
4	■			✚
5	■	✚		

(C) Sequence-Symmetry

Patient	Index on Exposure						
	-3	-2	-1	0	1	2	3
1				■	✚		
2				■			✚
3			✚	■			
4				■			
5				■	✚		

(D) Self-Controlled Case-Series

Patient	Timeline (days)																			
	1	2	3	4	5	6	7	8	9	10	11	12	13	14	15	16	17	18	19	20
1						■	✚			■				■			■			
2							■			✚					■			■		
3																✚	■			
4	■			✚			■				■									
5					■	✚					■		■						■	

■ Days patient takes the medicinal product
☐ Days patient does not take the product
▨ Exposure effect period
✚ Case-defining outcome
┌─┐ Time used for within-person comparison

FIGURE 4.2.3
Illustration of within-person comparisons using different self-controlled design approaches.

Alternative ways to operationalize case-crossover PASS could involve use of multiple reference windows to increase power, use of windows of different length, and variations on the duration of washout period, induction period, or exposure effect. Regardless of how the within-person time is sampled for comparison, to implement within-person comparisons, a matched analysis should be conducted using Mantel–Haenszel, McNemar's estimate (ratio of discordant pairs), or a conditional logistic or Poisson regression model. One way to set up the data for analysis is with a statistical software program would be to create two observations for each individual, one for each within-person time window being compared. Three variables are necessary for conditional regression models: a patient identifier, an indicator of whether or not the outcome occurred within each window, and an indicator of whether or not a patient was exposed within each window.

By comparing observed to expected probability of exposure, we measure how unusual it would be to see the observed frequency of exposure during the index period if there were truly no effect of exposure on outcome. However, the within-person comparison relies on the ability of the sampled reference window to capture the usual or expected probability of exposure within individuals. In the context of PASS, case-crossover studies typically are unidirectional, where all person-time is sampled prior to the case-defining outcome. This design is subject to bias from violations of the assumption that exposure probability remains stable over time. Sister methods to assess the presence of and adjust for population-level and prognosis-related trends in exposure have been developed (see methodological considerations in later section) (Suissa, 1995; Wang et al., 2011a,b).

Self-Controlled Risk Interval

The self-controlled risk interval is an exposure-indexed self-controlled design frequently applied in vaccine safety studies (Baker et al., 2015). These typically apply unidirectional self-controlled risk-interval designs, where within-person comparisons are based on person-time after exposure. The observed rate of events during an exposure effect risk window is compared with the expected rate of events within individual where the latter is estimated using person-time after the exposure effect on the outcome of interest is presumed to be over. An effect estimate and confidence intervals can be obtained with matched Mantel—Haenszel, McNemar's estimate, conditional logistic or Poisson regression. The data could be set up as reference windows are not identical, an additional variable capturing the duration of the window is necessary.

When designing self-controlled risk-interval PASS, researchers must consider how to parameterize risk window and reference window. The risk window captures person-time prior during which exposure could potentially have an effect on the outcome. The reference window includes person-time following exposure when exposure is not expected to be able to have an effect on the outcome. It may include person-time between exposure and the start of the window of the hypothesized effect of exposure on the outcome (induction period). Multiple reference windows may be sampled within individual to increase power. Application of this design has also involved use of risk window and reference window of different lengths, with the conditional analysis accounting for the variable person-time contribution. Inclusion of washout periods allows potential carryover effects of exposure to subside in between compared windows.

Because the self-controlled risk-interval approach is exposure-indexed, we align the start of exposure for each patient at time 0 (Fig. 4.2.3B). Given our assumptions about the exposure effect period, we choose to operationalize our within-person comparison as a comparison between an exposure risk window (person-time during which exposure could have an effect on outcome) and a reference window (person-time during which exposure is not expected to be able to have an effect on the outcome). For each case, we define the risk window as the day after exposure and the reference window as 3 days after exposure begins. This allows a washout of 1 day in between the exposure risk window and reference window to allow potential carryover effects of exposure to subside.

Again, because this design uses within-person comparisons, only patients who crossover in exposure and have an outcome within the compared windows contribute to the effect estimate. The observed rate of outcome during the exposure risk window is compared with the expected probability of outcome if there were no effect of exposure on outcome. The expected rate is estimated by the rate of outcome observed in the reference window. A simple way to operationalize the self-controlled risk interval is to use one exposure risk window and a reference window after the hypothesized exposure effect has dissipated, where both windows are of the same length. The OR can be estimated as a ratio of discordant pairs (i.e., ratio of cases with crossover in exposure and outcome during the risk window to cases with crossover in exposure and outcome during the reference window).

Similar to case-crossover design, the self-controlled risk-interval approach can be operationalized with multiple reference windows or windows of different duration and appropriate washout, induction, or exposure effect periods depending on study questions. As described before, the analysis should take into account the matched nature of the data to conduct a within-person comparison. However, this design can be biased if preexposure person-time is used to estimate the expected rate of outcome and the probability of exposure is event-dependent, i.e., occurrence of an outcome influences the individuals future probability of exposure or censors follow-up (Whitaker et al., 2006; Farrington et al., 2009).

Sequence Symmetry Analysis

The sequence symmetry analysis is a simple-to-implement screening method that can be used to examine hypotheses quickly as part of signal detection in pharmacovigilance activities (Petri et al., 1988; Hallas, 1996). This approach identifies all individuals who have both the exposure of interest and the outcome of interest after the start of follow-up. The start of follow-up may be after the start of available data to impose a washout period for identifying incident exposure. The outcome may be another prescription, a diagnosis, or other evidence for a health status change. Only individuals who have both the exposure and the outcome during follow-up contribute to the effect estimate, and only the first occurrence of exposure and outcome is counted. Therefore, all patients have both exposure and outcome, but the observed sequence may be either exposure→outcome or vice versa. The allowable gap between the two items in the sequence may be fixed. In other words, one can choose to specify that the exposure and outcome of interest must occur within 3, 6, or 12 months of each other (Wahab et al., 2013).

In theory, if there is no relationship between the exposure and the outcome, there should be equal number of patients exposed before the outcome as after the outcome. The crude sequence ratio estimate is calculated by dividing the number of patients who have outcome after exposure by the number with outcome before exposure (i.e., ratio of patients with sequence exposure→outcome to patients with sequence outcome→exposure). The degree to which the sequence ratio departs from unity reflects the relative magnitude of the association between exposure and outcome. However, this approach may be biased if the probability of either exposure or outcome changes over time. Confidence intervals may be obtained from the number of sequences and the binomial distribution (Morris and Gardner, 1988; Hallas, 1996).

Fig. 4.2.3C depicts operationalizing sequence symmetry analysis. We choose to require that outcomes must be within 1 day of exposure to count as part of a sequence. Based on this definition, patient 2 and patient 4 are not able to contribute sequences; patient 1 and patient 5 contribute to the numerator; and patient 3 to the denominator. This design can be biased when there are changes in probability of exposure or outcome over time, as these shifts will influence the probability of observing each sequence.

Self-Controlled Case-Series

The self-controlled case-series was first developed for the evaluation of adverse reactions to childhood vaccinations (Farrington et al., 1995). This approach identifies all cases within a study period defined by age and/or calendar time boundaries and classifies the exposure status of all person-time within those boundaries. The observed rate of outcome during exposed time is compared with the expected rate of outcome, as estimated using person-time classified as not exposed within each individual. Thus, this approach typically involves within-person comparisons using person-time both before and after the case-defining event.

In the same manner as the self-controlled risk-interval approach, researchers must consider how to parameterize exposure risk window and reference window. The exposure risk window should encompass all time during which exposure could potentially have an effect on the outcome. In the simplest case, the reference window includes all remaining person-time in the study period not attributed to the exposure risk window. However, more complex categorization of exposure can be helpful to evaluate carryover effects. For example, defining postexposure periods to evaluate the duration of carryover effects. Similar to self-controlled risk-interval approach, which includes person-time after the outcome, this design can be biased when the probability of exposure changes after the outcome. Use of preexposure windows can assist with evaluation and adjustment of bias due to event-dependent exposure.

Operationalizing study windows in self-controlled case-series is depicted in Fig. 4.2.3D. We define the study period using both age and calendar time boundaries. In this example, we choose to define the study period as calendar days 1–20 for patients 12–15 month of age. Based on this definition, patient 1 and patient 4 contribute less than 20 days of person-time because patient 1 ages in and patient 4 ages out within the calendar time boundaries of the study period. All case-defining events occurring during the study period are included, and the person-time within the study period is categorized as either within the exposure effect period or outside of the exposure effect period. Note that although only individuals that have outcomes and crossover in exposure status contribute to the effect estimate; individuals without outcomes may still contribute to estimated age or other effects (Whitaker et al., 2006).

The observed rate of outcome is compared with the within-person expected rate if there were no effect of exposure on outcome. The latter is estimated by the rate of outcome during person-time outside of the exposure effect window. The self-controlled case-series is typically analyzed via conditional Poisson regression with an offset for time. The conditioning is necessary to conduct within-person comparison (Whitaker et al., 2006).

METHODOLOGICAL CONSIDERATIONS

There are many methods developed to assess the presence of and adjust for population-level and prognosis-related trends in exposure and time-varying confounding in self-controlled study designs. The following are few approaches to consider when using self-controlled designs for PASS.

Population Trends in Exposure Over Time

A potential source of bias for designs that use within-person comparisons is the presence of population-level trends in exposure (Suissa, 1995; Hallas, 1996). This source of bias is especially important for PASS, where uptake of newly authorized medicinal products may result in increasing probability of exposure over time before reaching a steady state. In unidirectional case-crossover studies, where referent windows are prior to the hazard window, an increasing probability of exposure over time would result in underestimation of the expected probability of exposure at the time that the outcome occurs. For sequence symmetry analyses, this trend could result in an excess number of patients with the sequence outcome → exposure.

For the case-crossover study, the *case–time–control* design was proposed to adjust for exposure time trend (Suissa, 1995). In this method, exposure time trends are estimated in a matched control population (Fig. 4.2.4). These controls must be matched to cases and calendar time and may be matched on age, sex, or other characteristics. The index window and the reference window for the matched controls are defined by the same calendar time windows as the case to which they are matched. One or more controls may be identified per case. Because there is no possibility of causal effect of exposure on outcome in the controls, the crossover OR among controls estimates the population-level exposure time trend over the same calendar period as the cases. The estimated magnitude of the association between the exposure and the outcome after adjusting for exposure time trends can be obtained by dividing the case-crossover OR by the control-crossover OR. Alternatively, the adjusted estimate can be obtained by fitting a conditional logistic regression model with the window (index vs. reference) as the dependent variable, and exposure plus an exposure by group (case vs. control) interaction termed as the independent variables. In the conditional model, the interaction term

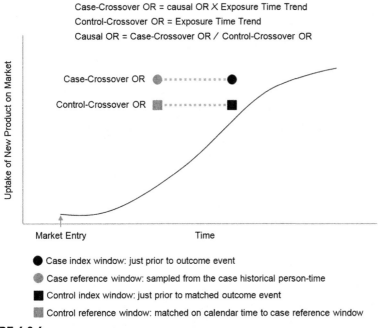

FIGURE 4.2.4
Population-level trends in exposure in case-time-control-crossover designs.

represents the association between exposure and outcome, above and beyond the effect of the exposure time trend.

For the case–time–control design to effectively adjust for population-level time trends, two assumptions must be met (Hernandez-Diaz et al., 2003). First, the time trend for the matched control population must represent the expected time trend for the cases. In other words, similar to a case–control study, the controls sampled to adjust for the exposure time trend should represent the source population for the cases. Second, the observed OR is the product of the causal OR for exposure on outcome and the exposure time trend OR. When either of these assumptions is not met, the case–time–control analysis may be biased either toward or away from the null.

The *case–case–time–control* design is implemented in the same way as the case–control design and is subject to the same assumptions; however, controls are sampled exclusively from "future" cases (Wang et al., 2011a). Because they are at risk for the event during historical person-time, they are eligible to be sampled as controls in the case–time–control design (Fig. 4.2.5). For example, a case on January 1, 2017 could use a future-case, occurring on January 1, 2018 as a matched control. The index window and the reference window for the future-case acting as a control would be matched to the windows defined for the case on January 1, 2017. For rare events, future-cases are unlikely to be sampled to match and act as a control to a case. However, future-cases may better represent crossover odds due to exposure time trends than age- and sex-matched population controls that may differ from cases in ways that are difficult to measure or match on.

The sequence symmetry analysis adjusts for population-level exposure time trends through use of a null-effect sequence ratio (Hallas, 1996). This ratio is estimated by assuming that there is no relationship between the exposure and the outcome. If a patient is exposed on day d, the probability of observing an outcome after day d is the number of outcomes after day d divided by the total number of outcomes in the entire study period. The overall probability of observing outcome after exposure if there were no relationship is calculated as the average across all day d weighted by the number of people exposed on day d. If the probability of observing outcome after exposure under the null is a, then the null sequence ratio is $a/(1 - a)$. Dividing the crude sequence ratio by the estimated null-effect sequence ratio provides an estimate that is adjusted for exposure time trends.

Healthy-User/Sick-Quitter Effects

Changes in prognosis may lead the patient or health-care professional to change treatment. In the context of PASS using large health-care databases, these are called "healthy-user" or "sick-quitter" effects (Glynn et al., 2001;

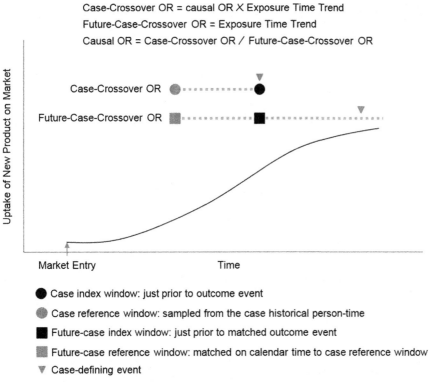

FIGURE 4.2.5
Population-level trends in exposure in case-case-time-control-crossover designs.

Wang et al., 2011a, 2013). For example, patients who know they are dying might discontinue use of lipid-lowering medications, opiates, or other treatments to alleviate symptoms. The changes in patient condition that lead to discontinuing or initiating such treatments are often difficult to capture in health-care databases. When the prognosis or indication for treatment is time-varying over the compared within-person time, this can result in bias in self-controlled analyses. Changes in prognosis are also often correlated with the ability to capture exposure using claims data. Because of lack of data linkage, medication exposure during inpatient or nursing home stays are not available in many US claims data sources. As patients become sicker, they are more likely to be hospitalized and more likely to have immeasurable time (Suissa, 2008).

In addition to mitigating population-level time trends, future-cases could adjust for some of the protopathic bias resulting from changes in treatment due to knowledge of or prodromal signs of an impending outcome (Ali, 2015). However, this adjustment would only occur if the prognosis-related crossover OR in future-cases reflects the expected crossover OR in current cases. When that assumption is not met, it could result in bias in any direction. An alternative way to use cases to estimate prognosis-related time trends would be to identify a negative control reference exposure and use the crossover OR for the negative control exposure to estimate the prognosis-related time trend and adjust the crossover OR for the exposure of interest. A negative control exposure should not have a causal effect on the outcome, be used for a similar type of indication as the exposure of interest (e.g., long-term preventive treatment vs. treatment for a short-term symptomatic condition), and be of the same modality (e.g., daily pill vs. injections). Ideally, the forces that influence the probability of exposure to the negative control over compared within-person time should be as similar as possible to that for the exposure of interest (Wang, 2013).

Event-Dependent Exposures

Self-controlled methods that sample person-time after the outcome have historically been applied to childhood vaccine safety studies, where there are scheduled point exposures for close to the whole population (Andrews et al., 2011; Greene et al., 2012). Timing of exposure to childhood vaccinations may be delayed temporarily, but generally, application of these self-controlled designs will not suffer from the same degree of confounding due to event-dependent prescribing that would be seen with PASS for other medicinal products, where there is often more patient and prescriber discretion in treatment timing and options. Prescribers may change prescribing based on the occurrence of an event. For example, having a bleeding outcome will likely reduce the probability of later exposure to anticoagulant agents, such as warfarin; or in a more extreme setting, death precludes exposure and if unaccounted for, would produce spuriously strong effect sizes.

When occurrence of an outcome temporarily interferes with probability of exposure, the presence and impact of such event-dependent exposure can be evaluated to some extent by including preexposure person-time (Whitaker et al., 2006, 2009). If the incidence rate in preexposure time differs from other unexposed person-time, this suggests that the occurrence of an event changes the probability of exposure. Removal or otherwise accounting for the person-time that does not represent the usual or expected rate of events when unexposed is warranted. In practice, it may be difficult to determine how long occurrence of an outcome influences probability of exposure. If the occurrence of an outcome has a more extreme impact (i.e., permanent contraindication or censors observation), extensions of the self-controlled case-series design have been developed, which involve reducing the studied population to cases who do not have an outcome before exposure, and left-censoring the study window to begin at the time of first exposure (Farrington et al., 2009;

Whitaker et al., 2009). For exposures that occur only once, the true exposure following outcome is known. For exposures that can recur, counterfactual exposure patterns are imputed based on prior exposure.

References

Ali, A.K., 2015. Biases related to prescribing decisions in retrospective database research in diabetes. Value Outcomes Spotlight 1 (4), 13−15.

Andrews, N., Stowe, J., Al-Shahi Salman, R., Miller, E., 2011. Guillain-Barre syndrome and H1N1 (2009) pandemic influenza vaccination using an AS03 adjuvanted vaccine in the United Kingdom: self-controlled case series. Vaccine 29 (45), 7878−7882.

Baker, M.A., Lieu, T.A., Li, L., et al., 2015. A vaccine study design selection framework for the post-licensure rapid immunization safety monitoring program. Am. J. Epidemiol. 181 (8), 608−618.

Consiglio, G.P., Burden, A.M., Maclure, M., McCarthy, L., Cadarette, S.M., 2013. Case-crossover study design in pharmacoepidemiology: systematic review and recommendations. Pharmacoepidemiol. Drug Saf. 22 (11), 1146−1153.

Farrington, C.P., 1995. Relative incidence estimation from case series for vaccine safety evaluation. Biometrics 51 (1), 228−235.

Farrington, P., Pugh, S., Colville, A., et al., 1995. A new method for active surveillance of adverse events from diphtheria/tetanus/pertussis and measles/mumps/rubella vaccines. Lancet 345 (8949), 567−569.

Farrington, C.P., Whitaker, H.J., Hocine, M.N., 2009. Case series analysis for censored, perturbed, or curtailed post-event exposures. Biostatistics 10 (1), 3−16.

Fireman, B., Lee, J., Lewis, N., Bembom, O., van der Laan, M., Baxter, R., 2009. Influenza vaccination and mortality: differentiating vaccine effects from bias. Am. J. Epidemiol. 170 (5), 650−656.

Gagne, J.J., Nelson, J.C., Fireman, B., Seeger, J.D., Toh, D., Gerhard, T., Rassen, J.A., Shoabi, A., Reichman, M., Schneeweiss, S., January 31, 2012. Taxonomy for Monitoring Methods within a Medical Product Safety Surveillance System: Year Two Report of the Mini-Sentinel Taxonomy Workgroup.

Glynn, R.J., Knight, E.L., Levin, R., Avorn, J., 2001. Paradoxical relations of drug treatment with mortality in older persons. Epidemiology 12 (6), 682−689.

Greene, S.K., Rett, M., Weintraub, E.S., et al., 2012. Risk of confirmed Guillain-Barre syndrome following receipt of monovalent inactivated influenza A (H1N1) and seasonal influenza vaccines in the Vaccine Safety Datalink Project, 2009−2010. Am. J. Epidemiol. 175 (11), 1100−1109.

Greenland, S., 1996. Confounding and exposure trends in case-crossover and case-time-control designs. Epidemiology 7 (3), 231−239.

Hallas, J., 1996. Evidence of depression provoked by cardiovascular medication: a prescription sequence symmetry analysis. Epidemiology 7 (5), 478−484.

Hallas, J., Pottegard, A., Wang, S., Schneeweiss, S., Gagne, J.J., 2016. Persistent user bias in case-crossover studies in pharmacoepidemiology. Am. J. Epidemiol. 184 (10), 761−769.

Hernandez-Diaz, S., Hernan, M.A., Meyer, K., Werler, M.M., Mitchell, A.A., 2003. Case-crossover and case-time-control designs in birth defects epidemiology. Am. J. Epidemiol. 158 (4), 385−391.

Horwitz, R.I., Feinstein, A.R., 1980. The problem of "protopathic bias" in case-control studies. Am. J. Med. 68 (2), 255−258.

Maclure, M., 1991. The case-crossover design: a method for studying transient effects on the risk of acute events. Am. J. Epidemiol. 133 (2), 144–153.

Maclure, M., 2007. 'Why me?' versus 'why now?'–differences between operational hypotheses in case-control versus case-crossover studies. Pharmacoepidemiol. Drug Saf. 16 (8), 850–853.

Maclure, M., Fireman, B., Nelson, J.C., et al., 2012. When should case-only designs be used for safety monitoring of medical products? Pharmacoepidemiol. Drug Saf. 21 (Suppl. 1), 50–61.

Madigan, D., Fireman, B., Maclure, M., October 4, 2011. Case-based Methods Workgroup Report. Mini Sentinel Methods Development. Available from: https://www.sentinelinitiative.org/sites/default/files/Methods/Mini-Sentinel_Methods_Case-Based-Report_0.pdf.

Morris, J.A., Gardner, M.J., May 7, 1988. Calculating confidence intervals for relative risks (odds ratios) and standardised ratios and rates. Br. Med. J. 296 (6632), 1313–1316.

Petri, H., De Vet, H.C.W., Naus, J., Urquhart, J., 1988. Prescription sequence analysis: a new and fast method for assessing certain adverse reactions of prescription drugs in large populations. Stat. Med. 7 (11), 1171–1175.

Suissa, S., 1995. The case-time-control design. Epidemiology 6 (3), 248–253.

Suissa, S., 2008. Immeasurable time bias in observational studies of drug effects on mortality. Am. J. Epidemiol. 168 (3), 329–335.

Taxonomy Project Workgroup (TPW), 2010. Taxonomy for Monitoring Methods within a Medical Product Safety Surveillance System: Report of the Mini-Sentinel Taxonomy Project Work Group.

Wahab, I.A., Pratt, N.L., Wiese, M.D., Kalisch, L.M., Roughead, E.E., 2013. The validity of sequence symmetry analysis (SSA) for adverse drug reaction signal detection. Pharmacoepidemiol. Drug Saf. 22 (5), 496–502.

Wang, S., Linkletter, C., Maclure, M., et al., 2011a. Future cases as present controls to adjust for exposure trend bias in case-only studies. Epidemiology 22 (4), 568–574.

Wang, S.V., Coull, B.A., Schwartz, J., Mittleman, M.A., Wellenius, G.A., 2011b. Potential for bias in case-crossover studies with shared exposures analyzed using SAS. Am. J. Epidemiol. 174 (1), 118–124.

Wang, S.V., Gagne, J.J., Glynn, R.J., Schneeweiss, S., 2013. Case-crossover studies of therapeutics: design approaches to addressing time-varying prognosis in elderly populations. Epidemiology 24 (3), 375–378.

Wang, S.V., Schneeweiss, S., Maclure, M., Gagne, J.J., 2014. "First-wave" bias when conducting active safety monitoring of newly marketed medications with outcome-indexed self-controlled designs. Am. J. Epidemiol. 180 (6), 636–644.

Whitaker, H.J., Farrington, C.P., Spiessens, B., Musonda, P., 2006. Tutorial in biostatistics: the self-controlled case series method. Stat. Med. 25 (10), 1768–1797.

Whitaker, H.J., Hocine, M.N., Farrington, C.P., 2009. The methodology of self-controlled case series studies. Stat. Meth. Med. Res. 18 (1), 7–26.

Yih, W.K., Kulldorff, M., Fireman, B.H., et al., 2011. Active surveillance for adverse events: the experience of the vaccine safety Datalink project. Pediatrics 127 (Suppl. 1), S54–S64.

Cohort and Nested Case—Control Studies

Beth L. Nordstrom

Evidera, Bethesda, MD, United States

INTRODUCTION

Many post-authorization safety studies (PASS) can be conducted with noninterventional, retrospective designs, using data that have already been collected in usual medical practice. These studies can offer savings in cost and timelines compared to prospective designs with primary data collection, although when essential measures are not typically taken in usual clinical practice, a prospective study is likely to be needed (Chapter 4.5 offers an introduction to common prospective designs used in drug safety research). The most common retrospective design is the cohort study, in which patients are followed through retrospective data from the start of an exposure period to search for the outcome of interest. As appropriate to the research questions and methods, additional analysis types may be performed within the context of a cohort study. One such analysis type is the nested case—control study, where cases and controls are selected from a predefined cohort.

Typically, PASS are initiated shortly after launch of a newly authorized medicinal product, when relatively few users of the product are available in the study data sources. These early analyses permit a timely view of safety signals but suffer from lack of statistical power. To overcome this limitation, PASS are often conducted using a rolling retrospective design, where sequential retrospective analyses are performed. Periodically, such as once or twice per year, an updated extract from the study data source is obtained. New patients and additional follow-up time on patients identified in prior extracts are added to the analysis in each round. Cohort and nested case—control studies can both be conducted in this manner.

COHORT STUDIES

For PASS, it is usually essential to define an inception cohort composed of new users of one or more medicinal products of interest (Ray, 2003). Because the risk of many adverse events varies with continued exposure to a product,

CONTENTS

Introduction 139

Cohort Studies .. 139
*Methodological
Considerations* 142

Nested
Case—Control
Studies 144
*Selection of Cases
and Controls* 144
*Methodological
Considerations* 146

References 148

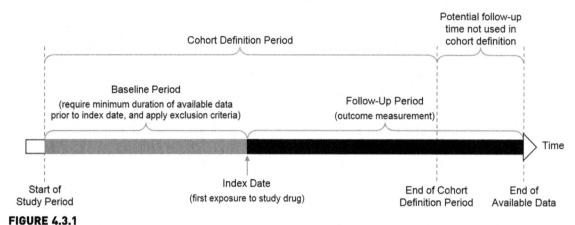

FIGURE 4.3.1

Cohort selection and time periods used in cohort studies.

beginning follow-up at the same point in exposure (i.e., the start) avoids bias that may arise if follow-up begins after some variable duration of exposure (Ali, 2013a). An index date is defined for each patient as the start date of the new medicinal product. Clinical events and treatment occurring before the index date are considered baseline information, which are used for describing and classifying patients risk status at the start of exposure.

Fig. 4.3.1 illustrates the key periods in a cohort study. Patients are selected based on first use of a study drug during a cohort definition period. This period will typically end sometime before the end of available data, to allow for some minimum duration of potential follow-up for patients. Note that no minimum is set for actual follow-up duration of each patient, which would bias the patient population by removing patients with fatal outcomes during the minimum follow-up period, and immortal time bias would arise (Ali, 2013a). For safety events that are expected to arise shortly after starting treatment, the cohort definition period can last until close to the end of available data (e.g., 30 days prior), but for longer-term outcomes, it may be important to cut off cohort entry at 6 months or even a year prior to the end of available data. See Fig. 3.1.2 for more information on cohort selection using large databases such as administrative claims, especially the application of enrollment requirement for cohort definition periods. Most PASS involve a comparison of safety outcomes between a newly authorized medicinal product and other treatments for the same condition. These comparisons provide context for the event rates observed in the newly authorized product: whether the rates are similar to those with previously authorized treatments or they are sufficiently elevated to suggest the new product may be unacceptably risky. Depending on the number of other treatments available for the same indication, the comparator group may comprise users of a single treatment or of any of a selection of treatments, e.g., pharmacologic or therapeutic class.

One notable issue with the study of safety in newly authorized products is that often patients with most severe disease, refractory to other treatments, are the first to be prescribed the new medicinal product (Schneeweiss et al., 2011). In addition, products that are believed to have a better risk profile with respect to some adverse events (e.g., cardiac events) may be preferentially prescribed to patients at higher risk of those events. A simple comparison of the event between patients prescribed the different products can then indicate an increase in risk of the event, but where that risk is driven by the very different underlying risks in the populations being prescribed each drug. These problems, often referred to as confounding by indication, are essential to address in the study design (Joffe, 2000; McMahon, 2003; Sjoding et al., 2015). Approaches to reduce confounding by indication include use of exposure propensity scores for matching, weighting, or stratifying analyses; traditional matching on individual variables rather than propensity scores and statistical adjustment via multivariable outcome modeling. Chapter 5.1 discusses exposure propensity scores, and Chapter 5.2 provides an overview of disease risk scores as approaches to prevent and mitigate biases in PASS.

As mentioned in Chapters 3.1 and 3.2, the retrospective study design limits the outcomes that can be examined to those that are routinely identified in usual medical settings. For example, results of a laboratory test that is not typically used in clinical practice would not be a valid outcome in a retrospective PASS. If a database containing diagnostic and procedure codes is used to define outcomes, the outcome should either have a well-validated definition using the same coding system or should be validated through a chart review or other form of confirmatory data. In health-care databases, multiple occurrences of an acute outcome in the same patient may be difficult to distinguish from ongoing care for an earlier occurrence of the outcome. For example, patients treated for venous thromboembolism may have repeat visits containing the thromboembolism diagnosis for months following the event. It is often unclear whether the later records represent the patient having received medical attention for the earlier event or the patient having experienced a new thromboembolic event. Careful examination of patient's medical chart may allow clear differentiation between these two possibilities, but diagnoses in databases are unlikely to contain clear indicators for new versus old events. In PASS, this can be especially troublesome if an outcome occurs both before and after the start of a study drug. For many studies, it is safest to exclude patients from the analysis if they have a recent history of the outcome. At a minimum, if such patients have to be included in the analyses, a stratified analysis should be considered to examine the association between the study drug and the outcome of interest separately in patients with completely new events versus those with a history of the event.

Covariates suffer from similar limitations to outcomes in retrospective database research, in that not all variables one might hope to examine will be visible in the data. Common concerns such as lifestyle factors (e.g., diet and exercise) are poorly represented in most data sources, even with access to full medical charts. Such information may be collected through patient surveys or other primary data collection tools, but this presents a large and at times, insurmountable hurdle for retrospective studies; for example, deceased patients cannot be included and would present a highly biased exclusion from a patient survey. Most PASS use as covariates, the information that can reasonably be gleaned from the chosen data source, with the hope that the available data—taken together—will serve as an adequate proxy for unmeasured confounders. Of course, all secondary use of data carry the standard caveat that residual confounding of the drug-outcome association may be present even in the adjusted results (Ali, 2013a).

Methodological Considerations

Two primary analytic approaches are used in cohort PASS: intention-to-treat (ITT) and time-on-treatment (TOT) analyses. Each of these approaches is illustrated in Fig. 4.3.2. ITT analyses follow patients from the start of a study drug through some follow-up duration, without regard to whether the patient

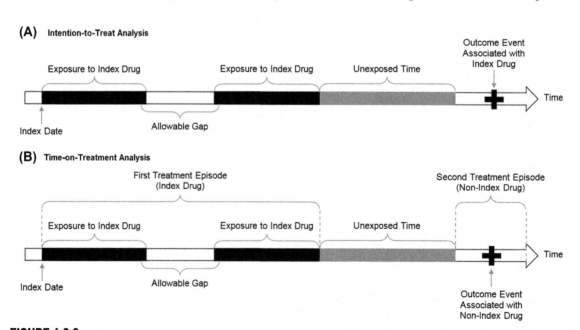

FIGURE 4.3.2

Illustration of intention-to-treat and time-on-treatment analyses in cohort studies.

remains on the index treatment (Hollis and Campbell, 1999; Hernan and Hernandez-Diaz, 2012). Discontinuation, switching, or adding another medicinal product may occur during the time included in the follow-up window. This design permits answers to research questions such as: what is the relative risk (RR) of outcome X in patients initiating product A versus product B? In ITT analysis, all follow-up time after the index date is used for outcome measurement.

For PASS with outcomes that should only occur during or very shortly after exposure to the product, the most common analysis is the TOT (also known as-treated or on-treatment analysis), looking at the first continuous episode of product use (Hernan and Hernandez-Diaz, 2012). To start, drug exposure is coded into episodes, typically allowing some maximum duration of gap time in exposure (e.g., when the patient's supply of medication has been exhausted, a refill is not obtained until some relatively short time afterward). This type of analysis can answer research questions aimed at identifying the RR of an outcome during exposure to one of the study drugs. Discontinuing, switching, or augmenting with another product for the same indication triggers the end of patient's follow-up in the analysis. TOT analyses can also be conducted with variable exposure during the follow-up period. These analyses map patient's exposure to each of the study drugs over time, assigning blocks of follow-up time to each product or combination of products. Compared to analyses that end follow-up at the end of the first continuous drug episode, they provide not only greater ability to examine all outcomes for patients but also can result in findings that are less clear in interpretation. If an outcome occurs 3 days after a patient switches from a long course of product A to product B, is the outcome associated with the recently and longer-used product A or the newly started product B? Both the current and recent uses of study drugs are generally mapped but teasing apart the relative contributions of each study drug to the risk of the outcome can be difficult. In TOT analysis, outcomes are examined within periods of exposure to each study drug an unexposed time.

Regardless of whether an ITT or TOT analysis is used, the statistical analyses generally need to allow for censoring. Kaplan—Meier plots of the outcome and corresponding Cox regression models are the most common analytic methods with tables report incidence rates and showing the proportion of patients who experienced the outcome. Comparative analyses should consider any special selection criteria such as matching, to ensure that the analyses are correctly specified for the selection methods and for the form of the data. Adjusted survival analysis models may use baseline characteristics alone, but in PASS with long-term follow-up, important covariates can change during follow-up period. Therefore, for some TOT analyses, the person-time of follow-up is coded into blocks of time with certain characteristics. The patient may change age, comorbidities, and exposure to treatments other than study drugs. Because it is complex and time-consuming to map out many changing variables over the follow-up period, these analyses generally include time-varying components for only a limited number of key confounders (Ali, 2013b).

NESTED CASE—CONTROL STUDIES

Nested case—control studies provide a more efficient data collection and analytic approach for some PASS (Essebag et al., 2005; Langholz and Richardson, 2009; Vandenbroucke and Pearce, 2012). Within a cohort of patients exposed to a study drug of interest (or depending on study design, one group may be untreated), all patients in the cohort experiencing the outcome are selected as cases. Controls are selected from among cohort members who have not had the outcome. The total number of patients in the analysis is thus substantially smaller than the full cohort size.

The most common situation where nested case—control analyses are used is when attempting to examine a large number of risk factors that change over time or factors that require additional data collection to obtain (Ernster, 1994; Essebag et al., 2003). The complexity and/or cost of conducting the analysis using a cohort study design may be prohibitive; the case—control approach allows for considerable streamlining of both timelines and cost. For example, a database analysis may include a large cohort of patients with certain key risk factors missing in the data. Information on the missing risk factors is sought through data collection (via chart review, survey, or other means) for only the subset of patients included in the nested case—control analysis. This allows evaluation of confounding by those key factors in the case—control analysis and estimation of the impact of residual confounding by the same factors in the larger cohort study.

Another common driver of selection of the nested case—control design is when an outcome has a long latency period, such as development of cancer (Chen et al., 2003; Wang et al., 2013; Boursi et al., 2015). A malignancy can be caused by a medicinal product with no sign of the event appearing for months or years after exposure to the product ends. The typical TOT analysis used with cohort studies would have to model a multitude of time-varying characteristics when the outcome event is a new diagnosis of cancer. The nested case—control design allows for lengthy look-back periods and complex exposure histories to be assessed more efficiently. Measures such as cumulative exposure to a product—which can be important predictors for development of cancer—are easily incorporated.

Selection of Cases and Controls

The cases in a nested case—control analysis are all individuals who experienced the event of interest during follow-up in the cohort study. Unlike in the cohort study design, the index date is not based on drug exposure. Instead, an index date is defined for each case as the date of the outcome event. Controls are selected from among the individuals in the cohort who have not experienced the outcome event and are considered to be still at risk of having the event. Depending on the number of available cases and the difficulty in obtaining the data needed for the case—control analysis, controls may be selected for cases at a 1:1 ratio or higher.

Most PASS allow patients to enter the study cohort throughout a relatively wide cohort selection period. In general, the most important aspect of timing of the outcome event is not calendar time, rather the time since the patient started the study drug. Therefore, controls are selected from among patients who are still under follow-up in the data and who have not had the outcome event as of the same time relative to drug start as a corresponding case event date. This criterion is illustrated in Fig. 4.3.3. If patient 1 has an outcome event at 10 days after initiating a study drug, then a control will be selected from among patients who are still under follow-up without having had the event, as of 10 days after they started a study drug. Patient 2 meets this criterion and so would be eligible to be selected as a control, but patient 3 ended follow-up on day 6 and so would be ineligible. However, patient 3 would be eligible as a control for cases occurring less than 6 days after drug start.

In addition to matching controls to cases on the basis of being at risk of the outcome on the case date, there may be additional matching criterion

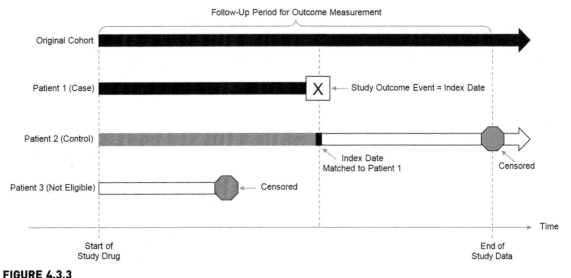

FIGURE 4.3.3
Selection of cases and controls for nested case-control studies.

that is desirable. Matching on calendar time may be appropriate for studies that span long periods. During the several years duration of typical PASS, the available treatments and patterns of care may change considerably, and those changes may lead to changes in overall risk of the outcome of interest. Thus, it may be prudent to match on calendar year to ensure that the control(s) for each case are selected from among patients who were at risk of the outcome during the same year. Matching on other potential confounders, such as age and sex, can provide a simple means of removing confounding by those factors, although it is important to match only on true confounders of the drug-event association to avoid overmatching, which can lead to biased results (Bloom et al., 2007). In addition, any variable that is used for matching cannot be examined in the analyses.

Methodological Considerations

Whereas in a cohort study most predictor variables are derived from a period prior to drug exposure (baseline period), the predictors in a nested case−control study focus on one or more periods preceding the case date. One of the advantages of the case−control design is that risk factors that arise during the follow-up period can easily be included in the analysis as simply yes/no flags, without having to code a large number of time-varying characteristics. Similarly, treatments received prior to the case date can be coded as binary variable, and if relevant, cumulative dose and duration of each treatment can be included as predictors. For the most part, there is no need to create time-varying covariates at all, although in some situations it may be desirable to have separate flags for treatment exposure during particular time windows, e.g., during the last month prior to the case date versus the 6 months prior to that.

Incidence rates of the safety outcome in PASS are derived from the cohort study, not directly from the nested case−control analysis. The primary analysis from the nested case−control design looks for predictors of the outcome (i.e., case vs. control status), with exposure to one of the study drugs of interest serving as the primary predictor. Therefore, exposure group is forced into the model, with confounders sought from among the other variables measured. For a matched case−control study, the most frequently used analytic approach is the conditional logistic regression. This method takes into account the matched nature of the data and produces odds ratios (ORs) for the drug-event association. If the outcome is rare, the OR is a good estimate of the RR. Alternatively, a Cox proportional hazards model can be constructed, with stratification by the matched case−control sets (Essebag et al., 2005).

Nested case−control analyses most often examine a single safety endpoint (Boxall et al., 2016; Muanda et al., 2017; Trifiro et al., 2017), although some consider a combination endpoint (Nowak et al., 2015) or conduct more than one nested case—control analysis to look at multiple endpoints (de Jong et al., 2017; Morales et al., 2017). This design is often used to study associations between exposures to medicinal products and subsequent development of cancer. For example, in a cohort of men diagnosed with diabetes in the United Kingdom CPRD database, a new diagnosis of prostate cancer was the outcome with pioglitazone antidiabetes medication as the primary exposure of interest (Boxall et al., 2016). Treatment-related variables in the logistic regression model included not only an indicator for ever having received pioglitazone but also for cumulative duration, cumulative dose, and time since initiation of pioglitazone. The findings for all of the treatment-related variables suggested no association between pioglitazone use and risk of developing prostate cancer. Similar approaches to drug exposure coding have been used in other studies (Morales et al., 2017; Trifiro et al., 2017), although for some exposures such as antibiotic use during pregnancy, a simple flag for ever versus never exposed may be sufficient (Muanda et al., 2017).

In contrast to the classic example of a single outcome of cancer, an entire series of nested case—control analyses were conducted, investigating many different outcomes among patients with relapsing-remitting multiple sclerosis treated with interferon-beta immunomodulator therapy (de Jong et al., 2017). The study used clinical and administrative health data from British Columbia. The outcomes examined ranged from various infections to depression and stroke. Interferon-beta exposure was coded as ever exposed, cumulative duration of use, and recentness of use. The findings revealed an increased risk of several outcomes with interferon-beta use, including stroke, migraine, depression, and hematologic abnormalities. When examining such a wide variety of endpoints, the selection of covariates for the models has to proceed with care. The inclusion of covariates that are not in fact confounders for the specific outcome analyzed can bias the results, at least in some instances (Li et al., 2016).

Combination treatments can be particularly tricky to study, as patients may receive dual-drug combinations immediately on initiation of treatment or may switch from a single drug to a combination and back again, perhaps repeatedly. The nested case—control design can help simplify the analysis of PASS for combination treatments. One such study investigated serious adverse events associated with fixed-dose combination antihypertensive products compared with single-pill free combinations (Nowak et al., 2015). The endpoint was hospitalization for any of several serious adverse events. This study was unusual for case—control analyses, in that all patients were treated with the same medicinal products; it was only the format of the combinations (fixed vs. free) that differed. Results showed that the fixed-dose combination carried a higher risk of serious adverse events than the free combinations.

References

Ali, A.K., 2013a. Methodological challenges in observational research: a pharmacoepidemiological perspective. Br. J. Pharmaceut. Res. 3 (2), 161—175.

Ali, A.K., 2013b. Causal inference from observational data with time-dependent confounding: application of marginal structural models for multi-category exposures. ISPOR Connections 19 (2), 11—13.

Bloom, M.S., Schisterman, E.F., Hediger, M.L., 2007. The use and misuse of matching in case-control studies: the example of polycystic ovary syndrome. Fertil. Steril. 88 (3), 707—710.

Boursi, B., Lurie, I., Mamtani, R., Haynes, K., Yang, Y.X., 2015. Anti-depressant therapy and cancer risk: a nested case-control study. Eur. Neuropsychopharmacol. 25 (8), 1147—1157.

Boxall, N., Bennett, D., Hunger, M., Dolin, P., Thompson, P.L., 2016. Evaluation of exposure to pio-glitazone and risk of prostate cancer: a nested case-control study. BMJ Open Diabetes Res. Care 4 (1) e000303.

Chen, K., Cai, J., Liu, X.Y., Ma, X.Y., Yao, K.Y., Zheng, S., 2003. Nested case-control study on the risk factors of colorectal cancer. World J. Gastroenterol. 9 (1), 99—103.

de Jong, H.J.I., Kingwell, E., Shirani, A., et al., 2017. Evaluating the safety of beta-interferons in MS: a series of nested case-control studies. Neurology 88 (24), 2310—2320.

Ernster, V.L., 1994. Nested case-control studies. Prev. Med. 23 (5), 587—590.

Essebag, V., Genest Jr., J., Suissa, S., Pilote, L., 2003. The nested case-control study in cardiology. Am. Heart J. 146 (4), 581—590.

Essebag, V., Platt, R.W., Abrahamowicz, M., Pilote, L., 2005. Comparison of nested case-control and survival analysis methodologies for analysis of time-dependent exposure. BMC Med. Res. Methodol. 5 (1), 5.

Hernan, M.A., Hernandez-Diaz, S., 2012. Beyond the intention-to-treat in comparative effectiveness research. Clin. Trials 9 (1), 48—55.

Hollis, S., Campbell, F., 1999. What is meant by intention to treat analysis? Survey of published randomised controlled trials. BMJ 319 (7211), 670—674.

Joffe, M.M., 2000. Confounding by indication: the case of calcium channel blockers. Pharmacoepidemiol. Drug Saf. 9 (1), 37—41.

Langholz, B., Richardson, D., 2009. Are nested case-control studies biased? Epidemiology 20 (3), 321—329.

Li, H., Yuan, Z., Su, P., et al., 2016. A simulation study on matched case-control designs in the perspective of causal diagrams. BMC Med. Res. Methodol. 16 (1), 102.

McMahon, A.D., 2003. Approaches to combat with confounding by indication in observational studies of intended drug effects. Pharmacoepidemiol. Drug Saf. 12 (7), 551—558.

Morales, D.R., Lipworth, B.J., Donnan, P.T., Jackson, C., Guthrie, B., 2017. Respiratory effect of beta-blockers in people with asthma and cardiovascular disease: population-based nested case control study. BMC Med. 15 (1), 18.

Muanda, F.T., Sheehy, O., Berard, A., 2017. Use of antibiotics during pregnancy and risk of spontaneous abortion. CMAJ (Can. Med. Assoc. J.) 189 (17), E625—E633.

Nowak, E., Happe, A., Bouget, J., et al., 2015. Safety of fixed dose of antihypertensive drug combinations compared to (single pill) free-combinations: a nested matched case-control analysis. Medicine 94 (49), e2229.

Ray, W.A., 2003. Evaluating medication effects outside of clinical trials: new-user designs. Am. J. Epidemiol. 158 (9), 915—920.

Schneeweiss, S., Gagne, J.J., Glynn, R.J., Ruhl, M., Rassen, J.A., 2011. Assessing the comparative effectiveness of newly marketed medications: methodological challenges and implications for drug development. Clin. Pharmacol. Ther. 90 (6), 777–790.

Sjoding, M.W., Luo, K., Miller, M.A., Iwashyna, T.J., 2015. When do confounding by indication and inadequate risk adjustment bias critical care studies? A simulation study. Crit. Care 19, 195.

Trifiro, G., de Ridder, M., Sultana, J., et al., 2017. Use of azithromycin and risk of ventricular arrhythmia. CMAJ (Can. Med. Assoc. J.) 189 (15), E560–E568.

Vandenbroucke, J.P., Pearce, N., 2012. Case-control studies: basic concepts. Int. J. Epidemiol. 41 (5), 1480–1489.

Wang, S.Y., Chuang, C.S., Muo, C.H., et al., 2013. Metformin and the incidence of cancer in patients with diabetes: a nested case-control study. Diabetes Care 36 (9), e155–156.

Enriched Studies

Jennifer B. Christian, Nancy A. Dreyer

IQVIA, Durham, NC, United States

CONTENTS

Introduction 150

Strengths and
Limitations of
Enriched
Studies 152

Evaluation of
Secondary Data
Sources for
Enriched
Studies 153

Operationalizing
Enriched
Studies 154

Methodological
Considerations .. 154

References 156

INTRODUCTION

Over the past 3 decades, there has been an explosion of new methods for designs and analyses that have strengthened the field of pharmacoepidemiology. These advances have led to the widespread use of safety surveillance programs leveraging existing data sources, such as the FDA Sentinel Program and the creation and implementation of high quality product and disease registries that are often recorded in the Registry of Patient Registries (Gliklich et al., 2014; FDA, 2016). There has also been a major increase over the past 15 years in the use of EMR in an effort to reduce medical errors and cost, consolidate health records, and increase the coordination and quality of medical care (Soper, 2002, Wang et al., 2003; Hillestad et al., 2005; Shekelle et al., 2006). Although there is no federal mandate that requires the use of EMR in the delivery of care, there are incentives for adopting "meaningful use" of certified EMR in clinical practice in the United States. To receive these monetary incentives, the use of EMR should result in health care that emphasizes prevention, efficiency, evidence-based medicine, and is patient-centered (HHS, 2010). The use of EMR in practice has significantly increased from 16% in 2003% to 52% in 2010, although the use of EMR varied by type of practice and clinician (Kokkonen et al., 2013). There are similar increases in the use of EMR in many parts of the world fueled by the growing use of clinical and nonclinical information systems, including patient administration, scheduling, and billing systems.

With the growing adoption of EMR in clinical practice, new opportunities have emerged for how existing data can be used for safety evaluations, spurring development of novel approaches to post-authorization safety studies (PASS) design, conduct, and evaluation. The term enriched studies is used to describe studies that combine existing (secondary) data such as EMR, claims, or established registries, with primary data collected directly from health-care providers and/or patients for study purposes (Mack et al., 2015). Enriched studies integrate and use elements of both existing health-related data and primary collection of data to optimize, guide, and enhance safety and effectiveness evaluations. Secondary data sources can be used to optimize the protocol, inform selection of investigative sites and patient recruitment strategies, and minimize the burden of primary data collection on patients and clinicians by using routinely collected clinical information from secondary sources. More detail on claims and EMR data sources is presented in Chapters 3.1 and 3.2, respectively.

The electronic data capture system is generally used as the backbone for important elements that are not reliably collected in existing data source, such as patient-reported outcomes and measurements that may not be routinely conducted, not reported in enough consistent detail to be useful, or recorded but not readily accessible. The benefits of this enriched approach are the efficiencies in identifying and recruiting patients, minimizing the burden of primary data collection by extracting baseline information from existing data sources and assembling valuable data from other data sources, such as wearables or biobanks, which can be used for better understanding clinical phenotypes and balancing important differences in populations across cohorts through statistical adjustments. Once these rich data are assembled and appropriately linked, there are numerous study designs and analytic methods that can be implemented, including nested case–control designs, prospective cohorts, and pragmatic trials.

Two notable examples of pragmatic trials that used an enriched approach include the Diuretic Comparison Project and ADAPTABLE (Aspirin Dosing: A Patient-centric Trial Assessing Benefits and Long-Term Effectiveness) study (Hernandez et al., 2015; Lederle et al., 2016). The former study was developed to optimize the use of EMR in the Veterans Affairs (VA) health system to perform large, inexpensive clinical trials that are integrated at the point of care. The primary clinical question being addressed is whether chlorthalidone reduces major adverse cardiovascular outcomes compared with hydrochlorothiazide in older veterans with hypertension. This trial involves finding eligible patients using the VA EMR system, with centralized recruitment, enrollment, and placement of notes and orders in the EMR. Collection of the outcomes is also centralized, and no local personnel are needed. The ADAPTABLE study is another example of a clinical trial that is designed to support real-world clinical decision-making. This 3-year clinical trial is intended to compare the effectiveness of two different daily doses of aspirin widely used in practice to prevent heart attacks and strokes in patients living with heart disease. Broad populations of patients are recruited, and the trial is conducted leveraging data from health systems to produce results that can be readily used to improve patient care.

PASS can be expensive, averaging more than $1.5–5.2 million USD per study (Rawlins, 2008). Therefore, the first question to consider when selecting an approach and allocating resources is to determine whether or not an existing database could be used to evaluate the safety question, without the need for primary data collection. Of the 189 PASS protocols that were submitted to the EMA's Pharmacovigilance Risk Assessment Committee between July 2012 and July 2015, ~42% were conducted using existing data, although the majority of these studies were to assess drug utilization rather than safety assessments (Engel et al., 2017).

Many studies, however, cannot fully evaluate the post-authorization use and safety of medicinal products from databases alone. Although some studies may indicate whether there is a potential safety signal, most often, further evaluation is needed to assess the severity of the event, how bothersome the safety event to the patient, the perceived benefits of the medicines relative to the safety event, validating and characterizing the safety event further with additional diagnostic measures not routinely or systematically recorded within databases. In addition, information is often missing on important confounders, especially those that characterize patient behaviors and beliefs that may influence the risk of having the specific safety event. Another important reason is to characterize the clinical phenotypes of individuals experiencing the safety events and to inform the clinical community as to the best candidates to receive the medicinal product.

STRENGTHS AND LIMITATIONS OF ENRICHED STUDIES

There are numerous advantages to using an enriched study design. The use of existing data reduces the burden of data collection on patients and clinicians, potentially increasing patient retention and simplifying, and possibly strengthening long-term follow-up of patients by minimizing the loss to follow-up that might be experienced simply through prospective data collection, also, enriched studies provide an opportunity to incorporate new assessments not otherwise feasible for observational studies based exclusively on existing data, such as daily diaries, activity trackers, wearable sensors, adherence monitors, and generic information. By using existing data for recruitment, the representativeness of the patient population can be demonstrated and further, it may increase the success of identifying and following the types of patients that may otherwise be to follow using existing data.

However, there are challenges to consider as well. Similar to other PASS, analytical plans that address missing data, confounding, and a careful review of the quality of data are needed. In addition, integration plans are needed that define a common data model to use in the study, and a prioritization of which data to use from which source of information prior to the study commencing. Institutional review boards and ethics committees may have additional concerns given the potential risk of personally identifiable information being obtained through linking numerous sources of data. Clearly written informed consent documents and standard operating procedures or work practices for ensuring the appropriateness of data handling are required. Moreover, careful processes for matching patients to other sources of information are used to reduce the likelihood of errors in linking data to the wrong patient(s). See Chapter 3.4 for more discussion on data pooling and linkage, and Chapter 5.4 for an introduction of data standardization and the application of common data models in analytic platforms.

EVALUATION OF SECONDARY DATA SOURCES FOR ENRICHED STUDIES

The concept of finding and accessing data may seem simple yet the execution can be quite challenging. First, finding appropriate data for the study can be difficult, and then securing appropriate access, even after ethical/institutional review, can add additional complexities. There are many constraints to data access that need to be evaluated, including whether applicants must be resident in the country, associated with academic institutions, the intended use of the data, whether the data partner will allow reidentification of health-care providers and/or patients, if they have a process for doing so, and whether the data will be transported for use outside of the country in which it was collected (largely an issue restricted to the European Union due to current privacy laws regarding cross-border transfer of data).

Assuming those hurdles can be overcome, the next set of questions that should be addressed concern whether patients in a particular health system have the exposure of interest, how frequently and up to date the information can be accessed and whether it is recorded routinely in the data source. For example, many EMR systems are used for ambulatory care. Detailed information about treatments received in hospitals or in outpatient infusion centers, for example, is not often also captured in an ambulatory care record keeping system, which make the process of study subject identification and full data acquisition much more laborious.

Similarly, some information about care performed in an ambulatory care system may not routinely be recorded in an EMR system. For example, consider testing for blood glucose levels in diabetes. Although appropriate care for patients with diabetes requires periodic testing of blood glucose levels through blood tests performed in an external laboratory, the test results may be made available to the health-care provider through a separate feed of laboratory data—one that is easily accessible to the physician during the patient encounter, but which may not be actually stored in the EMR.

OPERATIONALIZING ENRICHED STUDIES

Once it has been determined that the records under consideration are likely to include patients with the exposures and/or outcomes of interest, and that such patients and their health-care givers can be identified, researchers will need to prepare a data request document that describes the target population, data elements, and period of interest. A key to success is to understand how the data are stored and to prepare a simple coding extraction form that provides transparent and clear guidance on the specific variables to extract and how to define them. Although it is important to understand how data are coded in any single database, this is critically important when more than one database is used to ensure that uniformity is applied across the different systems and data are integrated appropriately.

A procedure needs to be well defined prior to study launch for linking data provided prospectively with that obtained from existing records, starting with a process of obtaining informed consent for record linkage. In some countries and locales, it may be acceptable to require agreement for data linkage to participate in the study, whereas in other countries and types of studies, it may be preferable to allow study participations to "opt in" or choose to participate but not be required to provide their agreement for data linkage.

Once the data are received, it is essential to review them to assure users that data extraction has been correctly performed, and whether there are sufficient data available for key variables of interest. Otherwise, prospective data collection may be used for key information that is not routinely captured.

METHODOLOGICAL CONSIDERATIONS

The primary aim of PASS is to quantify and assess safety risks or their absence (either known or for which there are uncertainties), to assess patterns of drug utilization that add knowledge on the safety profile of the medicinal product or to measure the effectiveness of risk minimization activities (EMA, 2016). Analyzing enriched studies involves integrating the data from various sources into a patient-level file to evaluate the primary, secondary, and exploratory objectives of the study. The added complexity of integrating numerous data sources requires a careful review of the integration process, including quality, transparency in the processes taken for extraction, and reproducibility checks and balances (Gini et al., 2016).

Once integration is achieved, the analysis considerations for enriched studies for the most part are similar to other PASS. There are special analytical considerations when data are available for some but not all of the study population (e.g., consider the impact of those who have chosen not to permit data linkage, i.e., opted out), or when there are multiple data sources that capture a specific variable of interest. For each of these issues, a clear and concise protocol and analytic plan should be written a priori to address how these concerns will be handled and main objectives will be analyzed.

Consider the situation where only a portion of the population has consented to have available health-care claims or EMR to be linked to their clinical study records. Depending on how these data were intended to be used in the study, there could be concern about systematic error in the final estimate of effect. For example, if an important confounder were being captured from these linkable data, this would be a concern that needs to be addressed analytically. On the other hand, if these data were to be used to capture a secondary or exploratory endpoint, such as patterns of drug utilization, then an analytical plan to handle the partial data collection would be needed. In either case, the analysis could be handled in a few different ways, including validation, calibration, sensitivity analysis, or as a substudy.

We will use the latter example of drug utilization to explain further. For validation, the entire population would need a measurement. For example, for adherence, we could have also measured adherence from a patient- or clinician-reported outcome across the entire study population. Then, in the sample with health-care claims, an analysis could be conducted to measure the differences in adherence reported from the patient or clinician compared with what was measured in the claims data. An assessment would also be made to compare the patient population who had claims available for linkage with the study population who did not have claims available to determine the applicability of these findings across the entire study population. Calibration techniques that quantify the extent and impact of bias would be used if significant differences were observed from the claims analysis. If the study population with claims was significantly different from the population without linkable claims, then stratified analyses should be reported in final study reports to evaluate results in these different populations. Sensitivity analyses that show how much bias could explain the observed results, either for key strata or for the entire study group, are very useful tools to guide interpretation of PASS results and are widely recognized as markers of high-quality research (Dreyer et al., 2016).

Another consideration that frequently occurs in enriched studies is the notion that specific variables of interest can be captured in a multitude of ways, and a decision must be made a priori as to how data will be pulled and analyzed. For example, comorbidities may be captured from the clinician and reported in the case report form, pulled from the medical record, and/or captured in a claims database. Depending on the importance of the information for the study purpose, the likelihood of being routinely captured and accessible from an existing data source, the quality of the data reported, and the frequency for which patients will have linkable files, the study team will need to decide on which record to use as the primary record and whether data on a variable should be collected from one or both sources (primary or existing data) for the purposes of the study. This hierarchy should be established prior to the start of the study so that there is consistency, transparency, and reproducibility in the data analysis. However, it is essential to recognize that enriched studies are generally full of surprises, and often data that are expected to be accessible from an EMR are not available for one reason or another. For example, data may be stored as image files or provided to clinicians alongside of the EMR and may not have been requested or sent as part of the data transfer.

With emerging technologies that routinely capture patient data, both through health systems and directly from patients, and the growing number of PASS required, enriched studies are likely to be increasingly used. These study designs take advantage of data routinely captured for efficiencies and cost-effectiveness to optimize, guide, and enhance drug safety and effectiveness evaluations, while also capturing the most relevant outcomes, such as whether patients actually feel better or worse and how their experiences impact their quality of life. Indeed, secondary data sources can be used to optimize the protocol, inform the site selection and recruitment strategies, and enhance evaluations. We are likely to see increases and improvements in user-friendly devices that capture meaningful patient data and tools to integrate information seamlessly with reduced risk of errors in the integration process. Still, careful implementation, integration, and analysis are required to ensure that enriched PASS are delivering high-quality, meaningful results and reducing the risk of errors that come with the complexity of numerous data sources.

References

Dreyer, N.A., Bryant, A., Velentgas, P., 2016. The GRACE checklist: a validated assessment tool for high quality observational studies of comparative effectiveness. J. Manag. Care Spec. Pharm. 22 (10), 1107–1113.

Engel, P., Almas, M.F., De Bruin, M.L., Starzyk, K., Blackburn, S., Dreyer, N.A., 2017. Lessons learned on the design and the conduct of Post-auhorization Safety Studies: review of 3 years of pharmacovigilance risk assessment committee (PRAC) oversight. Br. J. Clin. Pharmacol. 83 (4), 884–893.

European Medicines Agency (EMA), 2016. Guideline on Good Pharmacovigilance Practices (GVP) – Module VIII: Post-authorisation Safety Studies. Doc. Ref. EMA/813938/2011 Rev 2. Available at: http://www.ema.europa.eu/docs/en_GB/document_library/Scientific_guideline/2012/06/WC500129137.pdf.

FDA's Sentinel Initiative, 2016. Available at: http://www.fda.gov/Safety/FDAsSentinelInitiative/default.htm.

Gini R, Schuemie M, Brown J, Ryan P, Vacchi E, et al. Data Extraction and Management in Networks of Observational Health Care Databases for Scientific Research: A Comparison among EU-ADR, OMOP, Mini-Sentinel and MATRICE Strategies. eGEMs. 2016;4:1,2. Available at: https://doi.org/10.13063/2327-9214.1189. Available at: http://repository.edm-forum.org/egems/vol4/iss1/2/.

Gliklich, R., Dreyer, N., Leavy, M., et al., 2014. Registries for Evaluating Patient Outcomes: A User's Guide, third ed. Agency for Healthcare Research and Quality, Rockville, MD.

Health, Human Services (HHS), Centers for Medicare and Medicaid Services, 2010. Electronic Health Records at a Glance. Available at: https://www.medicare.gov/manage-your-health/electronic-health-records/electronic-health-records.html.

Hernandez, A.F., Fleurence, R.L., Rothman, R.L., 2015. The ADAPTABLE trial and PCORnet: shining light on a new research paradigm. Ann. Intern. Med. 163 (8), 635—636. https://doi.org/10.7326/M15-1460.

Hillestad, R., Bigelow, J., Bower, A., et al., 2005. Can electronic medical record systems transform health care? Potential health benefits, savings, and costs. Health Aff. 24, 1103—1117.

Kokkonen, E.W.J., Davis, S.A., Lin, H.C., Dabade, T.S., Feldman, S.R., Fleischer, A.B., 2013. Use of electronic medical records differs by specialty and office settings. J. Am. Med. Inf. Assoc. 20 (e1), e33—e38.

Lederle, F.A., Cushman, W.C., Ferguson, R.E., Brophy, M.T., Fiore, L.D., 2016. Chlorthalidone versus hydrochlorothiazide: a new kind of veterans affairs cooperative study. Ann. Intern. Med. 165 (9), 663—664.

Mack, C.D., Brinkley, E., Parmenter, L., Dreyer, N.A., 2015. Enriched real-world research: combining existing and new data collection for powerful studies. Pharm. Outsourcing. Available at: http://www.pharmoutsourcing.com/Featured-Articles/180633-Enriched-Real-World-Research-Combining-Existing-and-New-Data-Collection-for-Powerful-Studies/.

Rawlins, M.D., 2008. The Harveian Oration of 2008-De Testimonio: On the Evidence for Decisions about the Use of Therapeutic Interventions. Royal College of Physicians, p. 25.

Shekelle, P.G., Morton, S.C., Keeler, E.B., 2006. Costs and benefits of health information technology. Evid. Rep. Technol. Assess. 132, 1—71.

Soper, W.D., 2002. Why I love my EMR. Family Pract. Manag. J. 9, 35—38.

Wang, S.J., Middelton, B., Prosser, L.A., et al., 2003. A cost-benefit analysis of electronic medical records in primary care. Am. J. Med. 114, 397—403.

Prospective Studies

Alejandro Arana[1], Anne Fourrier-Reglat[2], Massoud Toussi[3]

[1]*RTI Health Solutions, Barcelona, Spain;* [2]*University of Bordeaux, Cedex, France;*
[3]*IQVIA, Cedex, France*

CONTENTS

Introduction 158

Prospective
Interventional
Studies 158

Prospective
Noninterventional
Studies 160

Methodological
Considerations .. 161

References 162

INTRODUCTION

A prospective study analyzes prospective experience of a cohort following the instant when the cohort is defined, e.g., the start of a medicinal product, which involves forming a cohort of subjects at the index date and observing them over a future period. Prospective studies need to be disambiguated with longitudinal studies where subjects, exposures, and outcomes are studied over time, and information is collected at multiple intervals (in contrast with cross-sectional studies where data collection is restricted to a single point in time). Longitudinal studies can be prospective or retrospective and can involve primary data collection or existing data.

Post-authorization safety studies (PASS) can be interventional or noninterventional in design. Prospective PASS can include either designs. In interventional studies, the choice of an exposure or an intervention that is assigned to subjects is determined by the investigators as per the study protocol. Noninterventional studies on the other hand include subjects treated with the medicinal product of interest under real-world conditions without control by the investigators, e.g., retrospective cohorts and case–control studies (see previous chapters on PASS study designs).

PROSPECTIVE INTERVENTIONAL STUDIES

Clinical trials are experimental studies that explore whether medicinal products, medical care procedures, or medical devices are efficacious. The purpose of clinical trials is research, so the studies follow strict scientific standards. These standards protect patients and help produce reliable study results. In clinical trials, a cohort of patients with a disease is divided into groups as determined by the investigators per the study protocol. Each group will receive a particular exposure or intervention and will be observed over time for the occurrence of outcomes. The idea behind group formation is to make groups that are equal in every aspect except in the exposure to attribute changes in occurrence of the outcome among subgroups to the discordant intervention (exposure). In addition to postmarketing (Phase IV) randomized clinical trials (RCT), prospective interventional designs that can be employed for PASS include pragmatic trials, large simple trials (LST), randomized database studies (RDS), and registry-based randomized trials.

RCT are considered the gold standard for demonstrating the efficacy of medicinal products and for obtaining an initial estimate of the risk of adverse outcomes. Assignment of exposure through randomization ensures even distribution of known and unknown risk factors among exposed and unexposed groups, providing strong internal validity. However, RCT are not free from limitations as generalization of results produced in a small, highly selected group of patients cannot be applied to the general population, and results for long-term exposure, or for events that occur with a very low frequency are not obtainable in RCT.

Pragmatic clinical trials (PCT) can be considered as clinical trials performed in populations that represent the patients by whom the medicinal product will be used. The idea is to evaluate benefits and risks of randomized treatments in patient populations and settings more representative of routine clinical practice (IMI, 2013). To be representative of routine clinical practice, PCT will include patients of all ages, with comorbidities and comedications (Collier et al., 2017). There are tools to support PCT designs and reporting, including guidance and checklists (Zwarenstein et al., 2008; Thorpe et al., 2009; Loudon et al., 2015).

LST are a kind of PCT whose objective is only focused on one or two questions in a broader patient population. It requires minimal data collection protocols that are focused on clearly defined outcomes. The saving in data collection can increase largely the sample size to detect small differences in effects with sufficient precision. LST can be designed to include the follow-up time that mimics normal clinical practice. If the safety research question allows it, LST are more efficient and less expensive than other large RCT. These designs are appropriate when the outcome is very rare or occurs with a long latency, e.g., thyroid cancer (Lesko and Mitchell, 1995; Strom et al., 2011).

RDS are born as a new strategy to produce studies with an acceptable balance between internal and external validity. Randomization minimizes confounding, the main fear in database studies, and large databases are representative of the target population. The idea would be to let a random function decide the exposure within the population in the database, e.g., EMR. RDS include randomization algorithms in computer-based patient records to determine exposure and using noninterventional methods to assess treatment effects. Patients included in the trial need to be enrolled in a health-care system with electronic records. Eligible patients may be identified automatically. Patient recruitment, informed consent, and proper documentation of information need to be addressed in accordance with the applicable legislation for RCT. Randomization will occur automatically when a patient is deemed suitable for inclusion. Database screening or record linkage can be used to detect and measure outcomes of interest, otherwise outcomes are assessed through normal process of care (van Staa et al., 2012, 2014). An extension of RDS, registry-based randomized trials use existing disease registries as the platform for the identification of subjects, randomization, and follow-up (Lauer and D'Agostino, 2013). As the RDS, these are hybrid designs that include randomization to determine exposure to medicinal products and assess outcomes through data routinely collected in registries (Frobert et al., 2013; Rao et al., 2014). See previous Chapter 4.4 for more discussion on enriched study designs.

PROSPECTIVE NONINTERVENTIONAL STUDIES

PASS are considered noninterventional if the medicinal product under investigation is prescribed in the usual manner according to the terms of the marketing authorization; the assignment of patients to a particular treatment is not decided in advance by a trial protocol but falls within current practice, and prescribing decision is clearly separated from the decision to include the patient in the study; and no additional diagnostic or monitoring procedures are applied to study patients, and pharmacoepidemiologic methods are used for the analysis of collected data.

In prospective cohort studies, researchers plan the design of the study and its execution before any of the subjects have developed any of the study outcomes. As opposed to retrospective cohort studies (see Chapter 4.3), the application of selection criteria and collection of exposure data on all patients has to occur before any of the subjects have developed any of the study outcomes. The members of the study cohort are then monitored through the future to record the development of any of the study endpoints. The monitoring can be conducted by different means, including regular medical practice as recorded in databases, medical examinations, clinical tests such as laboratory or imaging, questionnaires, home interviews, phone interviews, or via mobile applications or the internet. Combination of these methods is often used.

Examples of prospective cohort studies include the Framingham Heart Study (FHS, 2018); the Rotterdam Study (Hofman et al., 2015); and the MONICA (Multinational Monitoring of Trends and Determinants in Cardiovascular Disease) project (Bothig, 1989). In these studies, researchers wanted to study risk factors for common chronic diseases. They identified a cohort of possible subjects who would be monitored for a prolonged period. Eligible subjects had to meet certain criteria and were not allowed to participate if they had certain characteristics listed in the exclusion criteria. The information collected from all study subjects in the same way to minimize measurement bias.

Prospective cohort designs are often used for PASS. After baseline information is collected, subjects in these designs are followed up in time, in which they might be exposed to a medicinal product at one time, but unexposed at another. This longitudinal follow-up allows researchers to relate events, change in exposure, and loss to follow-up to the index date of starting study drug. By having individual data on these details for each subject, researchers can calculate and compare event incidence rates for each exposure group. Prospective cohorts are also useful for the evaluation of multiple adverse events within the same study. For instance, postmarketing safety studies (PMSS) that monitor the safety profile for newly authorized medicinal products are often required by Japan Pharmaceuticals and Medicinal Devices Agency (Takahashi et al., 2016).

In PMSS, it may be difficult to recruit sufficient number of patients who are exposed to the medicinal product of interest when studying an orphan product or when new product does not penetrate the market as expected. Like RCT, prospective cohort designs are not useful to study very rare outcomes. The identification of patients for prospective cohort studies may come from large automated databases (Arana et al., 2010) or from data collected specifically for the study at hand (Takahashi et al., 2016). In addition, these studies may be used to examine safety concerns in special populations (e.g., older persons, children, patients with comorbid conditions, or pregnant women). Through oversampling of these patients or by stratifying the cohort, sufficient numbers of patients exist.

METHODOLOGICAL CONSIDERATIONS

Cohort studies can be either closed or open. A closed cohort is one with fixed membership where the number of subjects at cohort entry cannot be increased once the study starts. The number of subjects may decline because of death or loss to follow-up, but no additional subjects are added. Children born to mothers exposed to thalidomide before the teratogenic effect was known would be considered members of a fixed or closed cohort that was defined by each event. In contrast, an open cohort is dynamic where members can leave or be added over time, e.g., patients enter the cohort when they are prescribed the study drug of interest and leave if they stop treatment with the drug (Arana et al., 2015).

Prospective cohort studies try to mimic RCT as much as possible and select a comparison group that differs with respect to the exposure of interest but is as similar as possible with respect to other factors that might influence the outcome. There are two key factors to consider when selecting a comparator in cohort PASS: the unexposed group (or exposed to another treatment) should be as similar as possible with respect to confounding factors; and data collection should be as accurate and as comparable as possible in all groups to avoid measurement bias. The notion of similarity of two groups shall be handled based on the context and with caution. Although it is of utmost importance in effectiveness evaluation studies, in PASS matching the exposed and unexposed groups may introduces selection bias in the unexposed patients. This is one of the reasons for which an internal comparison group with the same inclusion and exclusion criteria is preferred. Alternatively, comparison with the general population can be used when no other comparator is easily available; however, it may differ from the exposed cohort in many ways, including age, sex, and health characteristics.

Additionally, selection bias can occur in prospective cohort studies because of differences in retention during the follow-up period between exposed and comparator groups after enrollment. When the observation period is long enough, it can be difficult to track subjects for the entire study as they may die, relocate, or lose interest in the study. Loss to follow-up introduces bias if it differs by exposure status and outcome. The following chapters discuss analytical approaches to reduce bias and confounding in PASS, including techniques to prevent selection bias, e.g., propensity score matching.

References

Arana, A., Wentworth, C.E., Ayuso-Mateos, J.L., Arellano, F.M., 2010. Suicide-related events in patients treated with antiepileptic drugs. N. Engl. J. Med. 363 (6), 542–551.

Arana, A., Johannes, C.B., McQuay, L.J., Varas-Lorenzo, C., Fife, D., Rothman, K.J., 2015. Risk of out-of-hospital sudden cardiac death in users of domperidone, proton pump inhibitors, or metoclopramide: a population-based nested case-control study. Drug Saf. 38 (12), 1187–1199.

Bothig, S., 1989. WHO MONICA Project: objectives and design. Int. J. Epidemiol. 18 (3 Suppl 1), S29–S37.

Collier, S., Harvey, C., Brewster, J., Bakerly, N.D., Elkhenini, H.F., Stanciu, R., Williams, C., Brereton, J., New, J.P., McCrae, J., McCorkindale, S., Leather, D., 2017. Monitoring safety in a phase III real-world effectiveness trial: use of novel methodology in the Salford Lung Study. Pharmacoepidemiol. Drug Saf. 26 (3), 344–352.

Framingham Heart Study (FHS), 2018. About the Framingham Heart Study. Available at: https://www.framinghamheartstudy.org/about-fhs/index.php.

Frobert, O., Lagerqvist, B., Olivecrona, G.K., Omerovic, E., Gudnason, T., Maeng, M., Aasa, M., Angeras, O., Calais, F., et al., 2013. Thrombus aspiration during ST-segment elevation myocardial infarction. N. Engl. J. Med. 369 (17), 1587–1597.

Hofman, A., Brusselle, G.G., Darwish Murad, S., van Duijn, C.M., Franco, O.H., Goedegebure, A., Ikram, M.A., Klaver, C.C., Nijsten, T.E., et al., 2015. The Rotterdam Study: 2016 objectives and design update. Eur. J. Epidemiol. 30 (8), 661−708.

Innovative Medicines Initiative (IMI), 2013. Glossary of Definitions of Common Terms. GetReal-Project No. 115546. Available from: http://www.imi-getreal.eu/Portals/1/Documents/01% 20deliverables/D1.3%20-%20Revised%20GetReal%20glossary%20-%20FINAL%20updated %20version_25Oct16_webversion.pdf.

Lauer, M.S., D'Agostino Sr., R.B., 2013. The randomized registry trial—the next disruptive technology in clinical research? N. Engl. J. Med. 369 (17), 1579−1581.

Lesko, S.M., Mitchell, A.A., 1995. An assessment of the safety of pediatric ibuprofen. A practitioner-based randomized clinical trial. J. Am. Med. Assoc. 273 (12), 929−933.

Loudon, K., Treweek, S., Sullivan, F., Donnan, P., Thorpe, K.E., Zwarestein, M., 2015. The PRECIS-2 tool: designing trials that are fit for purpose. BMJ 350, h2147.

Rao, S.V., Hess, C.N., Barham, B., Aberle, L.H., Anstrom, K.J., Patel, T.B., Jorgensen, J.P., Mazzaferri Jr., E.L., Jolly, S.S., Jacobs, A., et al., 2014. A registry-based randomized trial comparing radial and femoral approaches in women undergoing percutaneous coronary intervention: the SAFE-PCI for Women (Study of Access Site for Enhancement of PCI for Women) trial. JACC Cardiovasc. Interv. 7 (8), 857−867.

Strom, B.L., Eng, S.M., Faich, G., Reynolds, R.F., D'Agostino, R.B., Ruskin, J., Kane, J.M., 2011. Comparative mortality associated with ziprasidone and olanzapine in real-wold use among 18,154 patients with schizophrenia: the ziprasidone observational study of cardiac outcomes (ZODIAC). Am. J. Psychiatry 168 (2), 193−201.

Takahashi, S., Hiramatsu, M., Hotta, S., Watanabe, Y., Suga, O., Endo, Y., Miyamori, I., 2016. Safety and antihypertensive effect of selara® (eplerenone): reults from a postmarketing surveillance in Japan. Int. J. Hypertens. 2016, 5091951.

Thorpe, K.E., Zwarenstein, M., Oxman, A.D., Treweek, S., Furberg, C.D., Altman, D.G., Tunis, S., Bergel, E., Harvey, I., Magid, D.J., Chalkidou, K., 2009. A pragmatic-explanatory continuum indicator summary (PRECIS): a tool to help trial designers. J. Clin. Epidemiol. 62 (5), 464−475.

van Staa, T.P., Goldacre, B., Gulliford, M., Cassell, J., Pirmohamed, M., Taweel, A., Delaney, B., Smeeth, L., 2012. Pragmatic randomised trials using routine electronic health records: putting them to the test. BMJ 344, e55.

van Staa, T.P., Dyson, L., McCann, G., Padmanabhan, S., Belatri, R., Goldacre, B., Cassell, J., Pirmohamed, M., Torgerson, D., et al., 2014. The opportunities and challenges of pragmatic point-of-care randomised trials using routinely collected electronic records: evaluations of two exemplar trials. Health Technol. Assess. 18 (43), 1−146.

Zwarenstein, M., Treweek, S., Gagnier, J.J., Altman, D.G., Tunis, S., Haynes, B., Oxman, A.D., Moher, D., CONSORT group, Pragmatic Trials in Healthcare (Practihc) group, 2008. Improving the reporting of pragmatic trials: an extension of the CONSORT statement. BMJ 337, a2390.

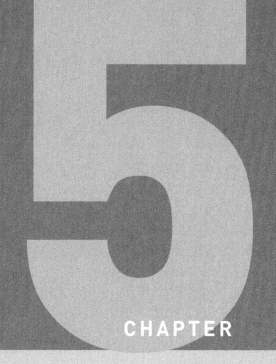

CHAPTER

Analytical Approaches for PASS

5.1 Exposure Propensity Scores 167
5.2 Disease Risk Scores 182
5.3 Instrumental Variables 197
5.4 Data Analytic Platforms 203
5.5 Proactive Safety Surveillance 209

Exposure Propensity Scores

John D. Seeger

Optum, Eden Prairie, MN, United States

INTRODUCTION

The labeled indication of a medicinal product offers insight into the patients to whom it is likely to be prescribed. Patients who have a condition, e.g., diabetes, will be the main recipients of a product, antidiabetes medication, and through routine prescribing practice, patients who are the recipients of the product will possess characteristics that might be expected among patients with the condition. These characteristics can be expected to differ somewhat from patients who are prescribed with other product, e.g., anticoagulant agent indicated for stroke prevention in atrial fibrillation. Of course, some patient characteristics will overlap between recipients of these two products and some patients will have both diabetes and atrial fibrillation, so that they might be suitable candidates for either or both products. However, the difference in indication of these two products will tend to produce differences in patterns of patient characteristics associated with their use. The epidemiology of the conditions will provide information regarding other aspects of the expected patient characteristics and inform about the relative numbers of patients who might be candidates to receive either products and the calendar years over which a comparison could be conducted.

The expected differences in characteristics between users of these products would suggest that initiators of the anticoagulant agent would generally not be suitable as a comparison group for initiators of the antidiabetes medication. In large part, this conclusion is driven by differences in covariate patterns among patients who receive either of these products, along with the implausibility that a clinician might make a choice between initiating treatment with both products in the same patient (these two products are not therapeutic alternatives). The scientific relevance of a comparison of two medicinal products that have different indications would tend to be limited. However, the difference in expected patient characteristics between the two products serves to illustrate some points that are important in making comparisons across products and to the use of exposure propensity scores (EPS) to address such

CONTENTS

Introduction 167

Confounding by Indication 169

Development of Exposure Propensity Scores 171

Strengths of Exposure Propensity Scores 173

Applications of Exposure Propensity Scores 175
Restriction 176
Stratification 176
Matching 176
Modeling 177
Weighting 178

Transparency 179

References 180

167

Post-Authorization Safety Studies of Medicinal Products. https://doi.org/10.1016/B978-0-12-809217-0.00005-2

differences in patient characteristics. A well-formed research question that is highly focused and specific seems to be a trivial consideration, but it has profound effects on a study that can be either positive (if the study question is well formed) or negative (if not) (Velentgas et al., 2013). Although the research question is important, it is possible to modify it in an iterative process in response to observations within the data to improve it and thereby improve the study.

EPS techniques represent a collection of tools that can be employed to address measured and known confounding variables. This is because the EPS are models built from measured variables that exist within a data source or that can be derived from variables that do. Patient characteristics that are not present in a database or are not included in the EPS model (perhaps by not being recognized as an important confounder) will not be accounted for by this technique. However, EPS offer a number of features that are useful in the context of research on the safety and effectiveness of medicinal products. Although many characteristics of patients initiating a medicinal product might be inferred from the labeled indication for the product, the practice of medicine further refines them through the process by which prescribers become accustomed to using a particular product, and this is influenced by both patient and prescriber factors, including local patient characteristics and preferences, regional practice patterns, national and international clinical guidelines, local and national opinion leaders, explicit and implicit guidance disseminated by training institutions, and individual experience.

Simply choosing two treatments that have the same or similar indications for use is not enough to ensure that the patients initiating the treatments are similar enough to be compared without addressing confounding that may arise through patient selection to one or the other of the treatments. The particular patients for whom a particular treatment might be prescribed can be identified as the end result of a complex prescribing process, and this selection extends considerably beyond whether or not the patient has a particular indication. For example, type 2 diabetes exists along a spectrum that extends from impaired glucose tolerance and prediabetes through long-standing diabetes with end-organ damage manifesting as vascular, neurologic, and renal complications. The various treatments for diabetes might be preferred at a particular stage or range of stages along this spectrum (Ali, 2015).

Further complicating this concept that indications exist along a spectrum that is not unidimensional. In addition to duration of diabetes, the degree of glucose elevation or lability might be thought of as a different dimension that affects how the duration of diabetes in a particular patient enters into the prescribing decision. For example, two patients who both have been recently diagnosed with diabetes might be prescribed different medications if they have different blood glucose or glycosylated hemoglobin (HbA1c) levels. In addition, patient symptomatology and history might represent another dimension of diabetes that also exists along a spectrum. Accordingly, two patients who each are at similar stages in their history of diabetes and who have similar blood glucose or HbA1c values might be prescribed different medications if they have differing histories with respect to hypoglycemia symptoms. Each of these dimensions and perhaps others are used by prescribers to define particular subtypes of diabetes indications, and these subtypes may receive different treatments, so that even among patients with a similar indication (e.g., type 2 diabetes) there can be substantial differences with respect to medicinal products used, and these differences are related to important disease or patient characteristics.

CONFOUNDING BY INDICATION

Beyond the indication and indication subtype for use of a medicinal product, an entire suite of demographic, clinical, and regional differences will influence prescribing decisions, and collectively they define the patients who would be candidates for the product. The set of variables used to prescribe a particular medicinal product and distinguish it from another will tend to be prognostic of a wide range of clinical outcomes that patients might experience, so that differences between initiators of two medicinal products with respect to these variables result in confounding. As a quantitative phenomenon, confounding is simply present or not but differs in magnitude depending on the amount of imbalance in the variable(s) between compared groups, the prevalence of the variable(s), and the strength of the variable(s) as risk factors for the outcome (Bross, 1966). Collectively, the characteristics that influence prescribing will have the effect of making almost any two products inappropriate comparators for one another, unless the resulting differences are accounted for in some way. The term *"confounding by indication"* is frequently applied to this phenomenon and refers to the confounding that arises from both measured and unmeasured differences between compared treatments that reflect the indication for the treatments, subtype of the indication, and correlated variables (Ali, 2013).

Confounding by indication is often of greatest concern when two medicinal products are compared that have different indications. In the most extreme forms, the indication and product selection are so tightly bound up with one another that disentangling one from the other becomes infeasible. The comparison of initiators of an antidiabetes medication to initiators of an anticoagulant is such an example where the difference in indication between the products might represent an insurmountable obstacle due to the potential for confounding that could not be addressed by accounting for measured variables. Sound inference regarding the beneficial or harmful effects of a medicinal product must address the potential for confounding that arises from any or all of the variables associated with both the indications for use and the actual use of a product, and a variety of analytical approaches can be used. Many of these approaches exploit variations in product choices that permit separating treatment effects from effects of other variables.

In the context of post-authorization safety studies (PASS), much of the potential confounding by indication depends on what the study product is compared to. Confounding is an inherently comparison-based phenomenon, so that a single group of patients who are users of an antidiabetes medication can be described and outcomes among them can be identified and presented quantitatively with no need to address confounding. It is only through comparison that confounding arises. However, comparisons can be either explicit or implicit. Without an explicit comparison group, often the comparison will be made to what would be historically expected for patients with the particular indication. Such a comparison can be affected by differences not only just in indication but also changes over time in the occurrence or coding of a particular outcome in health-care databases (see Chapters 3.1 and 3.2 for a discussion about claims and electronic medical record [EMR] data sources for PASS). Thus, a more reasonable comparison in antidiabetes medication PASS would be between two antidiabetes medications that are used for patients at similar stages of diabetes or for patients with similar comorbidities or concomitant medications. Alternatively, one might select such similar patients from among a combined group of patients receiving a number of different antidiabetes medications.

With an anticoagulant product, there exists a natural comparison in warfarin, the standard of stroke prevention in atrial fibrillation (Reynolds et al., 2004). As other newer oral anticoagulants became available, a comparison between two of the newer products may be feasible, but there may remain advantages in comparing each of the newer products to a common reference. The question sometimes arises why not compare all products that are available for a particular indication to determine which one is the "best" in terms of effectiveness or safety profile. There are two important reasons that such a question might be replaced with a series of pairwise comparisons. First, there would be different sets of patients who would be candidates for each of the products, so that the set of patients who would be candidates for all products might be small and might be different than the set of patients who would be candidates for any individual pair of products. Furthermore, the variables that might be confounders for one pair of products could differ from that between a different pair. It seems unreasonable to have a single model that accounts for confounding that might exist between all pairs of products, even if the medicinal products are used for similar indications.

Although the concept of new user cohorts is seemingly independent from the use of EPS in PASS, these two concepts are mutually reinforcing. Applications of EPS benefit from seeking to mirror the prescribing process (or treatment selection process), and considerations of prescribing are naturally associated with the initiation of treatment. With prescribing, a conscious choice is made to select a particular medicinal product instead of potential alternatives. Accordingly, accounting for confounding between two treatments requires consideration of factors that influence selection of one product relative to another. In selecting a particular product for a particular patient, the patient should be a candidate for either of the products because comparing two products for a patient who is not a candidate for one or the other violates the principle that patients with any set of covariates included in a study should have a nonzero chance of receiving either product (i.e., positivity assumption). This consideration also makes clear why the comparison of new users of one medicinal product to ongoing users of another product would not be appropriate. The treatment selection process is an active one, involving the patient and prescriber, which results in a new prescription, and this will almost always differ from the decision-making involved in continuing a medicinal product a patient is already taking. Patients receiving a new prescription will differ from those remaining on established treatment when the products are used for the same or similar indications even when the patients otherwise appear similar. Thus, the comparison of an anticoagulant and warfarin must find patients who are new users of either medication and it is a serious error to compare new users of an anticoagulant with continuers of warfarin (Schneeweiss et al., 2013).

DEVELOPMENT OF EXPOSURE PROPENSITY SCORES

The comparison of groups of patients defined by receipt of one or another medicinal product who differ from one another is not a novel concept, and EPS techniques have not fundamentally altered the challenges involved in making comparisons across exposures. However, EPS offer certain advantages that make them particularly well suited for PASS where there tend to be many confounding variables that can be identified and relatively few patients who experience the outcome being studied, particularly when the outcome represents an unexpected or an adverse effect of the treatment.

The five standard techniques used to mitigate confounding in PASS are restriction, stratification, matching, modeling, and weighting. Each represents a form of conditioning on a variable or set of variables so that the resulting effect estimate accounts for differences in the variable(s) being conditions (Kurth and Seeger, 2008). These techniques can be applied in several different ways either in the design or analysis stages of PASS. However, each of these techniques experiences challenges when the number of confounding variables increases, and these challenges may render the techniques infeasible or reduce their utility as means to address confounding.

As a solution to these concerns of comparing groups in the context of multiple confounders, the EPS are offered as a balancing score formed by summarizing a vector of covariates as a single variable (Rosenbaum and Rubin, 1983). If a comparison between exposure groups is made that condition on the EPS, then it will be balanced (in expectation) with respect to all components of the score. This leads to the powerful realization that it is possible to create a single model incorporating numerous potential confounders that predict selection of one exposure relative to another and use the predicted value from that model for each individual as a way to achieve control of potentially numerous confounders. Subject to this assumption that there is no unmeasured confounding, and the correct functional form has been used in developing the EPS model that summarizes the confounders, then conditioning on the EPS will enable estimation of exposure effect not only just unconfounded by the score but also unconfounded by any variable that is a component of the EPS. Any technique that assigns to individuals as a single predicted value from a set of characteristics will work as long as the technique appropriately reflects the contribution of each variable to that predicted value. Prediction modeling tools can be applied, with logistic regression being most common. Alternatively, tree-based classification methods may offer an advantage in situations, involving strong interactions between variables.

The concept of collapsing variables to arrive at a summary score goes beyond predicting exposure. It is also possible to collapse variables that predict outcome, and a number of disease prediction models have been developed, such as the Framingham risk score, a model that predicts 10-year probability of myocardial infarction from a set of variables. It is possible to enter age, gender, blood pressure, blood cholesterol level, and smoking status into a risk calculator based on the Framingham risk score and arrive at a single value that reflects the individual's probability of having a myocardial infarction in the next decade. This single value represents the joint contribution of each of the components, and different people could arrive at the same value through different combinations of variables; but if two people have the same predicted probability of myocardial infarction, it does not matter (in terms of the predicted probability) how they reached that level.

EPS are similar to disease risk scores in that they collapse several variables into a single value and different combinations of variables can produce a particular value. A detailed discussion and comparison between disease risk scores and EPS is provided in Chapter 5.2. In terms of confounder control, it will not matter how two different people achieved the same EPS. The theory underpinning EPS indicates that conditioning on the score will remove confounding from the suite of variables from which it is derived.

In the two-stage process of developing EPS, the first stage is to develop the score, and this must involve a selection of what variables (and in what form) to include. To address confounding, the score should include confounders and be cautious about inclusion of variables that are related to exposure but are not related to the outcome. Such variables increase the discrimination of the EPS model without being confounding variables, and their inclusion will decrease efficiency without adding any confounder control (Brookhart, 2006). Similarly, careful consideration should be applied to variables that are related to outcome, but not exposure. The contribution of these variables to exposure might be subtle and estimated imprecisely, so that imbalances in the variable may remain even after inclusion in the EPS. Such variables may be better accounted for through inclusion in the second stage of the EPS approach (the outcome model). Indeed, a metric has been proposed to aid investigators in determining whether a variable might be included in the EPS model or the outcome model (Hirano and Imbens, 2001).

STRENGTHS OF EXPOSURE PROPENSITY SCORES

In PASS, the numbers tend to be arranged in a manner that favors the use of EPS because there are many potential confounders, many patients who receive the medicinal product being studied, yet few patients who experience the relevant outcome. EPS offer a clear advantage in this scenario because the modeling of exposure occurs without use of the outcome variable, a rarely occurring outcome will not limit the development of an EPS model as it might be a model that is developed to predict the outcome. The EPS model does not even include the study outcome—it is based solely on the exposed and comparator patients and the variables thought to be confounders. Rare outcomes, as are common in pharmacoepidemiology, are typically well suited to EPS techniques (Borah et al., 2014).

Another advantage of the EPS relative to other techniques is the explicit modeling of indications for use, a feature that both enhances thinking about cofounding and how to control it. By explicitly modeling, the selection of the medicinal product, all of the variables that might represent the indication or correlates of it might be considered in an open and transparent manner. The two-stage method of EPS separates treatment selection and the variables associated with it from the outcome. Although the risk factors for a particular outcome may be incompletely understood, the process by which one medicinal product is chosen over another for a patient can be understood more fully. Because a product has to be chosen through a joint decision-making process, involving the prescriber and the patient, all of the factors that enter into this decision regarding treatment selection are, in principle, knowable. The prescriber can outline their decision-making, and published prescribing guidelines can be consulted to identify factors that prescribers in general will use. Other influences on prescribing, such as reimbursement policies or patient preference, are also knowable and measurable.

Additionally, EPS can make the area of common support between the exposures explicit. An intuitive approach to understanding this is that the overlap in the EPS represents patients with combinations of demographics, comorbidities, concomitant medications, procedures, and other health-care utilization indices where prescribers can be observed to sometimes prescribe one or the other of the compared exposures. Similarly, in ranges of the EPS where there is no overlap in the score, prescribers appear to always choose one or the other of the exposures. Such areas of nonoverlap might mean that clinical opinion is uniform in situations. This lack of apparent equipoise can be a useful caution in the conduct of PASS. Assessing the degree of overlap in EPS distributions represents an important diagnostic tool as it illustrates the clinical uncertainty between the two medicinal products. Accordingly, a finding of little overlap in EPS between products is not a limitation of the EPS method, rather a useful checkpoint highlighting the amount of clinical uncertainty, which would affect essentially any analysis comparing the two products, and is made explicit through EPS.

The degree of overlap can be judged in relation to the expected overlap. If the products are used for patients with similar indications, then there should be extensive overlap in the EPS. If there is not, this suggests something wrong with the EPS. For example, a variable that is strongly correlated with one of the products, then a decision can be made regarding whether the degree of overlap suggests a problem that might be resolved by refining or restructuring the question (Walker, 2013).

Other strengths of the EPS include that it tends to be robust to model misspecification relative to a single-stage model, depending on how the EPS is used (Drake and Fisher, 1995). Also, EPS offer a natural scale for assessing exposure effect heterogeneity (Glynn et al., 2006). EPS can be thought of as a summary measure of the strength of indication for one product relative to the comparator, so that stratifying (as by quintiles) the analysis will show the effect of the exposure relative to the comparator when prescribed to patients with most clear indications (the top stratum) for the product, when prescribed to patients with the most clear indications for the comparator (the bottom stratum), and across the strata in between. Such an analysis directly addresses the clinically intuitive expectation that the medicinal product should work best when prescribed to the most ideal candidates, and this assessment may be more useful than stratifying by age or gender in assessing heterogeneity.

Of course, assessing heterogeneity can include the EPS along with demographic and clinical characteristics.

As discussed in Chapter 4.5, EPS can be useful for prospective PASS where study outcome have not yet occurred. In such settings, it is infeasible to build an outcome model, but it may be feasible to build a model of exposure and use that EPS model to match study cohorts that could be followed for outcomes that will only reveal themselves at some point in the future. Cohorts matched using EPS in this manner can even be used to evaluate the effect on an outcome that was not envisioned at the outset of the study.

The restriction of covariate space and included covariate patterns leads to another advantage of the EPS technique: a restriction on the plausible ranges for unmeasured confounders. In the context of EPS matching, it offers straightforward approaches to address unmeasured confounding through sampled data collection, EPS calibration, or application of sensitivity analyses that assume an unmeasured confounding variable and its characteristics (Stürmer et al., 2005; Schneeweiss, 2006; Schneeweiss et al., 2007).

Randomized clinical trials (RCT) with two groups offer both simplicity and power by balancing two groups (exposure and comparator) with respect to any patient characteristics, both measured and unmeasured, allowing for the direct comparison of the two groups using standard statistical techniques. Clinicians, researchers, and regulators rely on RCT for decision-making, and there is generally a good reason for this. As mentioned in a Chapter 4, the findings provided by RCT are typically not subject to alternative explanations or at least the range of alternative explanations in the context of RCT are more limited than they are in noninterventional research. EPS analyses can adopt some of the features of RCT by identifying new user cohorts that are contemporaneous with one another, so that the most serious threat to a valid comparison is likely to arise from confounding. It is this construction of PASS where EPS appear particularly useful.

APPLICATIONS OF EXPOSURE PROPENSITY SCORES

The second stage in EPS analysis is to use the score to address confounding, and there are five distinct ways to do this: restriction, stratification, matching, modeling, and weighting. Each can address confounding, so the choice between them depends on other features. Certain ways to use EPS lend themselves more readily to transparency than others. For example, matching on EPS is intuitive and provides a transparent view of the groups to be compared along with those removed from the comparison. These two points address both the internal validity of the comparison and the external validity of the medicinal product users being compared.

Restriction

Restriction offers a straightforward approach to addressing confounding that is simple to understand. If the studied population included only males, then males make up 100% of both the treated and comparison groups, so that after applying this restriction, gender cannot confound the comparison. Restriction can be applied to more than one variable, but such multivariable restriction carries with it the risk of substantially reducing the sample size available for making the comparison. This represents a classic tradeoff between validity and comparison (the more similar the groups are by restricting on more variables, the better) and precision of the result (the smaller the sample contributing to the effect estimate, the wider the confidence intervals). Restriction can be applied to the summary of covariates represented by the EPS rather than on the individual variables and provides something of an advantage in doing so. For example, restricting to patients in the top quintile of the EPS will tend to provide good balance on patient characteristics and retain more patients than a similar restriction on each of the variables included in the EPS. In this way, trimming the EPS is a particular application of restriction (Stürmer et al., 2005). By trimming off ranges of the EPS above and below the asymmetric cutoff points suggested, the exposure and comparison groups will be more similar in each of the characteristics included in the EPS, and the sample size will be larger than applying the trimming on each of the variables separately.

Stratification

The application of EPS is similar to stratification with any continuous variable, requiring the investigator to define strata cutoff points (such as at quintile cutoff points) and then form subgroups based on those cutoff points. Within each stratum, the average EPS among exposure and comparison patients will be similar (certainly more similar than the mean was among the full population). In this way, balance is improved on the EPS and because the score is a summary of all the variables that go into its construction, then all of the components of the EPS will also show improved balance.

Matching

Matching on EPS leads to an intuitive presentation of the data because there will be two groups that should exhibit similar distributions of most covariates. Using EPS as a matching variable (particularly with 1:1 matching) will result in well-balanced comparison groups and can lead to straightforward outcome analyses, including a crude comparison of outcomes. Matching on EPS has the effect of balancing all the variables that are part of the score. This property of EPS is readily apparent after matching and permits some balance metrics to be applied. Applications of EPS for multicategory exposure groups have been proposed (Ali et al., 2015).

Matching on EPS can be accomplished using a number of existing matching algorithms. Simple algorithms might involve random sorting of exposure and comparison patients and then selecting exposed patients one at a time, serially checking EPS of the exposed patient to the comparison patients and outputting a pair whenever the two EPS are within a predefined distance (caliper). An algorithm that progressively expands the caliper for matching has been developed (Parsons, 2001), and this algorithm will tend to provide more matches that are also better matched (closer EPS) than fixed caliper matching algorithms. However, this variable caliper approach has the potential to include matches that have EPS that differ by as much as 10%, and this might be too large for certain variables in EPS, so guidance on the maximum caliper to be used in matching was developed (Austin, 2011).

Some additional considerations arise for matching ratios other than 1:1. A 1:2, 1:3, 1:4, or other matching ratios might be considered to increase statistical power, particularly when the number of patients initiating the medicinal product is constrained but there are many potential comparators from which to choose. These other than 1:1 ratios can be obtained by running the matching algorithm multiple times. Important considerations arise when matching in ratios other than 1:1 that increase the complexity of the outcome analysis. The second, third, or other match will tend to be a less good match than the first match, so there will be some decrease in the balance obtained with the additional matches, and this decrease in balance comes along with increased challenge presenting the balance obtained by matching in a single table, reducing the intuitive appeal of matching where it is easy to see balance across the compared groups. Also, a variable ratio match will tend to introduce better balance but increased complexity (Wang et al., 2014). In PASS, matching without replacement is generally preferred to prevent patients from being present multiple times in the analysis, and thereby contributing undue influence on the results.

Sometimes an additional matching requirement beyond EPS might be imposed for variables such as age, gender, or calendar time that are important to balance and where the investigator does not want to depend on the EPS to achieve balance. In addition to the intuitive assessment of balance obtained by matching, there are a range of quantitative balance metrics that have been proposed with the most accepted being the absolute standardized difference for individual variables (Austin, 2009; Stuart et al., 2013).

Modeling

As with any covariate, EPS can be included in an outcome model as an adjustment variable. Doing so will have the advantage that all subjects contribute to the analysis, and the properties of the EPS remain, so that adjusting for the single EPS variable will have the effect of adjusting for all of the components of the score. However, there are some additional considerations when using the EPS as an adjustment variable. First, the functional form of the EPS needs to be carefully assessed. Because the score is a composite of many variables, some of which are continuous and some are categories, the form of the association between EPS and study outcome might take on many different forms other than a single linear term. It might be a curvilinear function, a step function, or a saw tooth function. Misspecifying the association between EPS and the outcome may lead to incomplete control of the confounding embodied in the EPS and may even lead to increased confounding in some settings.

Another potential problem with the modeling approach is that it may hide the fact that there exists limited overlap in EPS. The model will produce an effect estimate, but limited overlap in EPS distributions may mean that the estimate is imprecise and may only come from a particular range of the EPS distribution (where the overlap exists).

Weighting

Weighting is a method of achieving balance through standardization. The process reweights individual patients in both the exposed and comparison groups to produce groups with essentially identical EPS distributions. These pseudo-populations are then compared with one another. Such comparisons are no longer confounded by characteristics of the EPS. There are three general versions of weighting approaches: inverse probability of treatment weighting (IPTW); standardized mortality/morbidity ratio (SMR) weighting; and matched weighting. Other weighting schemes are possible, but there offer many useful considerations. The weights applied under each of these approaches lead to different populations being compared and therefore provide answers to different questions.

By applying IPTW, the comparison is between treating everyone who receives either of the medicinal products with just one of the products and treating the same group (everyone who receives either of the products) with the alternative. By contrast, the SMR weighting compares those who receive one of the products to what would have happened if those people had received the alternative. The matched weighting answers yet another question and compares patients who receive one product in the overlap between the two products and those in the same region of EPS who receive the alternative. Each application of weighting has a potential advantage in that these approaches use all of the patients in the study. However, seeking to include all patients will sometimes include patients whose data are of questionable value, which can result in extreme weights that may be hidden in the analysis (Seeger et al., 2017).

TRANSPARENCY

In the setting of PASS, the EPS technique presents a number of advantages that are worth noting. First is that the EPS can address numerous differences between compared groups in straightforward ways. Second is that the EPS fits into the treatment selection and the intuitive understanding of clinicians who might prescribe the compared medicinal products. It becomes easy for clinical reviewers to determine whether EPS applied in a particular setting account for all of the variables known to go into the prescribing decision. In this way and in the application of EPS technique, transparency is an important aspect.

Because PASS benefit from transparency in methods, an emphasis will be made on analytic approaches and data displays that permit reviewers to assess aspects of balance obtained, the sensitivity of the results to the particular application of this method, and assessing potential unmeasured confounding. Sensitivity of results to particular application of EPS can be addressed by applying the EPS a number of different ways. However, when this is done, it should be made explicit what EPS methods were applied and what the results were from each approach tried. The PASS protocol should anticipate the use of different EPS approaches and specify which would be the primary approach and which would be secondary or supplemental. The use of EPS weighting, particularly with IPTW, can be sensitive to individuals with large weights and will benefit from additional EPS approaches that are less sensitive to influential individuals such as matching on EPS.

Noninterventional PASS must always consider the possibility of alternative explanations for the observed result. Residual confounding is just one of the possible alternative reasons for an observed result. Unmeasured confounding must abide by the same mathematical rules that apply to measured confounders. Invoking the term unmeasured confounder does not grant extraordinary powers to the variable or set of variables in question. These variables must still exert their confounding influence through an imbalance in prevalence or distribution across compared groups coupled with being a predictor of the outcome, so that the compared groups have a different risk of outcome that is not causally related to the exposure. Unmeasured confounding can be addressed either through sampled data collection on the hypothesized confounding variable or through sensitivity analyses that assume characteristics of the unmeasured confounder and quantify the effect of the unmeasured variable on the study effect estimate. Application of EPS (especially when used to match comparison groups) focuses these unmeasured confounder techniques on a subset of the population where the effect is most directly relevant. By restricting the subjects that are in the comparison groups, EPS matching limits the number of subjects from which external information would need to be obtained to address the unmeasured confounding. It also narrows the range of plausible values that would need to be applied in sensitivity analyses to address unmeasured confounding. Chapter 8 introduces the EU PAS Register as a means to improve transparency in PASS protocols and final study reports.

References

Ali, A.K., 2013. Methodological challenges in observational research: a pharmacoepidemiological perspective. Br. J. Pharmaceut. Res. 3 (2), 161–175.

Ali, A.K., 2015. Biases related to prescribing decisions in retrospective database research in diabetes. Value Outcomes Spotlight 1 (4), 13–15.

Ali, A.K., Hartzema, A.G., Winterstein, A.G., Segal, R., Lu, X., Hendeles, L., 2015. Application of multi-category exposure marginal structural models to investigate the association between long-acting beta-agonists and prescribing of oral corticosteroids for asthma exacerbations in the Clinical Practice Research Datalink. Value Health 18 (2), 260–270.

Austin, P.C., 2009. Balance diagnostics for comparing the distribution of baseline covariates between treatment groups in propensity score matched samples. Stat. Med. 28, 3083–3107.

Austin, P.C., 2011. Optimal caliper widths for propensity-score matching when estimating differences in means and differences in proportions in observational studies. Pharm. Stat. 10, 150–161.

Borah, B.J., Moriarty, J.P., Crown, W.H., Doshi, J.A., 2014. Application of propensity score methods in comparative effectiveness and safety research, where have we come and where should we go? J. Comp. Effect Res. 3, 63–78.

Brookhart, M.A., Schneeweiss, S., Rothman, K.J., Glynn, R.J., Avorn, J., Stürmer, T., 2006. Variable selection for propensity score models. Am. J. Epidemiol. 163, 1149–1156.

Bross, I.D.J., 1966. Spurious effects from an extraneous variable. J. Chron. Dis. 19, 637–647.

Drake, C., Fisher, L., 1995. Prognostic models and the propensity score. Int. J. Epidemiol. 24, 183–187.

Glynn, R.J., Schneeweiss, S., Sturmer, T., 2006. Indications for use of propensity scores and review of their use in pharmacoepidemiology. Basic Clin. Pharmacol. Tox. 98, 253–259.

Hirano, K., Imbens, G.W., 2001. Health Services & Outcome Research Methodology.

Kurth, T., Seeger, J.D., 2008. Propensity score analysis in pharmacoepidemiology. In: Pharmacoepidemiology and Therapeutic Risk Management. Harvey Whitney Books, Cincinnati, OH.

Parsons, L.S., April 22–25, 2001. Reducing bias in a propensity score matched-pair sample using greedy matching techniques. In: SAS Users Group International (SUGI) 26 Proceedings, pp. 214–226. Available from: http://www2.sas.com/proceedings/sugi26/proceed.pdf.

Reynolds, M.W., Fahrbach, K., Hauch, O., Wygant, G., Estok, R., Cella, C., Nalysnyk, L., 2004. Warfarin anticoagulation and outcomes in patients with atrial fibrillation: a systematic review and metaanalysis. Chest 126, 1938–1945.

Rosenbaum, P.R., Rubin, D.B., 1983. The central role of the propensity score in observational studies for causal effects. Biometrika 70, 41–55.

Schneeweiss, S., 2006. Sensitivity analysis and external adjustment for unmeasured confounders in epidemiologic database studies of therapeutics. Pharmacoepidemiol. Drug Saf. 15, 291–303.

Schneeweiss, S., Patrick, A.R., Stürmer, T., Brookhart, M.A., Avorn, J., Maclure, M., Rothman, K.J., Glynn, R.J., 2007. Increasing levels of restriction in pharmacoepidemiologic database studies of elderly and comparison with randomized trial results. Med. Care 45, S131–S142.

Schneeweiss, S., Huybrechts, K.F., Gagne, J.J., 2013. Interpreting the quality of health care database studies on the comparative effectiveness of oral anticoagulants in routine care. Comp. Effect. Res. 3, 33–41.

Seeger, J.D., Bykov, K., Bartels, D.B., Huybrechts, K., Schneeweiss, S., 2017. Propensity score weighting compared to matching in a study of dabigatran and warfarin. Drug Saf. 40, 169–181.

Stuart, E.A., Lee, B.K., Leacy, F.P., 2013. Prognostic score-based balance measures can be a useful diagnostic for propensity score methods in comparative effectiveness research. J. Clin. Epidemiol. 66 (8 Suppl.), S84–S90.

Stürmer, T., Schneeweiss, S., Avorn, J., Glynn, R.J., 2005. Adjusting effect estimates for unmeasured confounding with validation data using propensity score calibration. Am. J. Epidemiol. 162 (3), 279–289.

AHRQ Publication No. 12(13)-EHC099. In: Velentgas, P., Dreyer, N.A., Nourjah, P., Smith, S.R., Torchia, M.M. (Eds.), January 2013. Developing a Protocol for Observational Comparative Effectiveness Research: A User's Guide. Agency for Healthcare Research and Quality, Rockville, MD. Available from: www.effectivehealthcare.ahrq.gov/Methods-OCER.cfm.

Walker, A.M., Patrick, A.R., Lauer, M.S., Hornbrook, M.C., Marin, M.G., Platt, R., Roger, V.L., Stang, P., Schneeweiss, S., 2013. A tool for assessing the feasibility of comparative effectiveness research. Comp. Effect. Res. 3, 11–20.

Wang, S.V., Schneeweiss, S., Rassen, J.A., 2014. Optimal matching ratios in drug safety surveillance. Epidemiology 25, 772–773.

Disease Risk Scores

**Richard Wyss[1], Robert J. Glynn[1], Justin Bohn[1], Charles Poole[2],
Joshua J. Gagne[1], Ayad K. Ali[3]**

[1]*Brigham and Women's Hospital and Harvard Medical School, Boston, MA, United States;*
[2]*University of North Carolina at Chapel Hill, Chapel Hill, NC, United States;*
[3]*Eli Lilly and Company, Indianapolis, IN, United States*

CONTENTS

Disclaimer/
Acknowledg
ments 182

Introduction 182

Development of
Disease Risk
Scores 183
*Same-Sample Disease
Risk Scores
Estimation................. 184*
*Historical Disease Risk
Scores Estimation..... 185*

Methodological
Considerations .. 186

Disease Risk Scores
Versus Exposure
Propensity
Scores 188
*Strengths of Disease
Risk Scores 189*
*Limitations of Disease
Risk Scores 190*

Empirical
Example 190

Future
Directions 192

References 193

DISCLAIMER/ACKNOWLEDGMENTS

Part of this chapter was published in Current Epidemiology Reports in
December 2016 (Curr Epidemiol Rep. 2016; 3:277−284).

INTRODUCTION

Controlling for large numbers of confounding variables is often necessary for
estimating valid exposure effects in post-authorization safety studies (PASS)
that utilize health-care databases such as administrative claims and electronic
medical record (EMR). Standard methods for confounding control have traditionally relied on multivariable regression models. Although useful for many
situations, correct use of these models can be challenging for PASS, involving
large numbers of covariates. In these settings, explicitly modeling the modification of exposure effects by baseline covariates to account for exposure effect
heterogeneity can be difficult and substantially increases the likelihood of
model misspecification (Cochran, 1969; Sturmer et al., 2006; Arbogast and
Ray, 2009). Challenges in identifying areas of nonoverlap in covariate support
across exposure categories can further create problems with estimation of exposure effects by regression models (Patorno et al., 2013). To address these challenges, methods that collapse the information of a large set of covariates into a
single value or summary score, and then use this summary measure to assess
areas of nonoverlap in covariate support, control for confounding, and evaluate effect modification have become increasingly popular.

As discussed in Chapter 5.1, exposure propensity scores (EPS) technique has
been the most widely used summary measure and has become a standard
tool for confounding control in pharmacoepidemiologic studies, including
PASS (Rosenbaum and Rubin, 1983; Sturmer et al., 2006). An alternative

summary score to EPS is the prognostic scores technique, often referred to as disease risk scores (DRS). Instead of summarizing covariate associations with exposure, DRS act as "prognostic balancing scores" by summarizing covariate associations with potential outcomes (Hansen, 2008).

The idea of using an outcome summary measure to control for confounding was introduced several decades before the advent of EPS (Belson, 1956; Peters, 1941). The proposed method included fitting a risk model within the control population and then using the predicted values from this fitted model as a way to reduce dimensionality when matching. Later, it was proposed to stratify on a "multivariate confounder score" by fitting an outcome model to the full study population as a function of baseline confounders and exposure, and then assigning risk scores after setting exposure status to zero (Miettinen, 1976).

Despite the early introduction of using risk summary measures for confounding control, their use was impeded in part because of a simulation study that examined their statistical properties, which demonstrated that adjustment for DRS can result in exaggerated statistical significance of effect estimates (Pike et al., 1979; Arbogast and Ray, 2009). However, after reexamining these findings, it was found that this exaggeration is small except when there is a very strong correlation between confounders and exposures (correlation coefficient exceeding 90%) (Cook and Goldman, 1989; Arbogast and Ray, 2009, 2011). These settings are uncommon in practice and result in poor exposure equipoise, limiting the ability to conduct valid analyses to begin with (Cook and Goldman, 1989; Arbogast and Ray, 2009; Patorno et al., 2013). It was further explained that this exaggerated statistical significance is not a property of DRS themselves, but a result of model misspecification and overfitting that can occur when fitting the DRS model (Hansen, 2008; Leacy and Stuart, 2014).

Recently, it was shown that DRS act as prognostic balancing scores that can yield valid effect estimates with causal interpretations. Due in part to this recent theoretical work, there has been an increased interest in the application of DRS for confounding control with a recent surge in the number of applications of DRS in drug safety research (Arbogast and Ray, 2009; Cadarette et al., 2010; Wyss et al., 2014, 2015; Kumamaru et al., 2016a,b). They have also become increasingly used in clinical medicine to direct treatment decisions and evaluate exposure effect heterogeneity (Teasdale and Jennett, 1974; Knaus et al., 1991; Gail et al., 1999; Lyden et al., 1999; Freedman et al., 2011; Wang et al., 2016).

DEVELOPMENT OF DISEASE RISK SCORES

A formal definition of DRS and their balancing properties requires first introducing notation from counterfactual theory for potential outcomes. The counterfactual framework is fundamental to causal inference and an understanding of DRS (Neyman, 1923; Rubin, 1974; Robins, 1986). According to the potential outcomes framework for a binary exposure (E), each individual is assigned two potential (counterfactual) outcomes corresponding to each possible treatment assignment. Let (O_1) represents the potential outcome had the individual exposed to the medicinal product of interest (E = 1) and (O_0) the potential outcome had the individual exposed to the comparator product (E = 0). In practice, only one of the potential outcomes is observed. Let O represents the observed outcome, which corresponds with either O_1 or O_0 depending on whether the individual received the exposure or the comparator products. Furthermore, let Z represents a set of measured baseline covariates with EPS(Z) the EPS and DRS(Z) the DRS, both as a function of the baseline covariate Z.

EPS(Z) is formally defined as the conditional probability of exposure E given a set of baseline covariates Z. As mentioned in Chapter 4, conditioning on EPS(Z) is sufficient to balance the distribution of baseline covariates Z across exposure groups. This type of covariate balance has been termed "propensity balance" (Hansen, 2008).

DRS(Z) is formally defined as any function that balances covariates with respect to the potential outcome under the control condition O_0. This form of covariate balance has been termed "prognostic balance" (Hansen, 2008). In other words, DRS do not control for confounding by balancing covariates across exposures, but with respect to O_0. If the outcome is binary, or if the function relating O_0 to Z follows a generalized linear model, then DRS(Z) is simply the expected value of O_0 given Z, which is equivalent to the predicted values from the regression function relating O_0 to Z. Because O_0 is not observed for all individuals in the study population, O_0 cannot be modeled directly within the full study cohort. Consequently, modeling DRS in practice has challenges and requires additional assumptions that are not shared by EPS.

Same-Sample Disease Risk Scores Estimation

DRS have traditionally been estimated using one of two methods that have been termed "same-sample estimation". The first is to fit a regression model only to individuals receiving the control or comparator medicinal product, where O_0 is observed, then extrapolate this model to predict the disease risk for all individuals within the full cohort (Peters, 1941). The second strategy involves fitting a regression model to all individuals in the study cohort as a function of baseline covariates and exposure; risk scores are then assigned to each individual after setting exposure status to zero (Miettinen, 1976).

Fitting DRS to the full cohort benefits from increased sample size but can be particularly sensitive to model misspecification because it requires having to accurately model the relationship between exposure and outcome, including any potential exposure effect heterogeneity (Hansen, 2008). Incorrectly modeling the modification of exposure by baseline covariates can result in estimated scores that are influenced by the magnitude of exposure effect. This dependence between the estimated scores and exposure effect can obscure the overall effect estimate and generate false signals of effect modification along the distribution of the estimated risk scores (Leacy and Stuart, 2014).

On the other hand, accurately modeling DRS using only the comparator cohort presents its own challenges. Fitting DRS to only the comparator group can substantially increase the potential for overfitting the model to the comparator population, which is particularly concerning for PASS, involving rare outcomes or small samples (Glynn et al., 2012). Overfitting the risk model to the comparator group will result in overestimating disease risk for high-risk comparator individuals, while underestimating disease risk for low-risk comparator individuals. This type of overfitting can itself lead to false signals of effect modification across levels of disease risk and biased effect estimates.

In other words, risk models that are fitted to only the comparator group are more sensitive to problems caused by overfitting and model extrapolation, whereas fitting DRS to the full population is generally more sensitive to model misspecification. The performance of these same-sample estimation strategies have been evaluated in simulation studies and showed that when the DRS model is correctly specified, modeling DRS using the full cohort tended to perform better in terms of confounding control compared with modeling DRS only within the comparator cohort (Arbogast and Ray, 2011). However, these studies did not consider scenarios, involving model misspecification, and generalizability was lacking in the results. Although using the full sample to model DRS may be optimal when DRS model is correctly specified, the assumptions necessary for full sample estimation of the DRS can be very strong. Correctly modeling exposure effect heterogeneity by baseline covariates can be difficult, particularly for large numbers of covariates. In general, it is recommended using only the comparator cohort when using same-sample estimation for DRS to avoid the strong assumptions required for modeling the relationship between the exposure and outcome and to avoid any problems that can arise from dependence between the estimated scores and the exposure effects (Hansen, 2008).

Historical Disease Risk Scores Estimation

Recently, alternative strategies for estimating DRS that use data from outside the defined study cohort have been proposed. Modeling DRS within a historical set of controls can circumvent the complications of same-sample estimation by avoiding having to explicitly model exposure effect heterogeneity and reducing the likelihood of overfitting the risk model to the comparator cohort

(Hansen, 2008). Using historical data to estimate DRS can be particularly advantageous for evaluating the safety of new medicinal products and evolving products (Glynn et al., 2012).

The use of historical data to fit the risk model has gained in popularity in drug safety research with a number of recent studies implementing this approach (Glynn et al., 2012; Wyss et al., 2015; Kumamaru et al., 2016a,b). However, this strategy can also be challenging as it requires strong assumptions that the effects of covariates on the outcome, disease surveillance, covariate and outcome definitions, and coding practices do not change over time or across populations. Although studies have illustrated that historical estimation of DRS can perform well in certain settings, other studies have also discussed challenges with generalizing a historically fitted risk model to the study population (Kumamaru et al., 2016a).

When estimating DRS, these challenges highlight the difficulty of using risk scores for confounding control and illustrate why previous studies have found that DRS adjustment can result in exaggerated statistical significance of effect estimates (Pike et al., 1979). However, when DRS can be accurately modeled, the prognostic balance that results from DRS adjustment is sufficient to remove bias caused by measured confounders (Hansen, 2008). Although an accurately modeled DRS is sufficient to remove confounding bias, there are some notable differences in both the types of causal effects that can be estimated and necessary assumptions for causal inference when using EPS versus DRS for confounding control.

METHODOLOGICAL CONSIDERATIONS

In Chapter 5.1 we mentioned that EPS can be implemented through a variety of techniques. Confounding control with DRS has also been implemented through similar techniques, including matching, stratification, or covariate adjustment (Arbogast and Ray, 2009; Tadrous et al., 2013; Connolly and Gagne, 2016; Kumamaru et al., 2016b). Unlike EPS, there is currently no theoretical justification or examples in the pharmacoepidemiologic literature that illustrate methods for weighting on DRS.

If the exposure effect is modified by baseline patient characteristics, different methods for implementing EPS can yield effect estimates that are generalizable to different populations. For example, population average exposure effect (AEE) can be estimated through IPTW or the average exposure effect among the treated (AET) through SMR weighting (see Chapter 5.1 for more details on these weighting strategies). Matching on EPS yields an effect estimate that is generalizable to the exposed within the matched population, which is equivalent to AET when the entire exposure group can be matched. By stratifying on

EPS and then taking a weighted average of the stratum-specific estimates, investigators can obtain an estimate for the AEE, AET, or some other subgroup of the population, depending on how the individual strata are weighted (Brookhart et al., 2013).

In contrast, adjustment based on DRS yields effect estimates that are generalizable to only the exposed population or subgroups of the exposed population (Hansen, 2008). For example, if interest lies in evaluating exposure effect across levels of disease risk through DRS stratification, then the effect estimate within each stratum would be generalizable to the exposed population within that stratum. Both stratification and matching on DRS could also yield an overall estimate of the AET. In the case of DRS stratification, this would be done through a weighted combination of the strata-specific estimates with weights reflecting the distribution of the exposed population across the defined strata. In the presence of effect modification; however, investigators cannot obtain an estimated of the AEE by conditioning on the DRS alone. Estimation of the AEE through DRS adjustment would require investigators to explicitly model effect modification by baseline covariates after conditioning on the DRS (Hansen, 2008).

To illustrate, consider the hypothetical study population shown in Fig. 5.2.1, consisting of an exposure, an outcome, and a single baseline covariate Z. In this example, Z is unassociated with the outcome within the unexposed population, which implies that baseline risk is balanced across exposure groups. However, the variable Z does modify the effect of exposure on the outcome and is also associated with exposure. If we calculate the unadjusted risk difference in this population, we obtain a value of 0.23. This value is equivalent to the adjusted risk difference (adjusting for Z) that is standardized to the exposed population (i.e., AET). However, the adjusted risk difference that is

(A) Z = 1

Exposed	Outcome		Total
	Yes	No	
Yes	12	8	20
No	3	27	30
Total	15	35	50

Risk in Exposed = 0.6
Risk in Unexposed = 0.1
Risk Difference = 0.5

(B) Z = 0

Exposed	Outcome		Total
	Yes	No	
Yes	8	32	40
No	1	9	10
Total	9	41	50

Risk in Exposed = 0.2
Risk in Unexposed = 0.1
Risk Difference = 0.1

(C) Total

Exposed	Outcome		Total
	Yes	No	
Yes	20	40	60
No	4	36	40
Total	24	76	100

Risk in Exposed = 0.33
Risk in Unexposed = 0.1
Risk Difference = 0.23
Adjusted Risk Difference (AET) = 0.23
Adjusted Risk Difference (AEE) = 0.3

FIGURE 5.2.1
Illustration of stratification on DRS in the presence of effect modification.

standardized to the full study population (i.e., AEE) is 0.3. In other words, balancing disease risk across exposure groups only allows for the estimation of exposure effects that are generalizable to the exposed population, or when evaluating exposure effects within subgroups defined by the DRS, the exposed population within the given subgroup (Hansen, 2008).

The DRS is more restricted in being able to produce estimates that generalize to various study populations but is less restricted in certain assumptions that are necessary for causal inference. A necessary condition for the application of EPS technique is positivity or the condition that there be no covariate patters at which the medicinal product under investigation is received or not received with certainty (Westreich and Cole, 2010). DRS require a weaker condition that there would be no values of disease risk at which the product of interest is received or not received with certainty (Hansen, 2008). This condition has been termed "risk positivity" (Wyss et al., 2017). Although prognostic balance does not allow for the identification of AEE that is generalizable to the full study population, DRS analyses can potentially include a larger proportion of the study population when estimating the AET and can potentially evaluate exposure effects within certain subgroups of the exposed population where EPS analyses may be problematic (Hansen, 2008; Wyss et al., 2015).

DISEASE RISK SCORES VERSUS EXPOSURE PROPENSITY SCORES

Despite challenges to modeling and evaluating the validity of DRS, DRS can have advantages over EPS in certain settings. Risk scores in general provide a natural measure to evaluate exposure effect heterogeneity. Health-care professionals are often concerned about the modification of exposure effects according to patient's baseline risk for the outcome (Kent et al., 2010; Burke et al., 2014). Disease management guidelines in clinical medicine often require benefit-risk assessments within categories of disease risk (Ridker et al., 2010). For example, the Framingham risk score is widely used to help clinicians identify patient populations that are more likely to benefit from medicinal products for cardiovascular disease. Other risk scores that are used to guide prescribing decisions include the Gail model for invasive breast cancer (Gail et al., 1999; Freedman et al., 2011), the National Institutes of Health stroke scale (Lyden et al., 1999), the Glasgow coma scale (Teasdale and Jennett, 1974), and the acute physiology and chronic health evaluation (APACHE) II score for disease severity (Knaus et al., 1991). Evaluating exposure effect heterogeneity across the distribution of DRS provides a straightforward approach for clinicians to identify subgroups of patients that are most likely to benefit from the medicinal product, thereby improving prescribing decisions made by clinicians.

During the early periods of medicinal product authorization, factors affecting disease risk are more likely to be stable over time than are factors affecting treatment, potentially simplifying the estimation of DRS compared to a time-varying EPS (Seeger et al., 2007; Glynn et al., 2012; Mack et al., 2013). Moreover, when EPS and DRS control for the same set of covariates, the overlap in the distribution of DRS across exposure groups will always be at least as great as—and potentially much greater than—the overlap in the distribution of the EPS across exposures (Wyss et al., 2015). This increase in overlap can be particularly beneficial in PASS for medicinal products during early periods of marketing authorization where the separation in EPS distributions can be particularly strong (Schneeweiss et al., 2011; Gagne et al., 2013; Franklin et al., 2014). In such settings, DRS matched or stratified analyses can potentially improve the precision of the effect estimate and provide a more accurate estimate of the AET by including a larger proportion of the exposed population in the analysis (Wyss et al., 2015).

DRS models are also less likely to be negatively impacted by the inclusion of instrumental variables (i.e., variables that affect exposure but are unrelated to the outcome except through exposure). Previous studies have shown that adjusting for instrumental variables can decrease the precision of effect estimates and increase bias in the presence of unmeasured confounding (Brookhart, 2006; Bhattacharya and Vogt, 2007; Myers et al., 2011; Pearl, 2011; Wooldridge, 2016). With EPS directly modeling exposure assignment, excluding instrumental variables from EPS models can be challenging, particularly when controlling for large numbers of confounding, e.g., via high-dimensional propensity scores (Schneeweiss et al., 2009). By modeling covariate associations with the outcome, excluding instrumental variables is more natural for DRS models, particularly when using a historical set of controls prior to the introduction of exposure to model the DRS (Wyss et al., 2014). Chapter 5.3 introduces instrumental variables as a means for bias mitigation in PASS.

As the use of DRS continues to increase, it is important to understand the limitations and challenges of estimating DRS in practice. Recognizing situations where application of DRS or EPS methods can be problematic or beneficial can help to improve the robustness of causal inference when using summary scores to control for confounding in PASS.

Strengths of Disease Risk Scores

Compared to EPS, DRS have many advantages. DRS provide a natural scale to evaluate exposure effect heterogeneity and help guide clinical decision-making for prescribing medicinal products. Also, DRS are more biological in nature and stable over time, which can allow investigators to use historical data from outside the study cohort to model the DRS. This can be advantageous in settings, involving newly authorized products, where there may be limited data available to estimate EPS.

Adjustments based on DRS require a less restrictive positivity condition; and as mentioned earlier, the overlap in the distribution of DRS across exposure groups will always be at least as great as—and likely greater than—the overlap in EPS distributions across exposures (Wyss et al., 2015). Consequently, DRS adjustments are less restrictive than adjustments based on EPS. PASS using DRS have the potential to compare a larger proportion of the population across exposure groups compared with EPS-based PASS and can even allow for the estimation of exposure effects within subgroups of the population where EPS adjustments may be difficult or infeasible (Hansen, 2008).

Furthermore, settings involving a rare exposure have limited impact on DRS but can limit the ability to accurately model EPS; and DRS models are less likely to be negatively affected by instrumental variables, in particular when using a historical set of controls prior to adding exposure to model the DRS (Wyss et al., 2014).

Limitations of Disease Risk Scores

There are disadvantages and challenges in using DRS for confounding control as compared with EPS. Accurately modeling DRS in practice is generally more challenging and requires additional assumptions compared with modeling EPS. EPS models can be evaluated directly in their ability to control for confounding by assessing covariate balance across exposure groups after EPS adjustment. However, the prognostic balance that results from DRS adjustment cannot be evaluated within the full study population, and evaluating DRS in their ability to control for confounding remains a challenge compared with evaluating the validity of EPS models (Hansen, 2006; Wyss et al., 2017).

Additionally, settings involving rare outcomes (as with most PASS) greatly limit the ability to model DRS, although using historical data could help to overcome this limitation. Also, it is important to understand that the prognostic balance that results from DRS adjustment allows for the estimation of exposure effects that are only generalizable to the exposed population (AET), or when evaluating exposure effects within subgroups defined by disease risk, the exposed population within the given subgroup (Hansen, 2008).

EMPIRICAL EXAMPLE

We provide the following empirical example comparing dabigatran, an oral anticoagulant agent, versus warfarin in preventing major bleeding events to illustrate the discussed concepts of DRS and highlight that accurately modeling DRS in practice is generally more challenging compared with modeling EPS.

In a longitudinal cohort of initiators of study drugs who were enrolled in an administrative claims database between 2010 and 2013 were identified. To illustrate DRS estimation approaches, two cohorts were assembled, the *concurrent cohort* (including all patients in the above time frame) and the *historical cohort* (including warfarin initiators between 2009 and 2010). Patient selection criteria were applied to both cohorts. Patients were followed in an intention-to-treat approach, where follow-up continued until the occurrence of the outcome of interest (major bleeding event), study termination (end of 2013), or end of enrollment, whichever came first. Baseline covariates were measured during 12-month period prior to study drug initiation.

We implemented two approaches for estimating DRS for comparison. For both approaches, we fit a logistic regression model for the probability of experiencing a major bleeding event, including terms for the main effects of the baseline covariates. For the first DRS estimation method, we fit the logistic model among historical warfarin initiators only. Coefficients from this model were then used to predict DRS for all patients (both dabigatran and warfarin initiators) in the concurrent cohort (historical DRS estimation). For the second estimation approach, we fit the logistic model within the concurrent population of warfarin initiators and then used this model to predict DRS for each patient in the study population (same-sample DRS estimation).

For comparison, we also constructed an EPS model by fitting a logistic regression model for the probability of initiating dabigatran in the concurrent cohort, including terms for the main effects of baseline covariates. All covariates included in the EPS model were the same as those in the DRS model, with the exception of two covariates due to extremely strong associations with exposure.

Covariate balance was checked by comparing absolute standardized mean differences in covariates between dabigatran and warfarin initiators, in unmatched and matched cohorts. We also evaluated the predictive performance of the fitted EPS and DRS models by calculating the C-statistic (discrimination) and Hosmer–Lemeshow (HL) P-value (calibration). Cox proportional hazards models were used to compare the rate of major bleeding events among study drugs. Dabigatran initiators were matched to warfarin initiators in a 1:1 manner using a caliper of 10% times the standard deviation of the EPS or DRS. Hazard ratios (HR) in the matched analysis were estimated with Cox proportional hazards models, including a single term for dabigatran initiation and without stratification on the matched set.

The overlap in the distribution of DRS, for both historical and concurrent DRS, was slightly greater than the overlap in EPS across study drugs. However, differences were small as illustrated by the size of the matched cohorts (cohort sizes based on EPS matching of 43,942 vs. 45,480 and 45,488 in historical DRS and concurrent DRS matching, respectively).

Table 5.2.1 Empirical Example on Disease Risk Scores Application

| Method | Sample Size | Major Bleeding Events Dabigatran Versus Warfarin | | Performance | |
		HR	95% CI	C-statistic	HL *P*-value
Unadjusted	79,112	0.63	0.58–0.68	n/a	n/a
EPS matched	43,942	0.81	0.74–0.89	0.70	0.08
DRS matched historical	45,480	0.76	0.69–0.84	0.65	<0.01
DRS matched concurrent	45,488	0.77	0.70–0.84	0.67	<0.01

EPS, *exposure propensity scores;* HL, *Hosmer–Lemeshow;* HR, *Hazard ratios*

As expected, after matching on EPS, covariates were approximately balanced across exposure groups, whereas DRS models did not balance covariates with respect to exposure. We emphasize that DRS is not expected to balance covariates across exposure groups, and we simply included DRS models for illustrative purposes. As previously discussed, DRS controls for confounding by balancing covariates with respect to the potential outcome under the control condition (in this study warfarin), which cannot be evaluated directly within the full study population. Therefore, we evaluated the fitted DRS models through their predictive performance.

Both DRS models resulted in poor predictive performance for major bleeding events (C-statistic of 0.65 and 0.67 for historical and concurrent models, respectively; and HL *P*-values <.01 for both models). The fitted EPS model had better predictive performance for modeling exposure assignment (C-statistic of 0.7 and *P*-value of .08). Matching on EPS resulted in an effect estimate that is more consistent with RCT compared with matching on either the historical or concurrent DRS (Table 5.2.1).

FUTURE DIRECTIONS

Combining EPS with DRS through joint subclassification or matching has been proposed as a way to improve the robustness of causal inference when using summary scores for confounding control (Hansen, 2008; Leacy and Stuart, 2014). Although initial inspections of the joint use of EPS and DRS seem promising, benefits and challenges of these approaches remain largely unclear, particularly in settings, involving large databases (see Chapter 3.4 on big data in PASS). Strategies for trimming on DRS or jointly trimming on both DRS and EPS may also improve the robustness of causal inference in PASS by restricting the analysis to a population where there is strong equipoise.

Although a number of studies have discussed strategies and advantages of trimming on EPS, more research is needed on the performance and recommendations for DRS trimming (Crump et al., 2009; Sturmer et al., 2010; Walker, 2013).

DRS may also have benefits in designs other than cohorts. One study showed that matching on DRS may be advantageous in nested case–control studies to improve the precision of effect estimates (Desai et al., 2016). Furthermore, DRS may also have benefits for regression discontinuity designs (Hansen, 2008; Bor et al., 2014), which have been proposed for interventional and noninterventional PASS, including proactive safety surveillance settings (O'Keeffe et al., 2014; Walkey and Bor, 2015). Research is needed on the benefits and limitations of applying DRS in these alternative study designs.

Finally, additional research is needed on the performance of different strategies for modeling DRS. As previously discussed, modeling DRS in practice can be challenging and has limitations that are not shared by EPS. Recent studies have proposed ways to improve the robustness of DRS estimation, including shrinkage methods to reduce the dimensionality of covariates to limit problems with model extrapolation when fitting high-dimensional DRS models within historical data (Kumamaru et al., 2016b). In addition, leave-one-out and repeated split-sample regression methods have been proposed to avoid problems with extrapolation when modeling DRS within the same comparator population that is used in the study analysis (Abadie et al., 2014). However, more applications of these strategies are needed to elucidate the benefits and limitations of these approaches. The optimal strategy for modeling DRS in time-to-event data remains unclear. More research is needed on the potential use of survival models for estimating disease risk in these setting.

References

Abadie, A., Chingos, M.M., West, M.R., 2014. Endogenous Stratification in Randomized Experiments. NBER Working Paper, p. 19742. Available from: https://www.princeton.edu/~erp/erp%20seminar%20pdfs/stratification%20(Abadi).pdf.

Arbogast, P.G., Ray, W.A., 2009. Use of disease risk scores in pharmacoepidemiologic studies. Stat. Methods Med. Res. 18 (1), 67–80.

Arbogast, P.G., Ray, W.A., 2011. Performance of disease risk scores, propensity scores, and traditional multivariable outcome regression in the presence of multiple confounders. Am. J. Epidemiol. 174 (5), 613–620.

Belson, W.A., 1956. A technique for studying the effects of a television broadcast. J. R. Stat. Soc. 5 (3), 195–202.

Bhattacharya, J., Vogt, W.B., 2007. Do Instrumental Variables Belong in Propensity Scores? NBER Technical Working Paper, p. 343. Available from: http://www.nber.org/papers/t0343.pdf.

Bor, J., Moscoe, E., Mutevedzi, P., Newell, M.L., Barnighausen, T., 2014. Regression discontinuity designs in epidemiology: causal inference without randomized trials. Epidemiology 25 (5), 729–737.

Brookhart, M.A., Wyss, R., Layton, J.B., Sturmer, T., 2013. Propensity score methods for confounding control in nonexperimental research. Circ. Cardiovasc. Qual. Outcomes 6 (5), 604–611.

Burke, J.F., Hayward, R.A., Nelson, J.P., Kent, D.M., 2014. Using internally developed risk models to assess heterogeneity in treatment effects in clinical trials. Circ. Cardiovasc. Qual. Outcomes. 7 (1), 163–169.

Cadarette, S.M., Gagne, J.J., Solomon, D.H., Katz, J.N., Sturmer, T., 2010. Confounder summary scores when comparing the effects of multiple drug exposures. Pharmacoepidemiol. Drug Saf. 19 (1), 2–9.

Cochran, W.G., 1969. The use of covariance in observational studies. J. R. Stat. Soc. Ser. C 18 (3), 270–275.

Connolly, J.G., Gagne, J.J., 2016. Comparison of calipers for matching on the disease risk score. Am. J. Epidemiol. 183 (10), 937–948.

Cook, E.F., Goldman, L., 1989. Performance of tests of significance based on stratification by a multivariate confounder score or by a propensity score. J. Clin. Epidemiol. 42 (4), 317–324.

Crump, R.K., Hotz, V.J., Imbens, G.W., Mitnik, O.A., 2009. Dealing with limited overlap in estimation of average treatment effects. Biometrika 96 (1), 187–199.

Desai, R.J., Glynn, R.H., Wang, S., Gagne, J.J., 2016. Performance of disease risk score matching in nested case-control studies: a simulation study. Am. J. Epidemiol. 183 (10), 949–957.

Franklin, J.M., Rassen, J.A., Bartels, D.B., Schneeweiss, S., 2014. Prospective cohort studies of newly marketed medications: using covariate data to inform the design of large-scale studies. Epidemiology 25 (1), 126–133.

Freedman, A.N., Yu, B., Gail, M.H., Costantino, J.P., Graubard, B.I., Vogel, V.G., McCaskill-Stevens, W., 2011. Benefit/risk assessment for breast cancer chemoprevention with raloxifene or tamoxifen for women age 50 years or older. J. Clin. Oncol. 29 (17), 2327–2333.

Gagne, J.J., Bykov, K., Willke, R.J., Kahler, K.H., Subedi, P., Schneeweiss, S., 2013. Treatment dynamics of newly marketed drugs and implications for comparative effectiveness research. Value Health 16 (6), 1054–1062.

Gail, M.H., Costantino, J.P., Bryant, J., Croyle, R., Freedman, L., Helzlsouer, K., Vogel, V., 1999. Weighing the risks and benefits of tamoxifen treatment for preventing breast cancer. J. Natl. Cancer Inst. 91 (21), 1829–1846.

Glynn, R.J., Gagne, J.J., Schneeweiss, S., 2012. Role of disease risk scores in comparative effectiveness research with emerging therapies. Pharmacoepidemiol. Drug Saf. 21 (Suppl. 2), 138–147.

Hansen, B.B., 2008. The prognostic analogue of the propensity score. Biometrika 95, 481–488.

Hansen, B.B., June 2006. Bias reduction in observational studies via prognosis scores. Technical Report No. 441. Statistics Department, University of Michigan, Ann Arbor, Michigan. Available from: http://dept.stat.lsa.umich.edu/~bbh/rspaper2006-06.pdf.

Kent, D.M., Rothwell, P.M., Ioannidis, J.P., Altman, D.G., Hayward, R.A., 2010. Assessing and reporting heterogeneity in treatment effects in clinical trials: a proposal. Trial 11, 85.

Knaus, W.A., Wagner, D.P., Draper, E.A., Zimmerman, J.E., Bergner, M., Bastos, P.G., et al., 1991. The APACHE III prognostic system. Risk prediction of hospital mortality for critically ill hospitalized adults. Chest 100 (6), 1619–1636.

Kumamaru, H., Gagne, J.J., Glynn, R.J., Setoguchi, S., Schneeweiss, S., 2016a. Comparison of high-dimensional confounder summary scores in comparative studies of newly marketed medications. J. Clin. Epidemiol. 76, 200–208.

Kumamaru, H., Schneeweiss, S., Glynn, R.J., Setoguchi, S., Gagne, J.J., 2016b. Dimension reduction and shrinkage methods for high dimensional disease risk scores in historical data. Emerg. Themes Epidemiol. 13, 5.

Leacy, F.P., Stuart, E.A., 2014. On the joint use of propensity and prognostic scores in estimation of the average treatment effect on the treated: a simulation study. Stat. Med. 33 (20), 3488–3508.

Lyden, P., Lu, M., Jackson, C., Marler, J., Kothari, R., Brott, T., Zivin, J., 1999. Underlying structure of the national Institutes of health stroke scale: results of a factor analysis. NINDS tPA Stroke Trial Investigators. Stroke 30 (11), 2347–2354.

Mack, C.D., Glynn, R.J., Brookhart, M.A., Carpenter, W.R., Meyer, A.M., Sandler, R.S., Sturmer, T., 2013. Calendar time-specific propensity scores and comparative effectiveness research for stage III colon cancer chemotherapy. Pharmacoepidemiol. Drug Saf. 22 (8), 810–818.

Miettinen, O.S., 1976. Stratification by a multivariate confounder score. Am. J. Epidemiol. 104 (6), 609–620.

Myers, J.A., Rassen, J.A., Gagne, J.J., Huybrechts, K.F., Schneeweiss, S., Rothman, K.J., Glynn, R.J., 2011. Effects of adjusting for instrumental variables on bias and precision of effect estimates. Am. J. Epidemiol. 174 (11), 1213–1222.

Neyman, J., 1923. On the application of probability theory to agricultural experiments. Essay on principles. Section 9 Stat. Sci. 5, 465–472.

O'Keeffe, A.G., Geneletti, S., Baio, G., Sharples, L.D., Nazareth, I., Petersen, I., 2014. Regression discontinuity designs: an approach to the evaluation of treatment efficacy in primary care using observational data. BMJ 349 g5293.

Patorno, E., Grotta, A., Bellocco, R., Schneeweiss, S., 2013. Propensity score methodology for confounding control in health care utilization databases. Epidemiol. Biostat. Public Health 10 (3).

Pearl, J., 2011. Invited commentary: understanding bias amplification. Am. J. Epidemiol. 174 (11), 1223–1227 discussion pg 1228-1229.

Peters, C.C., 1941. A method of matching groups for experiment with no loss of population. J. Educ. Res. 34 (8), 606–612.

Pike, M.C., Anderson, J., Day, N., 1979. Some insights into Miettinen's multivariate confounder score approach to case-control study analysis. Epidemiol. Community Health 33 (1), 104–106.

Ridker, P.M., Macfadyen, J.G., Nordestgaard, B.G., Koenig, W., Kastelein, J.J., Genest, J., Glynn, R.J., 2010. Rosuvastatin for primary prevention among individuals with elevated high-sensitivity c-reactive protein and 5% to 10% and 10% to 20% 10-year risk. Implications of the Justification for Use of Statins in Prevention: an Intervention Trial Evaluating Rosuvastatin (JUPITER) trial for "intermediate risk". Circ. Cardiovasc. Qual. Outcomes 3 (5), 447–452.

Robins, J.M., 1986. A new approach to causal inference in mortality studies with sustained exposure periods. Math. Model. 7, 1393–1512.

Rosenbaum, P.R., Rubin, D.B., 1983. The central role of the propensity score in observational studies for causal effects. Biometrika 70, 41–55.

Rubin, D.B., 1974. Estimating causal effects of treatments in randomized and nonrandomized studies. J. Educ. Psychol. 66, 668–701.

Schneeweiss, S., Rassen, J.A., Glynn, R.J., Avorn, J., Mogun, H., Brookhart, M.A., 2009. High-dimensional propensity score adjustment in studies of treatment effects using health care claims data. Epidemiology 20 (4), 512–522.

Schneeweiss, S., Gagne, J.J., Glynn, R.J., Ruhl, M., Rassen, J.A., 2011. Assessing the comparative effectiveness of newly marketed medications: methodological challenges and implications for drug development. Clin. Pharmacol. Ther. 90 (6), 777–790.

Seeger, J.D., Kurth, T., Walker, A.M., 2007. Use of propensity score technique to account for exposure-related covariates: an example and lesson. Med. Care 45 (10 Suppl. 2), S143–S148.

Sturmer, T., Joshi, M., Glynn, R.J., Avorn, J., Rothman, K.J., Schneeweiss, S., 2006. A review of the application of propensity score methods yielded increasing use, advantages in specific settings, but not substantially different estimates compared with conventional multivariable methods. J. Clin. Epidemiol. 59 (5), 437–447.

Sturmer, T., Rothman, K.J., Avorn, J., Glynn, R.J., 2010. Treatment effects in the presence of unmeasured confounding: dealing with observations in the tails of the propensity score distribution—a simulation study. Am. J. Epidemiol. 172 (7), 843–854.

Tadrous, M., Gagne, J.J., Sturmer, T., Cadarette, S.M., 2013. Disease risk score as a confounder summary method: systematic review and recommendations. Pharmacoepidemiol. Drug Saf. 22 (2), 122–129.

Teasdale, G., Jennett, B., 1974. Assessment of coma and impaired consciousness. A practical scale. Lancet 2 (7872), 81–84.

Walker, A.M., Patrick, A.R., Lauer, M.S., Hornbrook, M.C., Marin, M.G., Platt, R., Schneeweiss, S., 2013. A tool for assessing the feasibility of comparative effectiveness research. Comp. Effect. Res. 2013 (3), 11–20.

Walkey, A.J., Bor, J., 2015. Risk-based heterogeneity of treatment effect in trials and implications for surveillance of clinical effectiveness using regression discontinuity designs. Am. J. Respir. Crit. Care Med. 192 (11), 1399.

Wang, S.V., Franklin, J.M., Glynn, R.J., Schneeweiss, S., Eddings, W., Gagne, J.J., 2016. Prediction of rates of thromboembolic and major bleeding outcomes with dabigatran or warfarin among patients with atrial fibrillation: new initiator cohort study. BMJ 353 i2607.

Westreich, D., Cole, S.R., 2010. Invited commentary: positivity in practice. Am. J. Epidemiol. 171 (6), 674–677 discussion 678–681.

Wooldridge, J.M., 2016. Should instrumental variables be used as matching variables? Res. Econ. 70, 232–237.

Wyss, R., Lunt, M., Brookhart, M.A., Glynn, R.J., Sturmer, T., 2014. Reducing bias amplification in the presence of unmeasured confounding through out-of-sample estimation strategies for the disease risk score. J. Causal Inference 2 (2), 131–146.

Wyss, R., Ellis, A.R., Brookhart, M.A., Jonsson Funk, M., Girman, C.J., Simpson Jr., R.J., Sturmer, T., 2015. Matching on the disease risk score in comparative effectiveness research of new treatments. Pharmacoepidemiol. Drug Saf. 24 (9), 951–961.

Wyss, R., Hansen, B.B., Ellis, A.R., Gagne, J.J., Desai, R.J., Glynn, R.J., Sturmer, T., 2017. The "Dry-Run" analysis: evaluating risk scores for confounding control. Am. J. Epidemiol. 185 (9), 842–852.

Instrumental Variables

Joseph A.C. Delaney[1], Ayad K. Ali[2]

[1]*University of Washington, Seattle, WA, United States;* [2]*Eli Lilly and Company, Indianapolis, IN, United States*

INTRODUCTION

One of the key issues in pharmacoepidemiologic studies is how to handle the subtle and difficult issues of bias due to factors such as confounding by indication and the healthy user effect (Blais et al., 1996; Bosco et al., 2010; Psaty and Siscovick, 2010). These biases are persistent features of any noninterventional PASS and call into question the validity of all estimates on intended effect. The traditional solution to this problem is an expensive and time-consuming instrumental variables (IVs) analysis—typically done as a double-masked placebo-controlled RCT (Miettinen, 1983). This strong instrument has the wonderful property of removing all confounding because of the allocation of the medicinal product and is likely the only viable approach for studying intended effects in pharmacoepidemiology.

But is randomization the only viable instrument to study the effects of medicinal products? Other areas of medicine have used instruments such as geography or calendar time in attempts to get the great properties of an instrument—namely that it is inherently unconfounded, and so the investigator does not have to worry about unmeasured confounding as a source of bias (Ertefaie et al., 2017). IV are variables that are associated with the exposure, are not associated with potential confounders—measured or unmeasured, and are associated with the outcome only through their association with the exposure itself and not directly (Ali, 2011). The classical exampling of IV analysis is an intention-to-treat (ITT) analysis of RCT (as randomization is associated with exposure, not with covariates, and associated with the outcome only through exposure to the randomized medicinal product).

If the confounders are measured and can be adjusted for, there is some ability to relax the assumption that the IVs are not associated with any confounding variables. However, if there is a possibility of measured confounding being present, then it is hard to rule out unmeasured confounding, making the

CONTENTS

Introduction 197

Instrumental Variable in Noninterventional Post-Authorization Safety Studies ... 198

Methodological Considerations .. 198

Limitations of Instrumental Variable 200

References 201

underlying (and unverifiable) assumption of a valid instrument even challenging. Once the investigator is willing to live with the risk of unmeasured confounding, other approaches are likely more statistically efficient.

INSTRUMENTAL VARIABLE IN NONINTERVENTIONAL POST-AUTHORIZATION SAFETY STUDIES

In noninterventional PASS, prescriber preference was proposed as an IV as an alternative to traditional randomization approaches, under the theory that (within a product class) there would be an inherently random element (Brookhart, 2006). The key feature was to extract this preference in a way that it was unrelated to the characteristics of the patient who was receiving the medicinal product. It is important to note that this approach is only optimal if there are only two alternative medicinal products under study, and selection bias can result if there are additional treatment options that are not being directly considered (Swanson et al., 2015a; Ertefaie et al., 2016).

The operationalization of prescriber preference was to use the last prescription given by the prescriber (to another patient) in a place of the actual exposure given to a patient. The insight here is that if physicians prefer one medicinal product in a class to another then, on average, their patients will show a slight imbalance toward the preferred product. This type of approach gives a weak instrument, as opposed to randomization, which gives a strong instrument. Survey approaches suggest that prescriber preference might work for some examples (Boef et al., 2016), it is impossible to generalize from specific examples to suggesting that these assumptions will always be met. It is also unclear if assumptions about patient preference (the existence of patients who take the opposite of the prescriber preference to be defiant) are likely to be met, and this complicates identifying the subgroup in which this association is likely to apply (Swanson et al., 2015b).

The exact strength of prescriber preference as a variable has been debated, although specific examples have been given where the instrument is strong enough for inference (Rassen et al., 2009b). Consequently, other investigators have suggested alternative IV. For example, clinic preference for medicinal product type may actually be a stronger instrument than prescriber preference (Pratt et al., 2010; Ionescu-Ittu et al., 2012). Still, the quest for perfect IV remains.

METHODOLOGICAL CONSIDERATIONS

The strength of IV can be determined by how closely associated the instruments are with the exposure experienced by the patient. In some types of randomization, this might lead to an absolute correspondence (like with a vaccine). In other forms, the association is diluted by adherence to medicinal products, becoming weaker as the level of adherence drops. The need to have the strongest possible instrument is one of the justifications for trying to optimize adherence in RCT. With a strong instrument, it is possible to analyze the instrument directly, as a proxy for the exposure. In RCT, this is known as ITT and will generally create a conservative bias in estimation.

However, the types of variables that are considered in noninterventional PASS are weak instruments. Generally, randomization is not called an instrument in studies of drug effects but forms its own specific subfield because of the importance of randomized studies to the approval process of medicinal products. The type of weak instrument considered in noninterventional studies is far weaker than in RCT. The difference in rates of product usage due to prescriber preference may be very low, as it is diluted by other factors, such as patient preference and the heterogeneity of indications. For example, although a specific prescriber might prefer a medicinal product, specific patients will present with medical histories that may suggest alternative treatments or have preferences of their own, perhaps based on previous successful therapy. This can make the instrument quite weak.

Therefore, it requires the use of specialized regression techniques to handle weak instruments, as direct analysis of the instruments will greatly dilute the size of the effect, beyond any useful level. The most basic approach to doing this type of analysis is to use two-stage least squares (2SLS) regression to correct for the weakness of the IV. One limitation of the 2SLS regression is that it can only estimate risk differences with IV and not relative risks. Other approaches do exist to handle dichotomous outcomes for relative measures, although they are less widely used (Rassen et al., 2009a).

A typical approach to conduct a 2SLS regression is to define two separate statistical models that, in conjunction, result in an estimate of the association between the exposure and the outcome of interest. The first model predicts the probability of a patient of a given prescriber being prescribed the product of interest, conditional on the IV, and a vector of baseline covariates. In this model, the IV represents the exposure assigned to the previous patient of the same prescriber and yields coefficients that quantify the association between the IV and the actual exposure in terms of adjusted risk difference.

The second model predicts the outcome of the patient conditional on the probability of exposure to the medicinal product of interest that is estimated in the first model and observed baseline covariates. The IV estimate of the effect of the exposure on the outcome is represented as adjusted risk difference (Abrahamowicz et al., 2011).

These two multiple linear regression estimates can be combined in a number of ways, including the straightforward approach of dividing the estimate from the second model by that of the first. Confidence intervals can be obtained by bootstrapping. Clearly, a very weak instrument could create an unstable estimate (Ionescu-Ittu et al., 2009).

LIMITATIONS OF INSTRUMENTAL VARIABLE

There are limitations with IV that has limited their popularity in pharmacoepidemiologic research, including PASS. Even designed instruments, such as randomization, may fail and may result in a biased estimate. This could happen if patient allocation was not truly masked or if there was an error in the assignment of patients such that they were no longer randomly assigned to exposures. Any bias in the estimate is at risk of being amplified by the correction for the weakness of the IV, as these approaches cannot distinguish between real signal and bias, thus, correction amplifies both signals (Ionescu-Ittu et al., 2009). Furthermore, the process of correcting for the weakness of the IV innately increases the variance of the estimate, making IV estimators inefficient compared to regular regression approaches (Ertefaie et al., 2017).

The other issue with IV is that it shifts the focus of how we assess whether estimates can be considered unbiased. For most PASS, we focus on whether confounding has been fully accounted for, even if it can be challenging to handle in studies of intended effect (Miettinen, 1983). In IV analysis, the scrutiny turns to whether or not a particular instrument meets the assumptions required to be an instrument. Whether an instrument meets the second or third conditions of our definition is not something that can be verified from the actual data set, although occasionally it can be disproven (Hernán and Robins, 2006). As a result, instead of focusing on whether all of the relevant confounders have been accounted for, one focuses on whether the instrument meets the key assumptions of being an IV or not. If one is wrong, then the impact can be greater than that of many confounding scenarios because of bias amplification, resulting in quite misleading estimates of association (Pearl, 2011).

Accordingly, the key element of evaluating PASS with IV is likely skepticism. Outside of the controlled case of randomization, the assumptions are moved from easy to evaluate to complex. The cases where there is a viable instrument available are limited and are generally cases of comparative effectiveness or safety, where the instrument can be used to compare two exposure groups.

References

Abrahamowicz, M., Beauchamp, M.E., Ionescu-Ittu, R., Delaney, J.A., Pilote, L., 2011. Reducing the variance of the prescribing preference-based instrumental variable estimates of the treatment effect. Am. J. Epidemiol. 174 (4), 494–502.

Ali, A.K., 2011. Analytical approaches to achieve quasi-randomization in retrospective database analysis. ISPOR Connections 17 (2), 10–11.

Blais, L., Ernst, P., Suissa, S., 1996. Confounding by indication and channeling over time: the risks of beta 2-agonists. Am. J. Epidemiol. 144 (12), 1161–1169.

Boef, A.G., le Cessie, S., Dekkers, O.M., Frey, P., Kearney, P.M., Kerse, N., Mallen, C.D., McCarthy, V.J., Mooijaart, S.P., Muth, C., Rodondi, N., Rosemann, T., Russell, A., Schers, H., Virgini, V., de Waal, M.W., Warner, A., Gussekloo, J., den Elzen, W.P., 2016. Physician's prescribing preference as an instrumental variable: exploring assumptions using survey data. Epidemiology 27 (2), 276–283.

Bosco, J.L., Silliman, R.A., Thwin, S.S., Geiger, A.M., Buist, D.S., Prout, M.N., Yood, M.U., Haque, R., Wei, F., Lash, T.L., 2010. A most stubborn bias: no adjustment method fully resolves confounding by indication in observational studies. J. Clin. Epidemiol. 63 (1), 64–74.

Brookhart, M.A., Wang, P.S., Solomon, D.H., Schneeweiss, S., 2006. Evaluating short-term drug effects using a physician-specific prescribing preference as an instrumental variable. Epidemiology 17 (3), 268–275.

Ertefaie, A., Small, D., Flory, J., Hennessy, S., 2016. Selection bias when using instrumental variable methods to compare two treatments but more than two treatments are available. Int. J. Biostat. 12 (1), 219–232.

Ertefaie, A., Small, D.S., Flory, J.H., Hennessy, S., 2017. A tutorial on the use of instrumental variables in pharmacoepidemiology. Pharmacoepidemiol. Drug Saf. 26 (4), 357–367.

Hernán, M.A., Robins, J.M., 2006. Instruments for causal inference: an epidemiologist's dream? Epidemiology 17 (4), 360–372.

Ionescu-Ittu, R., Delaney, J.A., Abrahamowicz, M., 2009. Bias-variance trade-off in pharmacoepidemiological studies using physician-preference-based instrumental variables: a simulation study. Pharmacoepidemiol. Drug Saf. 18 (7), 562–571.

Ionescu-Ittu, R., Abrahamowicz, M., Pilote, L., February 2012. Treatment effect estimates varied depending on the definition of the provider prescribing preference-based instrumental variables. J. Clin. Epidemiol. 65 (2), 155–162.

Miettinen, O.S., 1983. The need for randomization in the study of intended effects. Stat. Med. 2 (2), 267–271.

Pearl, J., 2011. Invited commentary: understanding bias amplification. Am. J. Epidemiol. 174 (11), 1223–1227.

Pratt, N., Roughead, E.E., Ryan, P., Salter, A., July 2010. Antipsychotics and the risk of death in the elderly: an instrumental variable analysis using two preference based instruments. Pharmacoepidemiol. Drug Saf. 19 (7), 699–707.

Psaty, B.M., Siscovick, D.S., 2010. Minimizing bias due to confounding by indication in comparative effectiveness research: the importance of restriction. J. Am. Med. Assoc. 304 (8), 897–898.

Rassen, J.A., Schneeweiss, S., Glynn, R.J., Mittleman, M.A., Brookhart, M.A., 2009a. Instrumental variable analysis for estimation of treatment effects with dichotomous outcomes. Am. J. Epidemiol. 169 (3), 273–284.

Rassen, J.A., Brookhart, M.A., Glynn, R.J., Mittleman, M.A., Schneeweiss, S., 2009b. Instrumental variables II: instrumental variable application-in 25 variations, the physician prescribing preference generally was strong and reduced covariate imbalance. J. Clin. Epidemiol. 62 (12), 1233–1241.

Swanson, S.A., Robins, J.M., Miller, M., Hernán, M.A., 2015a. Selecting on treatment: a pervasive form of bias in instrumental variable analyses. Am. J. Epidemiol. 181 (3), 191–197.

Swanson, S.A., Miller, M., Robins, J.M., Hernán, M.A., 2015b. Definition and evaluation of the monotonicity condition for preference-based instruments. Epidemiology 26 (3), 414–420.

Data Analytic Platforms

Stephanie Reisinger[1], Javier Cid[1], Ayad K. Ali[2]

[1]*Evidera, Bethesda, MD, United States;* [2]*Eli Lilly and Company, Indianapolis, IN, United States*

INTRODUCTION

Health-care data have been used for secondary analysis in drug safety studies and in broader epidemiological research for decades. In recent years, the volume and variety of health-care data available for secondary analyses and real-world evidence generation is exploding, both in the United States and across the globe. In the United States, which includes administrative claims and electronic medical records (EMR). Such wealth of data is partially catalyzed by the widespread implementation of "meaningful use" regulations that offer financial incentives for health-care providers and hospitals when they use EMR to achieve specified improvements in care delivery (Blumenthal and Tavenner, 2010). As discussed in Chapter 3.2, EMR provide patient data collected at the point of care in near real-time, blurring the boundary between retrospective and prospective study designs, and sometimes allowing the combination of both (see Chapter 4.4 for an overview of enriched studies combining both primary and secondary data). In addition, many EMR systems also include previously untapped sources of real-world data, such as free-form text found in physician notes, or imaging data in therapeutic areas where images are used in diagnosis and treatment. This offers another important source of data for noninterventional PASS.

Such explosive growth in the availability of real-world data has created significant opportunities and substantial challenges, putting pressure on traditional analytic approaches. Traditional analyses include bespoke analysis programs that are developed for each study and each database. This approach is not well suited for a rapidly evolving "big data" environment for a number of reasons. The first is inefficiency; the volume of analyses that can be done using a traditional approach is constrained by the number and knowledge of programmers writing the analytic code. In addition, heterogeneity inherent in these data sources introduces the potential for errors that could result in biased results, unless programs are carefully designed and meticulously coded (Ryan et al., 2010). Furthermore, custom programs create a lack of transparency

CONTENTS

Introduction 203

Common Data Models and Modular Analysis Programs 204

Data Analytic Platforms and Transparency 205

Limitations of Data and Analysis Standardization . 207

References 207

203

as assumptions related to patient and clinical event selection, which are important for interpreting PASS results, are embedded deep within the code. Moreover, custom coding often produces results that are not reproducible or meaningfully comparable across heterogeneous data sources. Chapter 3.4 discusses the concept of big data and its application in PASS.

COMMON DATA MODELS AND MODULAR ANALYSIS PROGRAMS

The issues described above are well known by investigators using databases to conduct PASS. In 2007, these limitations came into sharp focus after the FDA Amendments Act (FDAAA) was enacted by the US Congress (FDA, 2011). Partially as a response to several high-profile drug safety issues, FDAAA mandated that the FDA creates a new national system for monitoring the safety of authorized medicinal products using sources of real-world health-care data. To meet the obligations set forth by FDAAA, the FDA and several other organizations began research into better ways to analyze large volumes of heterogeneous health-care data. The FDA Sentinel Initiative (Sentinel, 2018a), the Observational Medical Outcomes Partnership (OMOP) (Stang et al., 2010), and the Observational Health Data Sciences and Informatics (OHDSI) collaborative (OHDSI, 2017a), where all established in the United States to address this issue. Similarly, both Innovative Medicines Initiative Pharmacoepidemiological Research on Outcomes of Therapeutics (Reyonlds et al., 2016), and Exploring and Understanding Adverse Drug Reactions project (Trifiro et al., 2009) were organized in part to develop novel ways to use heterogeneous real-world data sources to better monitor the safety of medicinal products across Europe. Chapter 5.5 discusses common proactive safety surveillance systems, including Sentinel with detail.

A common focus of research across all of these projects is the development and use of standards to enable more efficient analysis of real-world data. Data standardization is accomplished through the development of Common Data Model (CDM), which imposes a standard data format and vocabulary across all data sources. Both OMOP CDM and Sentinel CDM were developed to support efficient analysis of heterogeneous data sources. In addition to standardizing the data format, a primary benefit of implementing a CDM is that Modular Analysis Programs (MAP) can be written to use the standard data format, and thus reused on any real-world database that has been transformed into the standard format. Furthermore, key patient selection and analysis variables within each standardized module can be parameterized, enabling nonprogrammer investigators to execute an analysis without requiring custom codes to be written. This modular approach also supports greater transparency because the parameters contain many of the key assumptions that were

Table 5.4.1 Example of Steps Involved in Modular Analysis Program and Associated User Parameters

Analysis Question
• How many female patients over age 60 who have been diagnoses with atrial fibrillation were treated with warfarin within 7 days of their diagnosis? • Of those patients, what percentage had a stroke in the 365 days following diagnosis?

Step	Modular Analysis Program	User Parameter
Step 1	Select all patients with demographic parameters	• Gender: female • Age: 60 years or greater
Step 2	Restrict the patients selected above to only those with diagnosis parameters	• Diagnosis: atrial fibrillation
Step 3	Further restrict the selection to those patients who were treated with exposure parameters within time frame parameters	• Exposure: warfarin • Time frame: 7 days after diagnosis
Step 4	Of those patients, what percentage were diagnosed with outcome parameters within time frame parameters	• Outcome: cerebrovascular accident • Time frame: 365 days after diagnosis

previously embedded in program codes. Both the Sentinel initiative and OHDSI collaborative have developed parameter-driven MAP as part of their respective research programs (Sentinel, 2018b; OHDSI, 2017b).

A simplified illustration of a standardized analysis using a CDM and MAP approaches is shown in Table 5.4.1 and Fig. 5.4.1. All of the demographic and clinical variables used in this example are commonly available in real-world health-care databases, e.g., claims and EMR. There are many types of analyses that lend themselves well to this type of modular approach that ranges between exploratory and descriptive analyses to comparative safety and effectiveness analyses.

DATA ANALYTIC PLATFORMS AND TRANSPARENCY

Data and program standardization have catalyzed a new breed of real-world data analytic platforms, enabling investigators to submit analysis parameters through a user-friendly interface, execute MAP across a variety of real-world data sources, and produce results rapidly without custom programming. These data platforms emphasize shortened analysis cycle times, generating results in minutes or hours for analyses that used to take days, weeks, or longer (i.e., rapid-cycle analytics). They also make it possible for stakeholders from diverse backgrounds to collaborate across a shared data and analytic infrastructure.

Step 1. Demographic Data

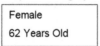

Step 2. Diagnosis Data

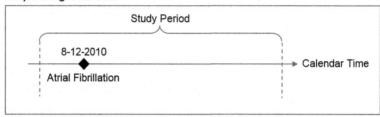

Step 3. Exposure Data

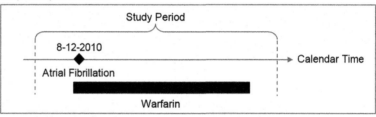

Step 4. Outcome Data

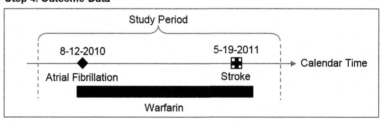

FIGURE 5.4.1

Illustration of modular analysis program applied to a patient record in CDM format.

Although the field is still in its infancy, there are several commercial organizations offering data analytic platforms built on public or proprietary data standards. In addition, the Sentinel system continues to be actively developed and used to monitor the safety of medicinal products authorized in the United States; as of January 2017, they have posted over 150 analysis results on their website that were generating using MAP and the Sentinel CDM (Sentinel, 2018b). The OHDSI consortium has taken a unique "open science" approach to building a standardized data analytic platform, inviting all organizational data investigators to collaborate, build, and share standard analytic modules based on the OMOP CDM. All of the OHDSI analysis modules, outputs, and results are posted on the OHDSI website with open source licensing, available for others to use and build on (OHDSI, 2017b).

LIMITATIONS OF DATA AND ANALYSIS STANDARDIZATION

Besides the inherent limitations that always accompany secondary use of health-care data for PASS, there are additional challenges related to data and analysis standardization that investigators should be aware of. Not all analyses can be standardized using the MAP described before; some analyses necessarily require custom programming because of the complexity of the research question. The data transformation process can be time-consuming and requires significant care to ensure that the source data are represented properly in the standardized format. In addition, data loss may occur during the transformation of the source data into the CDM if the model does not support all of the data elements included in the source data.

Despite these limitations, when used appropriately, standardized data analytic platforms offer a transparent approach to analysis of large health-care databases, making the use of real-world data for noninterventional PASS more efficient, with results that can be easily replicated and meaningfully compared.

References

Blumenthal, D., Tavenner, M., 2010. The "meaningful use" regulation for electronic health record. N. Engl. J. Med. 363, 501−504.

Food, and Drug Administration (FDA), 2011. Food and Drug Administration Amendments Act (FDAAA) of 2007. Available from: https://www.fda.gov/regulatoryinformation/lawsen forcedbyfda/significantamendmentstothefdcact/foodanddrugadministrationamendmentsactof 2007/default.htm.

Observational Health Data Sciences and Informatics (OHDSI), 2017a. Available from: http://www. ohdsi.org.

Observational Health Data Sciences and Informatics (OHDSI), Software, 2017b. Available from: http://www.ohdsi.org/analytic-tools/.

Reyonlds, R.F., Kurz, X., de Groot, M.C.H., Schlienger, R.G., Grimaldi-Bensouda, L., Tcherny-Lessenot, S., Klungel, O., 2016. The IMI PROTECT project: purpose, organizational structure, and procedures. Pharmacoepidemiol. Drug Saf. 25, 5−10.

Ryan, P.B., Welebob, E., Hartzema, A.G., Stang, P.E., Overhage, J.M., 2010. Surveying U.S. observational data sources and characteristics for drug safety needs. Pharm. Med. 24 (4), 231−238.

Sentinel, 2018a. Available from: https://www.sentinelinitiative.org.

Sentinel. Routine Querying Tools (Modular Programs), 2018b. Available from: https://www. sentinelinitiative.org/sentinel/surveillance-tools/routine-querying-tools.

Stang, P.E., Ryan, P.B., Racoosin, J.A., Overhage, J.M., Hartzema, A.G., Reich, C., Welebob, E., Scarnecchia, T., Woodcock, J., 2010. Advancing the science for active surveillance: rationale and design for the Observational Medical Outcomes Partnership. Ann. Intern. Med. 153 (9), 600–606.

Trifiro, G., Fourrier-Reglat, A., Sturkenboom, M.C., Díaz Acedo, C., Van Der Lei, J., 2009. The EU-ADR project: preliminary results and perspective. Stud. Health Technol. Inform. 148, 43–49.

Proactive Safety Surveillance

Joshua J. Gagne[1], Sengwee Toh[2], Ayad K. Ali[3]

[1]*Brigham and Women's Hospital and Harvard Medical School, Boston, MA, United States;*
[2]*Harvard Medical School and Harvard Pilgrim Health Care Institute, Boston, MA, United States;*
[3]*Eli Lilly and Company, Indianapolis, IN, United States*

INTRODUCTION

For decades, regulatory agencies have relied on spontaneous adverse event reports for the purposes of monitoring the safety of authorized medicinal products (Woodcock et al., 2011). Spontaneous reporting systems (SRS) capture case reports that describe adverse events that may be due to the use of one or more medicinal products. These programs are generally considered "passive" in that the agencies set up the infrastructure to receive reports and then wait for manufacturers, health-care professionals, patients, or others to submit individual reports of suspected product-related adverse events. The passive nature of these systems is both a strength and limitation. On one hand, SRS enable regulators to identify previously unsuspected signals of harm related to medicinal products as they are used in the post-authorization setting, without a prior hypothesis. On the other hand, regulators have no control over what gets reported, which can be subject to stimulating reporting and other reporting phenomena (Gagne, 2014). Even today, SRS contribute to most regulatory decisions concerning safety of medicinal products (Lester et al., 2013).

Increasingly, claims and electronic medical record (EMR) databases that are often used for post-authorization safety studies (PASS) are being harnessed for proactive safety surveillance programs (PSSP). Individually, these databases often capture routinely collected data on hundreds of thousands or millions of patients who use prescription products. Collectively, these databases comprise information on hundreds of millions of patients. Such data typically include adjudicated, time-stamped insurance claims for prescription products dispensed at pharmacies (prescriptions issued in the case of EMR), and transactional records of diagnoses made and procedures performed in various health-care settings (Schneeweiss and Avorn, 2005). Chapter 3.1 discusses claims databases, and Chapter 3.2 provides an overview of EMR databases for PASS.

CONTENTS

Introduction 209

Vaccine Safety
Datalink 210
*Governance and
Data*............................ *211*
Example *212*

Sentinels 213
*Governance and
Data*............................ *214*
Example *214*

The Canadian
Network for
Observational Drug
Effect Studies 215
*Governance and
Data*............................ *216*
Example *216*

The Asian Pharmaco
epidemiology
Network 217
*Governance and
Data*............................ *217*
Example *218*

References 218

In general, PSSP are defined as having the following characteristics (Aronson et al., 2012; Huang et al., 2014): designed for post-authorization safety surveillance of medicinal products; have one main goal of rapidly generating post-authorization safety information; use secondary electronic health-care data that are generated from routine practice (i.e., real-world data); and use distributed data network (DDN) structures. By leveraging routinely collected health-care data on tens or hundreds of millions of patients, PSSP can quickly characterize serious adverse effects of medicinal products. The DDN allows investigators to analyze multiple databases without the need for pooling the data into a central repository (Brown et al., 2010; Toh et al., 2013). Chapter 3.4 discusses the concept "big data" and its application in PASS.

In addition to the characteristics described above, PSSP can facilitate sequential surveillance of medicinal products (Gagne, 2013). Once a new product is authorized for marketing, each database within a DDN prospectively captures data describing the use of the product. To characterize associated outcomes as quickly as possible, analyses can also be performed prospectively, in a sequential manner, as the data accrue (Gagne et al., 2012). To further expedite analyses within the DDN, certain PSSP have developed semiautomated programs, in which standardized code can be quickly and repeatedly deployed across the DDN (Connolly et al., 2017). Using few inputs, these modularized programs can perform all steps in a typical study, from cohort identification to confounding adjustment to effect estimation and testing (Gagne et al., 2014).

The following is an overview of key PSSP around the world and examples of safety questions that they have examined. We discuss opportunities and challenges to conducting surveillance in DDN, and compare and contrast key attributes to existing PSSP, including data sources (e.g., claims or EMR), data structure (e.g., common data model [CDM] or common protocol), and governance. The list of systems, examples, and features are not intended to be exhaustive. We focus on the US Centers for Disease Control and Prevention (CDC) Vaccine Safety Datalink (VSD) (McNeill et al., 2014), the US FDA Sentinel System (Platt et al., 2012), the Canadian Network for Observational Drug Effect Studies (CNODES) (Suissa et al., 2012), and the Asian Pharmacoepidemiology Network (AsPEN) (AsPEN, 2013).

VACCINE SAFETY DATALINK

Established in 1990 by the CDC, the VSD is the earliest form of PSSP (CDC, 2017). In the 1980s, computerized health-care information emerged as a promising data source for evaluating the use and outcomes of medicinal products, including pharmaceuticals, biologicals, and vaccines (McNeill et al., 2014). During the late 1980s, the CDC conducted pilot studies to evaluate the use of these nascent data for studying the safety of vaccines and recognized their value in complementing individual reports of vaccine-related adverse events (Walker et al., 1987; Griffin et al., 1988; Walker et al., 1988). Setting its sights on continuous vaccine safety surveillance, the CDC began planning for the VSD in 1989 (Chen et al., 1997). Initially focused on the safety of childhood immunizations (Chen et al., 1997), VSD has expanded to monitor the safety of vaccines administered during pregnancy (Kharbanda et al., 2017), vaccines used in older adults, and the influenza vaccine, for which new versions are produced each year (Li et al., 2016).

Chapter 7.3 provides a detailed discussion of PASS for vaccines, including common data sources and study designs used in vaccine safety research. The results of VSD are intended to inform health-care professionals and public health officials, and national immunization policy.

The objectives of the VSD are to conduct research on important vaccine safety questions in large populations; conduct vaccine safety studies that come from questions or concerns in the medical literature or from other vaccine safety systems, such as the Vaccine Adverse Event Reporting System, which is the US FDA SRS for vaccines; monitor possible adverse events when new vaccines are licensed or when there are new vaccine recommendations; and provide information to committees who make vaccine recommendations in the United States (CDC, 2017).

Governance and Data

VSD is funded by the CDC and involves nine health-care organizations around the United States. Collaborating sites provide data, and investigators at each site also provide clinical, methodological, and data management expertise. Each of the VSD collaborating sites is an integrated health delivery system that provides a continuum of health services, including care from inpatient, outpatient, and emergency department settings. Focusing on integrated systems help ensure that both vaccine exposure and medical outcomes are captured with little missing information.

Using a DDN, each site maintains its electronic data in a standardized format known as CDM. Chapter 5.4 provides an overview of CDM and discusses its utility in rapid-cycle analytics. The VSD CDM comprises separate tables for demographic, enrollment, immunization, inpatient, outpatient, death, and cause of death information. Tables are linked by a unique deidentified patient number. The immunization table is populated from detailed information from EMR data at each site and includes information on the type of vaccine administered and date of vaccination. Often, additional data are also available, including manufacturer, lot number, and site of vaccination (Chen et al., 1997). The inpatient and outpatient tables are populated with automated diagnosis and procedure codes. Certain tables are updated weekly, allowing near real-time surveillance for select vaccine adverse events (Curtis et al., 2011). This ability to conduct rapid-cycle analysis is critical for evaluating the safety of certain vaccines, such as the influenza vaccine, which has a short immunization season.

The CDM enables a lead site to develop an analysis program that can be shared with and executed at each site, with minimal modification. The key benefits of the CDM approach are that it ensures that each site implements the same design and analysis and reduces programming errors that might occur if each site developed its own programming code. As mentioned in Chapter 4, the main disadvantage of the CDM approach is that it requires each collaborating site to convert its data into the CDM on an ongoing basis, which creates additional work for the sites and the opportunity for errors, though the latter can be ameliorated with careful checks of the data following conversion.

In addition to providing vaccine exposure information, the ability to access written or EMR is critical for validating the medical outcomes that are identified in the administrative data. Across the DDN, VSD sites have cumulative information on more than 21 million individuals who have collectively received over 134 million vaccine doses. Currently, VSD collects data on nearly 10 million individuals on an annual basis, including data for more than 2 million children, more than 2 million women of reproductive age, and more than 100,000 live births annually (Kharbanda et al., 2017).

Example

The VSD played an important role in evaluating the safety of thimerosal, a commonly used mercury-containing preservative in vaccines. In 1999, the US FDA estimated that infants who were immunized according to the recommended schedule could receive mercury exposure in excess of limits set by the US Environmental Protection Agency. Several groups, including the Public Health Service and the American Academy of Pediatrics, called on manufacturers to remove thimerosal from all infant vaccines and recommended that studies be conducted to elucidate potential long-term safety risks of thimerosal exposure. In response, the CDC used the VSD to evaluate the relationship between thimerosal exposure and neuropsychological functioning (Thompson et al., 2007). The study included more than 1000 children between the ages of 7 and 10 years and used the computerized immunization records and EMR in conjunction with personal immunization records, and parent interviews to assess exposure to mercury from the prenatal period through the first 7 months of life. Analyses of 42 neuropsychological outcomes did not support a causal association between early life exposure to mercury from thimerosal-containing vaccines and neuropsychological functioning at the age of 7−10 years.

The VSD has also been used for rapid-cycle analysis of seasonal vaccines. In early 2009, the United States experienced a pandemic of influenza due to a novel H1N1 virus. Several vaccines were developed and rapidly approved to combat the outbreak, including monovalent inactive vaccine and a live attenuated vaccine, which were in addition to a seasonal trivalent inactivated vaccine and a live attenuated influenza vaccine. The CDC used the VSD to prospectively monitor the safety of these vaccines during the 2009–10 flu season (Lee et al., 2011). With multiple study designs, the analysis evaluated more than 1.3 million doses of the monovalent inactive vaccine, 250,000 doses of live attenuated vaccine, 2.7 million doses of the seasonal trivalent inactivated vaccine, and 150,000 doses of the live attenuated influenza vaccine. On March 31, 2010, a signal was observed for Bell's palsy in association with monovalent inactive vaccine with one particular study design. However, further analyses did not substantiate the finding. Overall, these analyses found no major safety issues with the H1N1 vaccine or the seasonal vaccines used during the 2009–10 flu season. The analyses also demonstrated the ability of the VSD to conduct rigorous, rapid-cycle analyses to inform regulatory and public health decision-making.

SENTINELS

Following the withdrawal of rofecoxib (a COX-II inhibitor nonsteroidal antiinflammatory drug) from the US market, the US Congress enacted the FDAAA of 2007, which mandated that the FDA perform proactive surveillance of regulated medicinal products using routinely collected electronic health information for at least 100 million people (Behrman et al., 2011). In response, the FDA established the Sentinel Initiative in 2008, which included the development of the Mini-Sentinel pilot program in the following year (Platt et al., 2012). Mini-Sentinel was a collaboration between the US FDA and more than two dozen academic and private organizations, which established the framework, data sources, analytic capabilities, policies, and procedures to conduct proactive surveillance of authorized medicinal products, including drugs, biologics, and medical devices across a large DDN. In 2016, the FDA officially launched the Sentinel System, which is the full-fledged PSSP built from the pilot program (Robb et al., 2012; Gagne et al., 2018).

The purpose of the Sentinel System is to complement the FDA Adverse Event Reporting System SRS by supporting the agency's ability to proactively monitor the safety of medicinal products in the post-authorization setting (FDA, 2017). Sentinel enables the FDA to pose a wide range of utilization and safety questions to a large network of routinely updated electronic health-care databases. The FDA has used results of these queries to inform regulatory decisions about authorized medicinal products, including the issuance of safety communications and label changes.

Governance and Data

The Sentinel is funded by the US FDA and involves a coordinating center, led by the Harvard Pilgrim Health Care Institute, and more than two dozen collaborating organizations around the United States (Forrow et al., 2012). Participating organizations provide scientific, technical, and organizational expertise, and 18 organizations contribute data to the Sentinel Distributed Database (SDD) as of February 2018 (Sentinel Initiative, 2018a). The SDD contained information on 223 million distinct patient identifiers between the years 2000 and 2016. This included 178 million distinct patient identifiers with both medical and pharmacy benefits, 425 million person-years of observation time, and 43 million unique individuals actively accruing data prospectively (Sentinel Initiative, 2018b). Although the SDD contains information for individuals of all ages, older patients are underrepresented in Sentinel as the largest data partners provide data from commercial insurance companies, which cover predominantly working-age individuals and their families. This limitation is being addressed by the inclusion of Medicare fee-for-service members in 2018. Analyses conducted in the SDD are designed to minimize the need to share identifiable patient information.

Sentinel uses a CDM similar to that of the VSD (Popovic, 2017). The CDM includes separate, linked tables for enrollment information, demographics, health-care utilization, pharmacy prescriptions, diagnoses, procedures, laboratory tests, and vital signs. Each data partner periodically extracts, loads, and transforms its updated data into the CDM and SDD. In addition to what is in the CDM, each data partner has the ability to reach back to patients' medical records, which is essential for medical record review to adjudicate health outcomes of interest, for example.

To date, Sentinel has focused mainly on what it refers to as signal refinement, defined as the assessment of predefined exposure-outcome pairs to determine whether there is evidence of association. Assessments within Sentinel range from descriptive analyses (Winiecki et al., 2015; Andrade et al., 2016; Mott et al., 2016; Taylor et al., 2017) to large protocol-based assessments with customized programming, including PASS (Toh et al., 2012; Yih et al., 2014; Toh et al., 2016; Yih et al., 2016). Sentinel has recently begun to develop and evaluate approaches to hypothesis-free screening for signal detection (Brown et al., 2013). By the end of 2017, more than 200 exploratory analyses and two dozen safety analyses had been conducted in Sentinel, the results of which were used to inform safety communications of six medicinal products by the FDA.

Example

The Sentinel PSSP recently completed several prospective analyses evaluating safety outcomes in relation to newly authorized prescription products. The first was what is sometimes referred to as a protocol-based assessment, in which the FDA, in collaboration with Sentinel Investigators and the Sentinel Operations Center, conducted customized analyses using de novo programming (Toh et al., 2018). Using a sequential study design, this assessment compared rates of myocardial infarction among initiators of saxagliptin, a dipeptidyl peptidase-4 (DPP-4) inhibitor used to treat type 2 diabetes mellitus, to rates among initiators of other antidiabetes medications. The sequential design involved seven interim analyses as initiators of saxagliptin and the comparator agents accrued in the SDD. The study used several methods to address confounding, including both exposure propensity scores (EPS) and disease risk scores (DRS). Across a total of 168 analyses, a signal of a higher rate of myocardial infarction with saxagliptin compared with pioglitazone (a thiazolidinedione antidiabetes medication) was raised in the fifth sequential analysis. However, the association subsided in subsequent analyses. Overall, the results suggested no increased risk of myocardial infarction with saxagliptin as compared with other antidiabetes medications. See Chapters 5.1 and 5.2 for more discussions on EPS and DRS as means to control for confounding in PASS.

Sentinel also recently completed a pilot sequential surveillance assessment using a set of preprogrammed modular tools (Chrischilles et al., 2018). These tools were used to conduct EPS-matched cohort analysis without the need for de novo programming. The assessment compared rates of stroke and bleeding among initiators of rivaroxaban, a nonvitamin K antagonist oral anticoagulants, versus warfarin, a vitamin K antagonist. The assessment involved two sequential analyses. A signal indicating a lower risk of ischemic stroke with rivaroxaban versus warfarin was observed in the first analysis. A signal for a higher rate of gastrointestinal bleeding with rivaroxaban was observed in the second period. This assessment advanced prospective analyses within Sentinel by demonstrating the ability of the modular program tools to facilitate sequential analysis.

THE CANADIAN NETWORK FOR OBSERVATIONAL DRUG EFFECT STUDIES

Established in 2011 and funded by the Canadian Institute of Health Research, CNODES is a network of researchers across Canada and administrative databases from eight Canadian provinces (CNODES, 2018). CNODES is one of five collaborating centers supported by the Drug Safety and Effectiveness Network (DSEN) of the Canadian Institute for Health Research. Queries from stakeholders are prioritized by the DSEN head office and sent to the CNODES coordinating center. CNODES teams conduct analyses of a DDN of Canadian and international databases and report both to stakeholders and via published literature.

CNODES is designed to provide rapid evidence about drug safety to Canadian stakeholders, including health-care professionals, patients, policy-makers, regulators, and Health Canada, in particular.

Governance and Data

CNODES uses data from eight Canadian provinces (Alberta, British Columbia, Manitoba, Newfoundland and Labrador, Nova Scotia, Ontario, Quebec, and Saskatchewan), the UK Clinical Practice Research Datalink (CPRD), and the Truven Health MarketScan database from the United States. The Canadian provincial databases provide claims and EMR data for ~35 million Canadians.

CNODES is currently developing a CDM based on the Sentinel CDM but has, to date, used a common protocol approach to the DDN. When a government stakeholder poses a question to CNODES, a research team is formed that includes an investigator and an analyst from each participating site. Rather than distributing a standardized piece of programming code, the study team develops a standardized protocol and a detailed technical specification that is distributed to participating sites. The investigator and analyst at each site write code based on the protocol and specifications that is then executed on the site's data. The results from each site are transmitted to the research team, which combines them using metaanalytic methods (Platt et al., 2016).

The use of a common protocol without a CDM ensures the active involvement of individuals who are most familiar with the data from each site and allows the sites to define study variables in ways that are specific to the content and formatting of each site. This allows the investigators and analysts at each site to accommodate differences in coding practices, data quality and completeness, and other idiosyncrasies in each database. However, the common protocol approach without a CDM requires each site to have the expertise and resources to implement each protocol.

Example

CNODES has addressed a number of medicinal product safety issues, including the safety of incretin enhancers used to treat type 2 diabetes mellitus. In particular, CNODES investigators examined whether DPP-4 inhibitors and glucagon-like peptide-1 (GLP-1) receptor agonists are associated with higher rates of acute pancreatitis, pancreatic cancer, and heart failure compared with oral antidiabetes medications (Azoulay et al., 2016a; Azoulay et al., 2016b; Filion et al., 2016). The analysis involved data from seven sites, including five Canadian provinces (Alberta, Manitoba, Ontario, Quebec, and Saskatchewan), the Truven Health MarketScan database, and the CPRD. Approximately 1.5 million patients were included in the analyses of each of the three outcomes. No increases in occurrence of any of the outcomes were observed with DPP-4 inhibitors and GLP-1 receptor agonists, as compared to oral antidiabetes medications.

In addition to signal evaluation studies, CNODES has also been used to evaluate the effectiveness of risk evaluation and mitigation strategies by assessing adherence to the risk mitigation requirements. Isotretinoin is an oral product that is widely used to treat severe acne, which is also a potent teratogen and should be avoided during pregnancy. To mitigate the risk, Health Canada requires informed written consent and two negative pregnancy tests before starting isotretinoin and use of two reliable forms of contraception during treatment with the product. Health Canada asked CNODES to evaluate the frequency of pregnancy during isotretinoin use and the outcomes of the pregnancies (Henry et al., 2016). Using data from British Columbia, Manitoba, Ontario, and Saskatchewan, more than 50,000 female users of isotretinoin were identified between 1996 and 2011. Less than a third of these individuals received prescriptions for oral contraceptives while receiving prescriptions for isotretinoin. Almost 1500 pregnancies were identified by 42 weeks after treatment, of which 90% were terminated spontaneously or by medical intervention. Of the 118 live births that were identified, 9% had evidence of congenital malformations. Chapter 2.2 provides detail on risk minimization activities and strategies to assess their effectiveness.

THE ASIAN PHARMACOEPIDEMIOLOGY NETWORK

The Asian Pharmacoepidemiology Network (AsPEN) is a voluntary, collaborative, multinational research network that developed through a series of conferences beginning in 2008 (AsPEN, 2013). AsPEN is recognized as a special interest group in the International Society for Pharmacoepidemiology. As a voluntary network, AsPEN does not receive dedicated funding to support its efforts. The purpose of AsPEN is to provide a mechanism to support the conduct of pharmacoepidemiological research and to facilitate timely identification and validation of emerging safety issues of medicinal products among the Asian countries (AsPEN et al., 2013b).

Governance and Data

Despite its name, the network includes databases from Australia, Sweden, and the Medicare program in the United States, in addition to databases from China, Hong Kong, Japan, Korea, Singapore, and Taiwan. Combined, these databases comprise information on ~220 million individuals.

As with other PSSP, raw data reside at each individual site and only summary data are sent to a coordinating center for each study. AsPEN does not maintain a general CDM but rather operates a modified DDN model. For each study, each participating site prepares a data file with a common structure so that a single, standardized analytic program can be written by the coordinating center and distributed to each site. This flexibility is particularly useful given the differences in coding systems and languages across the participating sites. An example of study-specific common data structure may resemble the VSD and Sentinel CDM by including separate, linked tables containing information on demographics, eligibility, pharmacy, inpatient encounters, inpatient diagnoses, and outpatient diagnoses and procedures.

Example

AsPEN collaborators conducted a sequence symmetry analysis to evaluate the association between antipsychotic use and acute hyperglycemia (Pratt et al., 2013). The investigators used a total of eight databases from six countries (Australia, Japan, South Korea, Sweden, Taiwan, and the United States). The sequence symmetry design enabled a simple analysis across the complex network of databases, requiring only three data elements—a patient identifier, a medicinal product code, and a product exposure date relative to the outcome of interest. The analysis found some suggestion of an increased risk of hyperglycemia with olanzapine antipsychotic treatment in two of the larger databases. The simplicity of and speed with which the sequence symmetry design could be implemented provided support for its use in PSSP such as AsPEN.

References

Andrade, S.E., Reichman, M.E., Mott, K., Pitts, M., Kieswetter, C., Dinatale, M., Stone, M.B., et al., 2016. Use of selective serotonin reuptake inhibitors (SSRIs) in women delivering liveborn infants and other women of child-bearing age within the US Food and Drug Administration's Mini-Sentinel program. Arch. Womens Ment. Health 19 (6), 969—977.

Aronson, J.K., Hauben, M., Bate, A., 2012. Defining 'surveillance' in drug safety. Drug Saf. 35, 347—357.

Asian Pharmacoepidemiology Network (AsPEN), 2013. Governance Structure for AsPEN. July 3, 2013. Available from: http://aspennet.asia/pdf/GovernanceStructuresForAsPEN.pdf.

AsPEN collaborators, Andersen, M., Bergman, U., et al., 2013b. The Asian Pharmacoepidemiology Network (AsPEN): promoting multi-national collaboration for pharmacoepidemiologic research in Asia. Pharmacoepidemiol. Drug Saf. 22, 700—704.

Azoulay, L., Filion, K.B., Platt, R.W., Dahl, M., Dormuth, C.R., Clemens, K., Durand, M., Hu, N., Juurlink, D., Paterson, J.M., Targownik, L., Turin, T., Ernst, P., Canadian Network for Observational Drug Effect Studies (CNODES) Investigators, 2016a. Association between incretin-based drugs and the risk of acute pancreatitis. JAMA Intern. Med. 176 (10), 1464—1473.

Azoulay, L., Filion, K.B., Platt, R.W., Dahl, M., Dormuth, C.R., Clemens, K.K., Durand, M., Juurlink, D.N., Targownik, L.E., Turin, T.C., Paterson, J.M., Ernst, P., Canadian Network for Observational Drug Effect Studies (CNODES) Investigators, 2016b. Incretin-based drugs and the risk of pancreatic cancer: a large multi-center observational study. BMJ 352 i581.

Behrman, R.E., Benner, J.S., Brown, J.S., McClellan, M., Woodcock, J., Platt, R., 2011. Developing te Sentinel System—a national resource for evidence development. N. Engl. J. Med. 364, 498–499.

Brown, J.S., Holmes, J.H., Shah, K., Hall, K., Lazarus, R., Platt, R., 2010. Distributed health data networks: a practical and preferred approach to multi-institutional evaluations of comparative effectiveness, safety, and quality of care. Med. Care 48 (6 Suppl.), S45–S51.

Brown, J.S., Petronis, K.R., Bate, A., et al., 2013. Drug adverse event detection in health plan data using the gamma Poisson shrinker and comparison to the Tree-based scan statistic. Pharmaceutics 5, 179–200.

Canadian Network for Observational Drug Effect Studies (CNODES), 2018. About CNODES. Available from: https://www.cnodes.ca/about/.

Centers for Disease Control and Prevention (CDC), Vaccine Safety Datalink (VSD), September 8, 2017. Available from: https://www.cdc.gov/vaccinesafety/ensuringsafety/monitoring/vsd/index.html.

Chen, R.T., Glasser, J.W., Rhodes, P.H., Davis, R.L., Barlow, W.E., Thompson, R.S., et al., 1997. Vaccine Safety Datalink project: a new tool for improving vaccine safety monitoring in the United States. The Vaccine Safety Datalink Team. Pediatrics 99 (6), 765–773.

Chrischilles, E.A., Gagne, J.J., Fireman, B., et al., January 10, 2018. Prospective surveillance pilot of rivaroxaban safety within the US Food and Drug Administration Sentinel System. Pharmacoepidemiol. Drug Saf. 4375. https://doi.org/10.1002/pds (Epub ahead of print).

Connolly, J.G., Wang, S.V., Fuller, C.C., et al., 2017. Development and application of two semi-automated tools for targeted medical product surveillance in a distributed data network. Curr. Epidemiol. Rep. 4, 298–306.

Curtis, L.H., Weiner, M.G., Beaulieu, N.U., Rosofsky, R., Woodworth, T.S., Boudreau, D.M., Cooper, W.O., Daniel, G.W., Nair, V.P., Raebel, M.A., Brown, J.S., October 2011. Mini-Sentinel Coordinating Center Data Core: Year 1 Common Data Model (CDM) Report. Available from: https://www.sentinelinitiative.org/sites/default/files/data/DistributedDatabase/Mini-Sentinel_Year-1-Common-Data-Model-Report_Data-Core-Activities_0.pdf.

Filion, K.B., Azoulay, L., Platt, R.W., Dahl, M., Dormuth, C.R., Clemens, K., Hu, N., Paterson, M., Targownik, L., Turin, T., Udell, J., Ernst, P., 2016. CNODES Investigators. A multicenter observational study of incretin-based drugs and heart failure. N. Engl. J. Med. 374 (12), 1145–1154.

Food, Drug Administration (FDA), November 21, 2017. FDA's Sentinel Initiative. Available from: https://www.fda.gov/Safety/FDAsSentinelInitiative/ucm2007250.htm.

Forrow, S., Campion, D.M., Herrinton, L.J., et al., 2012. The organizational structure and governing principles of the Food and Drug Administration's Mini-Sentinel pilot program. Pharmacoepidemiol. Drug Saf. 21 (Suppl. 1), 12–17.

Gagne, J.J., Glynn, R.J., Rassen, J.A., et al., 2012. Active safety monitoring of newly marketed medications in a distributed data network: application of a semi-automated monitoring system. Clin. Pharmacol. Ther. 92, 80–86.

Gagne, J.J., 2013. You can observe a lot (about medical products) by watching (those who use them). Epidemiology 24, 700–702.

Gagne, J.J., 2014. Finding meaningful patterns in adverse drug event reports. JAMA Intern. Med. 174, 193405.

Gagne, J.J., Wang, S.V., Rassen, J.A., Schneeweiss, S., 2014. A modular, prospective, semi-automated drug safety monitoring system for use in a distributed data environment. Pharmacoepidemiol. Drug Saf. 23, 619–627.

Gagne, J.J., Houstoun, M., Reichman, M.E., Hampp, C., Marshall, J.H., Toh, S., 2018. Safety assessment of niacin in the US Food and Drug Administration's Mini-Sentinel System. Pharmacoepidemiol. Drug Saf. 27, 30–37.

Griffin, M.R., Ray, W.A., Fought, R.L., Foster, M.A., Hays, A., Schaffner, W., 1988. Monitoring the safety of childhood immunizations: methods of linking and augmenting computerized data bases for epidemiologic studies. Am. J. Prev. Med. 4 (2 Suppl.), 5–13.

Henry, D., Dormuth, C., Winquist, B., Carney, G., Bugden, S., Teare, G., Lévesque, L.E., Bérard, A., Paterson, J.M., Platt, R.W., 2016. Occurrence of pregnancy and pregnancy outcomes during isotretinoin therapy. CMAJ 188 (10), 723–730.

Huang, Y.L., Moon, J., Segal, J.B., 2014. A comparison of active adverse event surveillance systems worldwide. Drug Saf. 37, 581–596.

Kharbanda, E.O., Vazquez-Benitez, G., Romitti, P.A., Naleway, A.L., Cheetham, T.C., et al., 2017. Identifying birth defects in automated data sources in the Vaccines Safety Datalink. Pharmacoepidemiol. Drug Saf. 26 (4), 412–420.

Lee, G.M., Greene, S.K., Weintraub, E.S., et al., 2011. H1N1 and seasonal influenza vaccine safety in the vaccine safety datalink project. Am. J. Prev. Med. 41 (2), 121–128.

Lester, J., Neyarapally, G.A., Lipowski, E., Graham, C.F., Hall, M., Dal Pan, G., 2013. Evaluation of FDA safety-related drug label changes in 2010. Pharmacoepidemiol. Drug Saf. 22, 302–305.

Li, R., Stewart, B., McNeil, M.M., Duffy, J., Nelson, J., Kawai, A.T., Baxter, R., et al., 2016. Post licensure surveillance of influence vaccines in the Vaccine Safety Datalink in the 2013–2014 and 2014–2015 seasons. Pharmacoepidemiol. Drug Saf. 25 (8), 928–934.

McNeill, M.M., Gee, J., Weintraub, E.S., et al., 2014. The Vaccine Safety Datalink: successes and challenges monitoring vaccine safety. Vaccine 32, 5390–5398.

Mott, K., Graham, D.J., Toh, S., Gagne, J.J., Levenson, M., Ma, Y., Reichman, M.E., 2016. Uptake of new drugs in the early post-approval period in the Mini-Sentinel distributed database. Pharmcaoepidemiol. Drug Saf. 25 (9), 1023–1032.

Platt, R., Carnahan, R.M., Brown, J.S., et al., 2012. The U.S. Food and Drug Administration's Mini-Sentinel program: status and direction. Pharmacoepidemiol. Drug Saf. 21 (Suppl. 1), 1–8.

Platt, R.W., Dormuth, C.R., Chateau, D., Filion, K., 2016. Observational studies of drug safety in multi-database studies: methodological challenges and opportunities. EGEMS (Wash DC) 4 (1), 1221.

Pratt, N., Andersen, M., Bergman, U., Choi, N.K., Gerhard, T., Huang, C., Kimura, M., Kimura, T., Kubota, K., Lai, E.C., Ooba, N., Osby, U., Park, B.J., Sato, T., Shin, J.Y., Sundstrom, A., Yang, Y.H., 2013. Multi-country rapid adverse drug event assessment: the Asian Pharmacoepidemiology Network (AsPEN) antipsychotic and acute hyperglycemia study. Pharmacoepidemiol. Drug Saf. 22 (9), 915–924.

Popovic, J.R., 2017. Distributed data networks: a blueprint for Big Data sharing and healthcare analytics. Ann. N. Y. Acad. Sci. 1387, 105–111.

Robb, M.A., Racoosin, J.A., Sherman, R.E., Gross, T.P., Ball, R., et al., 2012. The US Food and Drug Administration's Sentinel Initiative: expanding the horizons of medical product safety. Pharmacoepidemiol. Drug Saf. 21 (Suppl. 1), 9–11.

Schneeweiss, S., Avorn, J., 2005. A review of uses of health care utilization databases for epidemiologic research on therapeutics. J. Clin. Epidemiol. 58, 323–337.

Sentinel Initiative, 2018a. Data Partners. Available from: https://www.sentinelinitiative.org/sentinel/data/data-partners.

Sentinel Initiative, 2018b. Snapshot of Database Statistics. Available from: https://www.sentinelinitiative.org/sentinel/data/snapshot-database-statistics.

Suissa, S., Henry, D., Caetano, P., et al., 2012. CNODES: the Canadian Network for Observational Drug Effect Studies. Open Med. 6, 134–140.

Taylor, L.G., Bird, S.T., Sahin, L., Tassinari, M.S., Greene, P., Reichman, M.E., et al., 2017. Antiemetic use among pregnant women in the United States: the escalating use of ondansetron. Pharmacoepidemiol. Drug Saf. 26 (5), 592–596.

Thompson, W.W., Price, C., Goodson, B., et al., 2007. Early thimerosal exposure and neuropsychological outcomes at 7 to 10 years. N. Engl. J. Med. 357 (13), 1281–1292.

Toh, S., Reichman, M.E., Houstoun, M., Ross Southworth, M., Ding, X., et al., 2012. Comparative risk of angioedema associated with the use of drugs that target the renin-angiotensin-aldosterone system. Arch. Intern. Med. 172 (20), 1582–1589.

Toh, S., Reichman, M.E., Houstoun, M., Ding, X., Fireman, B.H., et al., 2013. Multivariable confounding adjustment in distributed data networks without sharing of patient-level data. Pharmacoepidemiol. Drug Saf. 22 (11), 1171–1177.

Toh, S., Hampp, C., Reichman, M.E., Graham, D.J., Balakrishnan, S., et al., 2016. Risk of hospitalized heart failure among new users of saxagliptin, sitagliptin, and other antihyperglycemic drugs: a retrospective cohort study. Ann. Intern. Med. 164 (11), 705–714.

Toh, S., Reichman, M.E., Graham, D.J., et al., 2018. Prospective postmarketing surveillance of acute myocardial infarction in new users of saxagliptin: a population-based study. Diabetes Care 41, 39–48.

Walker, A.M., Jick, H., Perera, D.R., Thompson, R.S., Knauss, T.A., 1987. Diphtheria-tetanus-pertussis immunization and sudden infant death syndrome. Am. J. Public Health 77 (8), 945–951.

Walker, A.M., Jick, H., Perera, D.R., Knauss, T.A., Thomson, R.S., 1988. Neurologic events following diphtheria-tetanus-pertussis immunization. Pediatrics 81 (3), 345–349.

Winiecki, S., Baer, B., Chege, W., Jankosky, C., Mintz, P., et al., 2015. Complementary use of passive surveillance and Mini-Sentinel to better characterize hemolysis after immune globulin. Transfusion 55 (Suppl. 2), S28–S35.

Woodcock, J., Behrman, R.E., Dal Pan, G.J., 2011. Role of postmarketing surveillance in contemporary medicine. Annu. Rev. Med. 62, 1–10.

Yih, W.K., Lieu, T.A., Kulldorff, M., Martin, D., McMahill-Walraven, C.N., et al., 2014. Intussusception risk after rotavirus vaccination in US infants. N. Engl. J. Med. 370 (6), 503–512.

Yih, W.K., Kulldorff, M., Sandhu, S.K., Zichittella, L., Maro, J.C., Cole, D.V., et al., 2016. Prospective influenza vaccine safety surveillance using fresh data in the Sentinel System. Pharmacoepidemiol. Drug Saf. 25 (5), 481–492.

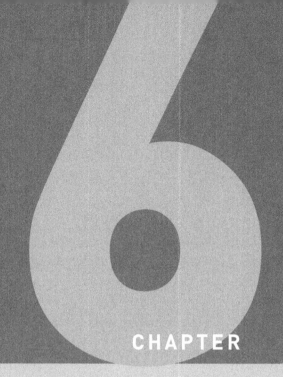

CHAPTER

Benefit-Risk Evaluation

6.1 Benefit-Risk Evaluation Frameworks 225
6.2 Post-Authorization Effectiveness Studies 242

Benefit—Risk Evaluation Frameworks

Lesley Wise

Takeda Pharmaceuticals, London, United Kingdom

INTRODUCTION

We are used to making decisions in our everyday lives. When we do this, we (usually subconsciously) balance benefits of that decision against risks involved in the decision. For example, we decide whether to take a raincoat when we leave the house. The risk if we do not take the coat is that we may get wet if it rains; the risk if we do take the coat is that we have to carry a coat and it may not rain. We are also used to everyday life to the differences between personal decisions (such as the raincoat) and community-based decisions such as those taken by the British Board of Film Classification. Benefit—risk decision-making also applies to the choice of whether or not to take a medicinal product (personal choice) and to the choice of whether or not to approve a product (community-based choice). This chapter will explore the development of frameworks that describe decisions on the approvability and use of medicines, and the issues that impact such benefit—risk decisions.

Benefit—risk evaluation frameworks for medicinal products have evolved over the last decade from purely descriptive frameworks to structured descriptive frameworks with some quantitative information, through frameworks that are in essence fully quantitative assessments with some descriptive text. This evolution has been driven by an increased focus on the need to better communicate both the decisions about authorizing medicinal products (CHMP, 2008; Brett et al., 2013; Pignatti et al., 2015) and also the management of the safety profile of products so that patients achieve maximum benefit and harms are minimized (Wise et al., 2009). Risk assessment is discussed in Chapter 2.1, followed by an overview of risk minimization approaches in Chapter 2.2.

As a consequence of this increased focus on benefit—risk management, regulatory authorities, pharmaceutical industry, and academia are now paying far more attention to benefit—risk assessment, and the quality and communication of those assessments together with increased transparency,

CONTENTS

Introduction 225

Stakeholders 226

Benefit Information 227
Presentation of Benefit Information 229

Risk Information 229
Presentation of Risk Information 231

Impact of Uncertainty 232

Preferences and Values 233

Risk Minimization Measures 233

Overall Benefit—Risk Assessment 235

Role of Post-Authorization Safety Studies in Benefit—Risk Assessment 236

Ongoing Benefit—Risk Evaluation 237

References 239

Post-Authorization Safety Studies of Medicinal Products. https://doi.org/10.1016/B978-0-12-809217-0.00006-4

provision of patient accessible information, and a focus on consideration of both benefits and risks in communications with stakeholders. For example, a major work package within IMI-PROTECT (Innovative Medicines Initiative—the Pharmacoepidemiological Research on Outcomes of Therapeutics by a European Consortium) addressed quantitative benefit—risk methods under a public—private partnership. It aimed to assess the utility of various benefit—risk methodologies and particularly how these assessments can be visualized (PROTECT Consortium, 2018a). Other approaches have been investigated by the Center for Innovation in Regulatory Science, most recently with the Unified Methodologies for Benefit—Risk Assessment initiative, which built on the benefit—risk assessment taskforce work and the work of the European Medicines Agency (EMA) in developing PROACT-URL (CIRS, 2018; PROTECT Consortium, 2018b). At the same time, regulators are working on guidance to improve the standardization of the assessments provided to them and that they provide back to the pharmaceutical industry. This is also being taken forward by an International Conference on Harmonization (ICH) Working Group established to provide direction to industry to help standardize the way that benefit—risk assessments are provided in the submission dossier. This updated guidance will also leave scope for new approaches, methods, and data sources, such as patient perspectives and preferences to capture emerging trends in benefit—risk assessment and management (Wise et al., 2009; Brett et al., 2013; Frey, 2015; MDIC, 2015).

Benefit—risk evaluations take place throughout the product life cycle, and different stakeholders may have different views on some parts of any particular evaluation. This chapter will illustrate the different aspects of benefit—risk assessment frameworks, how the information and assumptions may be described or displayed, and identify the types of scenarios when different types of frameworks may be appropriate. The impact of emerging information from post-authorization safety studies (PASS) and other sources on the continuous review of the benefit—risk profile will also be considered. Specific methodologies are discussed in detail in other publications (Wise, 2011; Leong et al., 2015; Jiang and He, 2016; PROTECT Consortium, 2018a).

STAKEHOLDERS

It is clear that different people place different weight on different attributes of benefits and risks of certain decisions. This is as relevant in decision-making about medicinal products as it is for other decisions and mandates the need for good communication from decision makers to those impacted by the decision. Throughout this chapter, the need for adequate and appropriate communication to and from four different groups of stakeholders (company, regulator, health-care professional, and patient/caregiver) will be considered as the importance they place on different attributes of benefit and risk is likely to differ.

Benefit—risk assessments do not take place in a vacuum; they take place in the context of the therapeutic space and alternatives (including nontherapeutic), stakeholder perspectives and preferences, and health-care systems/social contexts. When a company makes a submission for a product authorization, this is usually underpinned by evidence on both benefits and risks from clinical studies where the new product was studied against either placebo or standard of care. Different stakeholders are likely to put different emphasis (or value) on the benefits and risks under evaluation (Coplan et al., 2011), and that emphasis will differ according to the type of medicinal product under consideration and the disease being treated (Wise, 2011; FDA, 2013). For example, for patients with an immediately life-threatening or life-changing condition (e.g., cancer), the benefits of the product are likely to be far more important than long-term risks, whereas for patients with a chronic—mainly silent—condition (e.g., hypertension), the adverse effects of treatment may be more important than the (unseen) benefits. In addition, health-care system providers are likely to approach therapy decisions with a "population focus" to the benefit and risk information, which may be very different to the view that the patient/caregiver or their health-care professional has.

The key attributes of any benefit—risk assessment framework include not only the benefit and risk but also uncertainty, and stakeholder preferences and values. Each of these will be discussed further below.

BENEFIT INFORMATION

Clinical trials are set up with a clear hypothesis (or more than one) to be tested, and objectives/endpoints to be measured. In general, these randomized controlled trials (RCT) measure efficacy parameters and/or surrogates for those parameters. The RCT can be the basis for applications for product authorization or extensions where the benefit of the product is related to but may not be the same as the endpoint(s) studied. For example, an antihypertensive agent may be tested in an RCT to assess the extent of blood pressure lowering and the time course of the effect. The efficacy endpoint will be related to the amount of blood pressure lowering achieved. However, this is not really the benefit of treatment with the medicinal product but is a marker for what is expected to be the benefit of lowering of the blood pressure (e.g., reduced risks of myocardial infarction and/or stroke). The long-term benefits of lowering blood pressure are not seen in a short-term RCT to show that the product does lower the blood pressure. On the other hand, a vaccine study can show the immediate benefit as measured by the proportion of patients treated with the vaccine who do not contract the disease but may not show longer-term impacts on population health and health resource use. Similarly, some of the benefits of an antibiotic may be shown by comparing "cure" rates.

From a health-care system perspective, there may be multiple options for benefits in a single assessment, some of which are "contained within each other." One example of this is the measure of joint activity developed by the American College of Rheumatology (ACR) and used for rheumatoid arthritis RCT. As can be seen below, patients achieving ACT 70 will automatically fulfill ACR 20 and ACR 50 (Pincus, 2005):

> the ACR Core Data Set includes seven measures—swollen joint count, tender joint count, patient assessment of global status, an acute phase reactant (erythrocyte sedimentation rate—ESR or C-reactive protein—CRP), health professional assessment of global status, physical function, and pain; the first four of these measures are included on the assessment. Improvement criteria for the ACR Core Data Set are based on improvement of at least 20% in both tender and swollen joint counts, and three of the five additional measures (ACR 20), and corresponding ACR 50 and ACR 70.

The key to conducting a benefit–risk assessment that is robust, transparent, and easily communicated is to concentrate on those distinct benefits (and risks) that are most important for treatment decisions.

In a typical benefit–risk assessment, there will only be a few important benefits associated with the product, and one of the tasks is deciding what those key benefits are. Ultimately the most important, or key, benefits of a product may be most easily identified by answering the following questions: *Why would the patient take this?* (specific benefits of this product on the disease and specific benefits of this product/formulation/delivery compared to other treatments) and *why would the health-care system implement this?* (especially in the case of a vaccine).

It is possible that a combination of RCT endpoints may not only provide the information for some of the benefits but also possible that some benefits, which may be very relevant to the patient or health-care professional, are not captured as primary or secondary RCT endpoints at all. For example, ease of administration, an oral versus an intravenous formulation, and lower side effects than an existing treatment are all types of benefits that may be important to a patient but are not easily translated into RCT endpoints. The incorporation of patient perspectives into benefit–risk assessments is increasingly common, but methodology for formal assessments of patient perspectives and preferences is still being developed (MDIC, 2015).

Presentation of Benefit Information

The first challenge for a benefit–risk assessment is identifying the most important benefits of the medicinal product. This is unlikely to be all benefits but will be a subset of them and may in fact be a combination of them. The ICH guideline on the clinical trial dossier has recently been revised to incorporate more guidance on the development of the benefit–risk section of the dossier. This revised guidance reached Step 4 of the ICH process in June 2016 (Frey, 2015) and noted the following as important for identifying the key benefits of a product:

> clinical importance of benefit (e.g., life-prolonging, curative, disease-modifying, symptomatic relief, improved patient compliance, functional or quality of life improvement, prevention of disease progression, prevention of infectious disease, or diagnostic); absolute difference in frequency of the effect in the study population versus the comparator(s); in some cases, also expressing the difference relative to the comparator may be informative (e.g., if the response rate is 20% in the product group and 8% in the control group, the absolute difference is 12% and the relative effect is 2.5).

As we consider the four groups of stakeholders, it is easy to see that there may be different perspectives on what constitutes the most important benefits, and therefore companies (who usually hold the data) need to be able to create these assessments with flexibility to adapt to the needs of different audiences.

As described above, to understand the impact of the benefits on the condition being treated, it is important to reflect this benefit in absolute terms. In addition, it is important that this difference is put into the context of the impact on the patient population being treated, or in the case of a vaccine, in the occurrence of the disease and associated complications.

The impact of surrogate endpoints on the understanding of benefit is also important and uncertainty around this needs to be reflected (De Gruttola et al., 2001; Garattini, 2010). Additionally, the benefits may not be equally apparent in all population subgroups, and therefore, identifying the key benefits in the key groups becomes important to decision-making. Beyond this, benefits can be shown in tabular or graphical form, and/or discussed in text.

RISK INFORMATION

Over the last two decades, the management of safety of medicinal products has undergone a change from fairly passive management to a more proactive identification of the most "important" risks, and management of those to maintain a positive benefit–risk for the product. A concept paper was agreed by the ICH to define a risk management guideline, which aimed to better define what was known about the safety profile of a medicinal product when it was authorized, in terms of the number of patients studied and the types of risks identified, as well as plans for obtaining further data and managing the known risks (ICH, 2004). Taken together, it was anticipated that such an approach would help to ensure that the safety profile of a product early in the post-authorization phase would be closely monitored to detect any new safety concerns early and also to ensure that the safety profile, as seen in RCT, was reflected in clinical use.

The guidance has been implemented in most ICH regions, with non-ICH countries also requesting similar documentation. As examples, the EMA implemented initial guidance and a template, which was revised in 2012 as part of the revisions to the European Union (EU) pharmacovigilance legislation (EMA, 2013). The EU risk management plan (RMP) document is required as part of a number of different national submission packages outside of the EU (e.g., Australia and Canada). See Chapter 2.1 for a detailed discussion of the RMP in the context of risk assessment.

In Japan, there is a guidance and template, which conforms with the ICH E2E guidance, although it differs somewhat from the EMA version, mainly in the extent of information provided on the current evidence based on which the risk assessment is based (PMDA, 2018).

In the United States, the FDA implemented the risk evaluation and mitigation strategy (REMS) approach, which provides the documentation for management of specific risks where additional risk minimization is considered necessary for the maintenance of a positive benefit—risk balance (FDA, 2018). Chapter 2.2 provides an overview of risk minimization and mitigation strategies. In the context of a benefit—risk assessment for a product, the term risk is used to apply to not only just adverse events associated with taking the product but also other unfavorable effects associated with the product. For example, there may be environmental impacts; risks to contacts of the treated patient (e.g., shedding of a viral vector) (Baldo et al., 2013; Anderson, 2016); or social impacts (e.g., addiction to opiates) (FDA, 2017). As with the discussion on the benefits, the benefit—risk assessment will be based on the key risks of the product. This will be a subset of all risks and will include the risks most likely to impact the overall benefit—risk assessment in terms of seriousness/severity, frequency, reversibility, tolerability, and impact on public health.

Therefore, the priority for the "risk" part of a benefit risk assessment is to identify the key risks from the broader list of adverse events and any other important unfavorable effects associated with the product.

The key risks of a product may be most easily identified by answering the following questions: *What might make the patient stop this product? What patients should not receive this product?* (exclusion of such patients may identify a subset of patients where the benefit–risk balance is positive) and *are there other important concerns?* (e.g., diversion, abuse, or illicit use).

As with the benefit information, when presenting information on risks for discussion in a benefit–risk assessment, it is important to understand the absolute risks and risk differences, as well as the frequency in the background population, if available. The variability of the risk in different subgroups and the nature of the risk in terms of temporality and time to resolution are important for providing the essential context for a benefit–risk assessment. The proposed approach to managing each key risk is also important together with an explanation of why the approach should be effective.

The perspectives of the four groups of stakeholders on risks will differ at least as much as perspectives on benefits. Although regulators may be focused on serious but very rare events, patients may be more concerned about more common events that impact their daily living (e.g., moderate gastrointestinal effects). Equally, if a medicinal product has a very serious side effect but a major benefit in terms of a serious/disabling disease, then some patients may be prepared to take what other stakeholders may view as an unacceptable risk. An example often used is that of natalizumab, a humanized monoclonal antibody for the treatment of multiple sclerosis. The product was authorized in the United States in 2004 and was suspended from the US market in 2005 following two cases of progressive multifocal leukoencephalopathy (PML) (FDA, 2005). However, the benefits of the product were considered by the multiple sclerosis community to be substantial, and natalizumab was reinstated with strict measures to ensure that patients are fully aware of the risk, and that regular examinations take place to detect PML early and stop treatment with the product (FDA, 2015b; EMA, 2016). This example highlights the need for all groups of stakeholders to be involved with benefit–risk discussions so that a range of perspectives can be understood and incorporated. Additionally, where restrictive measure or regular monitoring may be needed, the view of the patient on the acceptability of this is needed.

Presentation of Risk Information
To understand the impact of the risks against the benefits, it is important to reflect the risks in absolute terms with the same denominator as the benefit if possible; for example, the absolute difference in adverse effect of interest in the treated group compared with the untreated group. This will help later in the benefit–risk assessment where these differences can be put into the context of the impact of the benefit on the patient population being treated with the

medicinal product. Beyond this, risks, as benefits, can be shown in tabular or graphical form, and/or discussed in text.

IMPACT OF UNCERTAINTY

The information on benefit and risks always has a certain level of uncertainty as we never fully know all the characteristics of a product. It is important to reflect that uncertainty within the benefit–risk assessment. For example, RCT involving a relatively small number of exposed patients will mean that there is uncertainty in both the benefit estimate and the risk estimate. The impact on the benefit estimate is that we will be less sure on the overall extent of the benefit and need to be aware that it may be smaller than we have seen or possibly larger. This is partially reflected in the confidence intervals around any point estimates for the study endpoints, but these do not provide the full assessment of uncertainty. Small studies may also have quite restricted populations both in terms of disease profile and also other demographic characteristics. There are additional uncertainties possibly incurred by the study duration, especially if the product is designed for chronic use or has life-time effects (e.g., vaccines) but has only been studied for a few months. The assumptions of generalizability of benefits from restricted populations or study durations to the general disease population need to be addressed in the benefit–risk assessment. This is additional to the uncertainty of real-world effectiveness compared with the efficacy seen in RCT.

Other sources of uncertainty that might need to be addressed for benefits include aspects of study design such as the comparator used, blinding, whether this is an interim analysis, completeness of data collection and follow-up, differential dropout rates (possibly seen when a product is effective and patients on placebo dropout), consistency of results across studies, and overall assessments of generalizability.

The impact of small study populations on the confidence surrounding the safety data is that we may be concerned about the risks that we have not yet had the opportunity to see either because the safety population is too small, too refined, or the studies were too short. This raises the level of concern about the safety profile in the context of the concern about the generalizability of the benefit information.

For discussing the impact of uncertainty on the risk profile, in addition to the above considerations, some other topics may also need to be addressed, such as the adequacy of risk assessment in terms of study size, duration, frequency of monitoring, any specific studies to address safety concerns (e.g., nonclinical studies or special investigations), and any impact of the comparator chosen on the observed safety profile.

PREFERENCES AND VALUES

The concepts of preferences and perspectives are implicit in all value judgments that we make every day, as illustrated with a simple decision on whether or not to take a waterproof coat on a commute to the office: *Risk and uncertainty* (70% chance it may rain); *outcome of risk if it happens* (if it rains I will get wet); *risk minimization* (I should take a coat); and *perspective and preference* (a coat is heavy, I will choose to get wet if it rains). Such decisions are also present in health care, including decisions to authorize medicinal products for human use.

One problem with perspectives and preferences is that they tend to be very individual and not easily reproducible, and therefore, there has been a great deal of effort to try to ensure that benefit–risk decisions are documented in such a way that the preferences are explicitly noted, at least during formal processes such as assessments for authorizations (Coplan, 2011). This is not so straightforward when it comes to individual patient decisions because each patient (and health-care professional) will have different perspectives and preferences. This means that transparency over those benefits and risks that are likely to impact the benefit–risk assessment is essential for communication between health-care professionals and their patients (Egbrink and IJzerman, 2014; MDIC, 2018).

Eliciting aggregate information on patient perspectives and preferences is not easily accomplished. It relies on eliciting the information either formally (via studies) or informally (via focus groups) from groups of patients. Such studies require methods that are different to the usual quantitative approaches applied during product development (Marshall et al., 2010; FDA, 2015a). Aside from the obvious challenges of ensuring that the sample is representative of the intended treatment population, it should be anticipated that the outputs of such studies will have very wide variability because the "typical patient" does not really exist. Each patient has their own underlying values and preferences, which are part of their perspective regarding treatment with the medicinal product (Hanger et al., 2000; Slot and Berge, 2016). However, some studies have identified common themes in patient perspectives, which could be helpful in the context of benefit–risk assessments.

RISK MINIMIZATION MEASURES

In some situations, specific measures may be put in place to address concerns over kay benefits or key risks. Usually, this is less for key benefits but may occur in special situations such as an accelerated assessment for a product that is seen to be a major advance in therapy but that may be based on interim data. In this case, the level of uncertainty is increased, and therefore, restrictions may be included, such as license that is conditional on the provision and assessment of the final data.

The situation is more common for risks, when there may be situations where important risks need to be addressed by the inclusion of additional measures to try to mitigate those risks or to further examine the study population/risk to develop and target risk minimization. See Chapter 2.2 for more details on risk minimization activities.

As an historical example, thalidomide is now known to cause phocomelia and other congenital abnormalities, as well as long-term health issues. In the late 1950s and early 1960s, thalidomide was used as a hypnotic and antiemetic, which seemed to have a low level of obvious side effects in patients, and was considered to be much safer in overdose than the available alternative—barbiturates. Then, as the product spread, including use in pregnancy, some obstetricians started to notice congenital anomalies in babies born to mothers who had taken thalidomide during pregnancy (Mcbride, 2016; Speirs, 2016). This was the start of the unfolding of what is described as the thalidomide disaster, which was responsible for the initiation of systems to monitor the safety of authorized medicinal products in many countries of the world (Waller, 2010).

Thalidomide was never authorized in the United States and was withdrawn from use in 1961 in Germany and the United Kingdom. However, it was authorized for use in Europe in 2008 in a very different population, patients with multiple myeloma, a type of bone marrow cancer that occurs mainly in people over 60 years (EMA, 2009b). This authorization for use is associated with a range of educational materials that are intended to minimize the risk of any fetal exposure to thalidomide (EMA, 2009a).

Another example, isotretinoin is an orally administered product used to treat acne, a disease often associated with teenage years. This product causes birth defects if taken during pregnancy, and unlike thalidomide, isotretinoin is used in a population where pregnancy may be more common. It is also covered by a very strict risk minimization program to prevent exposure during pregnancy (MHRA, 2013).

The success of these programs is pivotal for the benefit–risk profile of the product to remain positive, and therefore their implementation and assessment of their effectiveness will be very important for periodic reassessments of benefit–risk balance during the product life cycle. It is here that the regulatory links are made between the documents detailing risk management commitments (based on ICH E2E) and those reassessing the benefit–risk balance (based on ICH E2C-R2).

OVERALL BENEFIT—RISK ASSESSMENT

Having identified the key benefits, key risks, associated uncertainties, and any measures intended in the management of the benefits and risks, it is then necessary to construct the benefit—risk assessment, which is a structured synthesis of the benefit, risk, and uncertainty information, incorporating value judgments on the part of the author (e.g., marketing authorization holder—MAH) and other parties. Furthermore, it may be necessary to provide different benefit—risk assessments depending on the audience to ensure that the perspectives and preference of each audience are reflected.

In terms of regulatory documents, the MAH assessment of the benefit—risk balance of the product is first presented in Section 2.5.6 of the clinical trial dossier in the submission package. This is covered by an ICH guidance document—ICH M4E, which was recently revised—ICD-M4E(R2) (Frey, 2015). This updated guidance provides an overall structure to be considered, in line with that discussed above, which is also in line with the ICH document on periodic benefit—risk evaluation reports (PBRER) in the post-authorization setting (ICH, 2012). The guidance sets out the expectation as follows:

> the purpose of this section is to provide a succinct, integrated, and clearly explained benefit-risk assessment of the medicinal product for its intended use. The benefit-risk assessment is based on a weighing of the key risks of the medicinal product.

As noted before, the benefit—risk assessment always takes place in a therapeutic context, which is important for the management of that benefit and of any associated risks. The therapeutic context includes the severity of the disease, the expected benefit of the product, the profile of other therapeutic options, the medical need, any specific measures to minimize risks, and the patient perspective (which is informed by all the above).

The structured synthesis of information can take a range of formats, from purely descriptive to a qualitative approach utilizing some quantitative information, possibly in the form of graphs or figures, to a fully quantitative assessment that explicitly models the impact of value judgments and preferences (Coplan et al., 2011; Leong et al., 2015; Jiang and He, 2016). Purely descriptive (narrative) benefit—risk assessments are usually best employed when there is relatively little if any quantitative information available, for example, an application for a generic version of a well-established medicinal product or for a "well-established use" application.

Descriptive approaches using quantitative information, which may be considered as semiquantitative approaches, provide the quantitative information in a structured way and possibly utilize some graphical displays. These approaches are well suited for applications for most products and are very flexible. A range of information in addition to the information on the key benefits and risks can be incorporated, including patient/stakeholder preferences and visualization of the impact of uncertainty. Both the EMA and FDA have tabular approaches to the display of the information and the assessment of the data, which ensures a consistency in assessment reports. However, it should be noted that the assessors' preferences and value judgments are still, to a certain extent, implicit in the assessment.

The fully quantitative methods incorporate explicitly the weightings, value judgments, and preferences of the person conducting the assessment, and also therefore, explicitly allow the impact of changes to those parameters to be evaluated. These methods are more complex to understand for the reader/stakeholder, and the amount of information required to complete these methods is greater. As discussed above, obtaining these preferences, values, and weightings is a difficult task. For this reason, fully quantitative models may be best reserved for special situations (e.g., a product with a clear benefit, but one major risk) or situations where there is a single stakeholder group. A good example of the use of these models was provided by the PROTECT project in the form of a number of case studies (PROTECT Consortium, 2018c).

However, as noted above, the key skills required for studying and validating stakeholder/patient preferences may not necessarily reside in traditional biostatistics groups, which tend to be oriented to quantitative sciences rather than qualitative sciences. Even the fully quantitative benefit—risk assessment will require input from qualitative research of patients' attitudes, preferences, and weights. Therefore, careful planning for these types of analyses is required.

ROLE OF POST-AUTHORIZATION SAFETY STUDIES IN BENEFIT—RISK ASSESSMENT

A positive benefit—risk assessment may depend on the success of programs to minimize key risks. Therefore, the implementation of these measures and assessment of their effectiveness will be very important in the periodic reassessments of benefit—risk monitoring during the product life cycle. Studies to assess the effectiveness of these measures are designated as PASS in the EU (EMA, 2013). As noted in Chapter 2.2, these assessments are also required as part of any REMS agreed in the United States. These studies traditionally measure knowledge and behavior of the target audience. For example, they will survey health-care professionals to assess whether the risk minimization measure is understood, and whether the measure is being adhered to. An alternative way to assess behaviors, but not knowledge, is to study drug utilization if the product is prescribed in a setting or way where that is possible (see Chapter 4.1 for a discussion on drug utilization studies and cohort event monitoring studies). From a study design and validity perspective, the product utilization approach can minimize the biases that may be present in a survey and are therefore more generalizable.

Other PASS approaches that may be relevant include long-term prospective studies to assess long-term safety if this has not been studied previously. Some designs may eventually lead to the capture of long-term comparative safety information across a class of products, which simultaneously inform the benefit—risk profile for a group of products in the same/similar indication (BSRBR Rheumatoid Arthritis Register, 2016). Enriched study designs that combine primary and secondary data are discussed in Chapter 4.4, and prospective study designs are discussed in Chapter 4.5.

The implementation and success of these measures is also closely tied with preferences and values expressed within and by the health-care system and the patient. Studies to elicit these preferences are also a form of PASS and/or may be directly related to the interpretation of results of a study to assess the success of risk minimization implementation. A full discussion of these methods is not in scope of this chapter, but the methods associated with implementation and communication sciences are gradually gaining ground in studies assessing risk minimization implementation and effectiveness (Smith and Morrato, 2014). As discussed earlier, this is an area where both pharmaceutical companies and regulatory authorities are developing their expertise as it relies on communication sciences that have not traditionally been areas of expertise of research and development organizations. The design of such studies should follow the principles laid out elsewhere in this book, and it is essential that the aims of the study are clearly aligned to the risk minimization measure being assessed, so that the results and the impact on the benefit—risk assessment are interpretable.

Noninterventional studies other than PASS, such as comparative effectiveness studies, e.g., post-authorization effectiveness studies (PAES), can provide useful information to be incorporated in the benefit—risk assessment of medicinal products. Chapter 6.2 provides an overview of PAES and discusses the overlaps between these studies and PASS.

ONGOING BENEFIT—RISK EVALUATION

Once a product is authorized by a regulatory agency, the benefit—risk profile continues to be assessed and managed as it becomes used in a larger exposed population. The major regulatory document for these assessments is the PBRER (ICH, 2012). Each PBRER requires a formal assessment of the benefit—risk of the product in a similar manner to that described above, which takes into account all the data for the product, and includes how effective the risk minimization measures are in reducing either the risk of an adverse event or the severity of the adverse event if it occurs. This assessment will consider the importance and the magnitude of the benefit seen (rather than those expected), and trade off against that the important risks in the context of their frequency and seriousness, and the context of the benefit.

These evaluations provide not only a summary of both the information on benefits and risks arising during the period of the review but also an interpretation of the information in the context of the cumulative information. This includes information from PASS, PAES, and spontaneous reports. Such an evaluation may include a new benefit identified in ongoing RCT and/or a new risk identified from RCT, PASS, or signal detection activities. It is expected to follow a similar format to the assessment of benefit–risk balance in the initial application (Frey, 2015). The evaluation may also conclude there is a reduction in uncertainty arising from a completed RCT or PASS that provides important reassurance over the observed benefit and/or risk profile in subpopulations and increasing the amount of safety data available. As the product life cycle is traversed, the key benefit-/risk-related activities of the product remain the same (i.e., signal detection, evaluation, management of potential and identified risks, and evaluation of risk minimization activities); the amount and type of data available to base the benefit-risk assessments on changes.

As more data accumulates, it may be possible to identify subgroups of patients who respond better to the product (or less well), and subgroups who have a greater risk of more serious adverse events. Trying to identify and characterize the subgroups is an important part of maximizing patient benefit and minimizing risk. In this context, the role of further studies of the product, including well-designed PASS, is clearly important.

Throughout this chapter, we have seen that the assessment of benefits and risks is something we all do all the time. In the context of medicinal products, this assessment is done at several levels. Regulators assess whether the potential benefits outweigh the potential risks for the average patient in the sought indication, and so decide whether a product should be authorized or not (population level). If the product is authorized and is made available for use, decisions are then made at the prescriber (and patient) level as to whether to prescribe it for an individual patient (this takes into account information on the benefits and risks of both treatment and nontreatment).

Clearly presented information on the benefits and risks, the context to which these are managed, and the degree of uncertainty about them, is essential to allow stakeholders to make informed decisions on what matters to them.

References

Anderson, E.J., 2016. Rotavirus vaccines: viral shedding and risk of transmission. Lancet Infect. Dis. 8 (10), 642–649.

Baldo, A., van den Akker, E., Bergmans, H.E., Lim, F., Pauwels, K., 2013. General considerations on the biosafety of virus-derived vectors used in gene therapy and vaccination. Curr. Gene Ther. 13 (6), 385–394.

Brett, H.A., Fairchild, A.O., Reed, J.F., 2013. Quantifying benefit–risk preferences for medical interventions: an overview of a growing empirical literature. Appl. Health Econ. Health Pol. 11 (4), 319–329.

BSRBR Rheumatoid Arthritis Register, 2016. Available from: http://www.rheumatology.org.uk/resources/bsr_biologics_registers/bsrbr_rheumatoid_arthritis_register/default.aspx.

Center for Innovation in Regulatory Science (CIRS), 2018. Unified Methodologies for Benefit-Risk Assessment (UMBRA) Initiative. Available from: http://www.cirsci.org/decision-making-frameworks/umbra-initiative/.

Committee for Medicinal Products for Human Use (CHMP). Reflection paper on benefit-risk assessment methods in the context of the evaluation of marketing authorisation applications of medicinal products for human use. March 2008. Available from: http://www.ema.europa.eu/docs/en_GB/document_library/Regulatory_and_procedural_guideline/2010/01/WC500069634.pdf

Coplan, P.M., Noel, R.A., Levitan, B.S., Ferguson, J., Mussen, F., 2011. Development of a framework for enhancing the transparency, reproducibility and communication of the benefit–risk balance of medicines. Clin. Pharmacol. Therapeut. 89 (2), 312–315.

De Gruttola, V.G., Clax, P., Demets, D.L., Downing, G.J., Ellenberg, S.S., Friedman, L., De Gruttola, V.G., 2001. Considerations in the evaluation of surrogate endpoints in clinical trials: summary of a National Institutes of Health Workshop. Contr. Clin. Trials 22 (22).

Egbrink, M., IJzerman, M., 2014. The value of quantitative patient preferences in regulatory benefit-risk assessment. J. Market Access Health Policy 2.

European Medicines Agency (EMA), 2009a. Conditions or Restriction With Regard to the Safe and Effective Use of the Medicinal Product to Be Implemented by the Member States. Available from: http://www.ema.europa.eu/docs/en_GB/document_library/EPAR_-_Conditions_imposed_on_member_states_for_safe_and_effective_use/human/000823/WC500037051.pdf.

European Medicines Agency (EMA), 2009b. Thalidomide Celgene. Available from: http://www.ema.europa.eu/ema/index.jsp?curl=pages/medicines/human/medicines/000823/human_med_001090.jsp&mid=WC0b01ac058001d124.

European Medicines Agency (EMA), 2013. Guideline on Good Pharmacovigilance Practices (GVP). Available from: http://www.ema.europa.eu/docs/en_GB/document_library/Scientific_guideline/2012/06/WC500129137.pdf.

European Medicines Agency (EMA), 2016. Tysabri - EMA Review. Available from: http://www.ema.europa.eu/ema/index.jsp?curl=pages/medicines/human/referrals/Tysabri/human_referral_prac_000049.jsp&mid=WC0b01ac05805c516f.

Food and Drug Administration (FDA), 2005. Postmarket Drug Safety Information for Patients and Providers - Public Health Advisory - Suspended Marketing of Tysabri (Natalizumab). Retrieved from: http://www.fda.gov/Drugs/DrugSafety/PostmarketDrugSafetyInformationforPatientsandProviders/ucm051761.htm.

Food and Drug Administration (FDA), 2013. PDUFA V Draft Implementation Plan: Structured Approach to Benefit-Risk Assessment in Drug Regulatory Decision-Making (Feb 2013). Available from: https://www.fda.gov/downloads/ForIndustry/UserFees/PrescriptionDrugUserFee/UCM329758.pdf.

Food and Drug Administration (FDA), 2015a. Patient Preference Information — Submission, Review in PMAs, HDE Applications, and De Novo Requests, and Inclusion in Device Labeling Draft Guidance for Industry, Food and Drug Administration Staff, and Other Stakeholders Preface Additional Copies. Available from: http://www.fda.gov/downloads/medicaldevices/deviceregulationandguidance/guidancedocuments/ucm446680.pdf.

Food and Drug Administration (FDA), 2015b. Tysabri: Approved Risk Evaluation and Mitigation Strategies (REMS). Available from: http://www.accessdata.fda.gov/scripts/cder/rems/index.cfm?event=IndvRemsDetails.page&REMS=63.

Food and Drug Administration (FDA), 2017. Shared System REMS for Extended Release and Long Acting Opioid Analgesics. Available from: http://www.accessdata.fda.gov/scripts/cder/rems/index.cfm?event=RemsDetails.page&REMS=17.

Food and Drug Administration (FDA), 2018. Approved Risk Evaluation and Mitigation Strategies (REMS). Available from: http://www.accessdata.fda.gov/scripts/cder/rems/.

Frey, P., 2015. ICH M4E(R2): Revised Guideline on Common Technical Document—Efficacy. Available from: http://www.ich.org/fileadmin/Public_Web_Site/ICH_Products/CTD/M4E_R2_Efficacy/M4E_R2__-_Step_2_-_Presentation_26Aug2015.pdf.

Garattini, S., 2010. Evaluation of benefit-risk. Pharmacoeconomics 28 (11), 981—986.

Hanger, H.C., Fogarty, B., Wilkinson, T.J., Sainsbury, R., 2000. Stroke patients' views on stroke outcomes: death versus disability. Clin. Rehabil. 14 (4), 417—424.

International Conference on Harmonization (ICH), November 2004. ICH Harmonized Tripartite Guideline. Pharmacovigilance Planning—E2E. Available from: http://www.ich.org/fileadmin/Public_Web_Site/ICH_Products/Guidelines/Efficacy/E2E/Step4/E2E_Guideline.pdf.

International Conference on Harmonization (ICH), 2012. ICH Harmonised Tripartite Guideline: Periodic Benefit-Risk Evaluation Report (PBRER). Available from: http://www.ich.org/fileadmin/Public_Web_Site/ICH_Products/Guidelines/Efficacy/E2C/E2C_R2_Step4.pdf.

Jiang, Q., He, W. (Eds.), 2016. Benefit-Risk Assessment Methods in Medical Product Development: Bridging Qualitative and Quantitative Assessments. Chapman and Hall.

Leong, J., Salek, S., Walker, S.R., 2015. Benefit-Risk Assessment of Medicines: The Development and Application of a Universal Framework for Decision-Making and Effective Communication, first ed. Springer.

Marshall, D., Bridges, J.F.P., Hauber, B., Cameron, R., Donnalley, L., Fyie, K., Johnson, F.R., 2010. Conjoint analysis applications in health — how are studies being designed and reported? Patient 3 (4), 249—256.

Mcbride, W.G., 2016. Thalidomide and congenital abnormalities. Lancet 278 (7216), 1358.

Medical Device Innovation Concortium (MDIC), 2015. Medical Device Innovation Consortium (MDIC) Patient Centered Benefit-Risk Project Report: A Framework for Incorporating Information on Patient Preferences Regarding Benefit and Risk into Regulatory Assessments of New Medical Technology. Medical Device Innovation Consortium (MDIC). Available from: http://mdic.org/wp-content/uploads/2015/05/MDIC_PCBR_Framework_Web1.pdf.

Medical Device Innovation Consortium (MDIC), 2018. Patient Centered Benefit-Risk Assessment. Available from: http://mdic.org/pcbr/.

Medicines and Healthcare Products Regulatory Agency (MHRA), 2013. Oral Retinoids: Pregnancy Prevention—Reminder of Measures to Minimise Teratogenic Risk. Available from: https://www.gov.uk/drug-safety-update/oral-retinoids-pregnancy-prevention-reminder-of-measures-to-minimise-teratogenic-risk.

Pignatti, F., Ashby, D., Brass, E.P., Eichler, H.G., Frey, P., Hillege, H.L., et al., 2015. Structured frameworks to increase the transparency of the assessment of benefits and risks of medicines: current status and possible future directions. Clin. Pharmacol. Therapeut. 98 (5), 522—533.

Pincus, T., 2005. The American College of Rheumatology (ACR) core data set and derivative "patient only" indices to assess rheumatoid arthritis. Clin. Exp. Rheumatol. 23 (5 Suppl. 39), S109—S113.

Pharmaceuticals and Medical Devices Agency (PMDA), 2005. History. Available from: https://www.pmda.go.jp/english/about-pmda/outline/0002.html.

PROTECT Consortium, 2018a. EU PROTECT Benefit-Risk Project. Available from: http://protectbenefitrisk.eu/.

PROTECT Consortium, 2018b. PrOACT-URL. Available from: http://protectbenefitrisk.eu/PrOACT-URL.html.

PROTECT Consortium, 2018c. PROTECT Case Studies. Available from: http://protectbenefitrisk.eu/casestudies.html.

Slot, K.B., Berge, E., 2016. Thrombolytic treatment for stroke: patient preferences for treatment, information, and involvement. J. Stroke Cerebrovasc. Dis. 18 (1), 17—22.

Smith, M.Y., Morrato, E., 2014. Advancing the field of pharmaceutical risk minimization through application of implementation science best practices. Drug Saf. 37 (8), 569—580.

Speirs, A.L., 2016. Thalidomide and congenital abnormalities. Lancet 279 (7224), 303—305.

Waller, P., 2010. An Introduction to Pharmacovigilance. Wiley-Blackwell, Wiley InterScience.

Wise, L., 2011. Risks and benefits of (pharmaco)epidemiology. Therapeut. Adv. Drug Safety 2 (3), 95—102.

Wise, L., Parkinson, J., Raine, J., Breckenridge, A., 2009. New approaches to drug safety: a pharmacovigilance tool kit. Nat. Rev. Drug Discov. 8 (10), 779—782.

Post-Authorization Effectiveness Studies

Stella Blackburn[1], Ayad K. Ali[2]

[1]IQVIA, Durham, NC, United States; [2]Eli Lilly and Company, Indianapolis, IN, United States

CONTENTS

Introduction 242

PAES in Europe . 244

PAES in United States 246

Examples of Required PAES .. 246

Future Directions 247

References 248

INTRODUCTION

Most medicinal products are authorized on the basis of the results of randomized controlled trials (RCT), which are intended to answer the question *"can the product work under ideal circumstances?"* Initial trials are usually conducted in a relatively small homogenous population in experienced research centers. If efficacy is seen, the population size in increased and inclusion criteria is broadened to increase the diversity of patients, but even so, they are never likely to include anywhere near the huge multiplicity of patients seen in ordinary health-care practice—particularly if one considers the global use of medicinal products.

Many factors can influence how a product performs, including genetics, age, sex, disease severity, comorbidities, and concomitant medications; so in the real-world, there will be a much greater heterogeneity of effect. In addition, the setting may also measure effectiveness. For example, in RCT, a research center may have access to a particular test that is not widely available outside of certain centers. If response is linked to the results of the test, use of the product in a wider setting where the test is unavailable will almost inevitably lead to a much lower overall response. Therefore, taking into account the different factors that may play a role in determining effect, the "effectiveness" of a product, as seen in routine clinical practice, is likely to be less than the "efficacy" seen under the idealized clinical trial setting.

Table 6.2.1 shows the differences between efficacy and effectiveness. Although authorization is usually based on efficacy, payers and health technology assessment bodies are more often interested in the effectiveness of a medicinal product because they are interested in whether it works in practice rather than the ideal setting of a clinical trial. Whereas effectiveness is looking at the effect across a population in the real-world (as opposed to the clinical trial world),

Table 6.2.1 Differences Between Efficacy and Effectiveness

Term	Definition
Efficacy	The extent to which a medicinal product does more good than harm under ideal circumstances. *"Can it work?"*
Effectiveness	The extent to which a medicinal product does more good than harm when provided under usual circumstances of health-care practice. *"Does it work in practice?"*
Personalized effectiveness	The extent to which a medicinal product does more good than harm to the patient when used under usual circumstances of health-care practice. *"Will it work for me/my patient?"*

the question that is often most important to patients and health-care professionals is whether the product will work in a particular individual. This is what we term "personalized effectiveness" and will depend on the combination of "benefit" factors, which affect effectiveness seen in the individual. The differences between efficacy and effectiveness have been somewhat muddied by the European Union (EU) legislation talks about "post-authorization efficacy studies (PAES)" (EC, 2010a,b). In some cases, it is clear that they probably do mean efficacy studies, but in others, it seems possibly that effectiveness may be the more likely target.

Until relatively recently, most post-authorization studies were primarily safety-based and intended to identify and characterize adverse reactions, i.e., post-authorization safety studies (PASS). However, it is increasingly apparent that it is also important to characterize "benefit or effectiveness factors" to predict who is likely to get most benefit from a product. After all, what is the point of taking a medicinal product and risking adverse events, if you are unlikely to benefit from it? As mentioned in Chapter 5, by combining both risk and benefit management, the benefit–risk balance can be maximized both at the population and at the individual level. Studying effectiveness is therefore important for a great many stakeholders.

There has also been an assumption that efficacy is relatively constant over time in an individual. However, there are a number of circumstances where that assumption could be wrong. We know that receptors can be upregulated and downregulated, and so this could change efficacy due to differing interaction with receptors. Most of the important systems in the body have built in feedback loops, so it is possible that these may adapt to alter the effect of a medicinal product targeting a particular system. Many biological products are proteins and so can induce antibodies over time (Felis-Giemza and Moots, 2015). There was a concern that the development of neutralizing antibodies could potentially not only block the product but also any endogenous

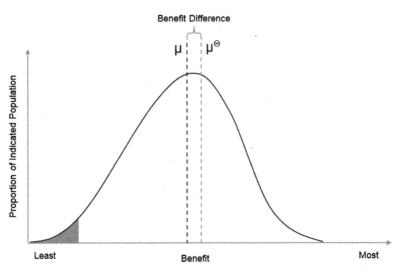

FIGURE 6.2.1
Illustration of benefit management for medicinal product in the indicated population.

hormone (e.g., erythropoietin) that it was augmenting. Although, theoretically, a gene therapy should provide a lifelong cure, this obviously is not proven and so long-term follow-up of effectiveness will be required—apart from the follow-up needed to rule out theoretical safety concerns.

The effectiveness of a medicinal product (or its benefit) in the real-world depends on a variety of factors. We characterize risk factors for adverse drug reactions so why not characterize "benefit" or "effectiveness" factors? Fig. 6.2.1 is a hypothetical mapping of the benefit of a product in the indicated (or target) population. It makes the assumption that there is a normal distribution with the population "average" benefit shown by μ. By removing those patients who show least benefit from the product, the mean is shifted from μ to $\mu^{\ominus}$ so the population benefit is increased. The shift is somewhat exaggerated in the diagram, but the principle remains the same.

Therefore, we will replace "efficacy" with "effectiveness" in PAES to use the term as "post-authorization *effectiveness* studies" throughout the book instead.

PAES IN EUROPE

The EU regulators identified a number of particular situations where it might be necessary to do PAES to confirm evidence seen pre-authorization. These tended to be situations whereby the data available at the time of the original authorization needed confirmation or where initial efficacy might change as a result of long-term use. The legislation dealing with these particular situations included the ability to compel a marketing authorization holder to do a study. The situations included medicinal products given a conditional authorization on the basis of unmet medical need and promising results from initial RCT; products given an authorization under exceptional circumstances; advanced therapy medicinal products; certain pediatric authorizations; and following a referral procedure (EMA, 2006; EC, 2006, 2007).

It was not until the pharmacovigilance legislation in the EU in 2010, whereby the ability to require PAES for any medicinal product, and not just the particular situations specified above, was added (EC, 2010a,b). The lawyers termed these studies "efficacy," but the recital in the legislation suggests that both efficacy and effectiveness can "impose" PAES for products outside of the specialized situations mentioned above (i.e., making it a condition of the marketing authorization). These are to conduct PAES

- where concerns relating to some aspects of the efficacy of the medicinal product are identified and can be resolved only after the product has been marketed or
- when the understanding of the disease or the clinical methodology indicates that previous efficacy evaluations have to be revised significantly.

Furthermore, the circumstances in which these PAES might be required are specified by the European Commission in its delegated regulation 357/2014 (EC, 2004):

- an initial efficacy assessment that is based on surrogate endpoints, which require verification of the impact of the product on clinical outcome or disease progression, or confirmation of previous efficacy assumptions;
- in the case of medicinal products that are used in combination with other products, the need for further efficacy data to clarify uncertainties that had not been addressed when the product was authorized;
- uncertainties with respect to the efficacy of a product in certain subpopulations that could not be resolved prior to marketing authorization and require clinical evidence;
- the potential lack of efficacy in the long term that raises concerns with respect to the maintenance of a positive benefit–risk balance of the medicinal product;
- benefits of a medicinal product demonstrated in RCT are significantly affected by the use of the product under real-world conditions, or, in the case of vaccines, protective efficacy studies have not been feasible;
- a change in the understanding of the standard of care for a disease or the pharmacology of a medicinal product that requires additional evidence on its efficacy; or

- new concrete and objective scientific factors that may constitute a basis for finding that previous efficacy evaluations might have to be revised significantly.

The European Medicines Agency (EMA) published a scientific guidance on PAES, which came into effect in June 2017 (EMA, 2015). Although the guideline states that studies may be randomized or nonrandomized, its stated preference is for randomized studies. However, this would not permit the study of effectiveness in real-world conditions, which is what is required for many stakeholders. It also calls into question as one of the premises of the legislation that the results should only be resolvable following marketing because RCT could presumably be carried out pre-authorization.

PAES IN UNITED STATES

The FDA can require post-authorization studies or RCT for medicinal products approved under the accelerated approval requirements or the Pediatric Research Equity Act (FDA, 2016). The FDA has a specific category for PAES when efficacy has been proven only on the basis of animal studies because the product cannot be ethically or feasibly tested in humans. Under the requirements, the marketing authorization holder must conduct post-authorization studies or RCT when such studies or trials are feasible and ethical (FDA, 2015).

In addition to required studies or trials, the FDA can also agree to post-authorization commitments with a marketing authorization holder to further define efficacy in RCT. These include evaluation of long-term effectiveness or duration of response, evaluate efficacy using a withdrawal design, and evaluate efficacy in a subgroup (FDA, 2011).

EXAMPLES OF REQUIRED PAES

The following are some examples of specific situations where PAES could be required or requested by regulatory authorities. Antidiabetes medications usually have the measurement of glycosylated hemoglobin (HbA1c) as a marker for average plasma glucose levels over a period. By keeping HbA1c levels as close to the normal range a possible, it is assumed that this will prevent the long-term effects of diabetes—namely, cardiovascular disease, renal failure, and vision impairment. However, to demonstrate the reduction in these adverse outcomes would require many years, so authorization is frequently based on HbA1c changes. PAES could be required to see whether reductions in HbA1c actually do lead to improved outcomes because the product could have deleterious effects on other risk factors as was seen with the thiazolidine-diones. Similarly, other surrogate endpoints might require confirmatory PAES are CD4 counts in HIV disease, and cholesterol and blood pressure as markers for cardiovascular disease.

Another example where PAES may be necessary is when efficacy has been proven with one dose but there are concerns that a different dose could provide a better effect or that certain subpopulations may not benefit equally. An example of this was ipilimumab cancer immunotherapy for patients with previously treated advanced melanoma. The dose of 3 mg/kg was approved by the EMA based on a clinically relevant overall survival (EMA, 2011). However, there was concern that women over the age of 50 might benefit less, and there was limited or no information on patients with active brain metastases or ocular melanoma. In addition, there was some evidence that a higher dose might be more effective, although there were concerns about the potential for higher toxicity. The EMA requested post-authorization research into subgroups of patients who might get greater or lesser benefit and also do a study comparing 3 mg/kg versus 10 mg/kg.

The actual strains of influenza virus involved in a pandemic are not known until the pandemic starts, so authorization is often based on a core pandemic dossier with a pandemic variation once the strains are known. A study on vaccine effectiveness is therefore required for pandemic vaccines in the EU.

As mentioned above, legislation gives regulatory authorities in certain jurisdictions, the ability to mandate or require PASS and PAES. However, pharmaceutical companies would be wise to plan research in this area both to provide evidence for other stakeholders and to improve the benefit—risk balance of their medicines. See Chapter 6.1 for an overview of benefit—risk assessments.

FUTURE DIRECTIONS

Prior to the ICH E2E guideline on pharmacovigilance planning (which introduced the concept of pharmacovigilance planning), post-authorization studies were limited in number (ICH, 2004). Since then, risk management planning is a mainstream activity with most innovative products planning studies, especially PASS into the identification and characterization of risks. Why not do the same to plan PAES? This can be started pre-authorization by both looking at variance in efficacy in the RCT population to see which factors predict greater efficacy and by looking at subpopulations who were, or who were not, studied.

By looking at the mechanism of action, it may be possible to predict populations who will benefit less. For example, if a product is a prodrug, deficiency or impaired function of the system metabolizing it to the active substance may limit efficacy. However, it is likely that the relatively small numbers of patients and the homogeneity of the trial population may mean the most identification of benefit factors cannot be really done until the product is used in a much larger, real-world population. But the planning of these studies and analyses can be done prior to authorization.

The cost of new medicinal products and the increased medical needs of an aging population mean that health-care systems are under strain, and the current system is probably unsustainable long term. Pay for performance agreements are already in place for a number of products in different jurisdictions. Patients do not want to be exposed to risk if they are unlikely to benefit from treatment. All these factors suggest that the current way of doing things needs to change. PAES are one of the tools that will help answer the questions regarding predictability of benefit.

In the past, authorization of a product was the end of research. PASS have already changed that paradigm. If we consider the life span of a medicinal product from first in man to when it is withdrawn, authorization is really only a milestone in that pathway, and other stakeholders make important decisions along the route. We need to change the way we think about evidence generation along that pathway, and PAES will be an important part of this.

References

European Commission (EC), 2004. Commission Delegated Regulation (EU) No 357/2014 Supplementing Directive 2001/83/EC of the European Parliament and of the Council and Regulation (EC) No 726/2004 of the European Parliament and of the Council as Regards Situations in Which Post-authorisation Efficacy Studies May Be Required. Available from: http://eur-lex.europa.eu/legal-content/EN/TXT/?uri=celex%3A32014R0357.

European Commission (EC), 2006. A Paediatric Use of a Medicinal Product in Accordance with Article 34(2) of Regulation (EC) No 1901/2006 of the European Parliament and of the Council. Available from: https://ec.europa.eu/health/sites/health/files/files/eudralex/vol-1/reg_2006_1901/reg_2006_1901_en.pdf.

European Commission (EC), 2007. A Marketing Authorisation Granted to an Advanced Therapy Medicinal Product in Accordance with Article 14 of Regulation (EC) No 1394/2007 of the European Parliament and of the Council. Available from: https://ec.europa.eu/health/sites/health/files/files/eudralex/vol-1/reg_2007_1394/reg_2007_1394_en.pdf.

European Commission (EC), 2010a. DIRECTIVE 2010/84/EU of The European Parliament and of the Council of 15 December 2010 Amending, as Regards Pharmacovigilance, Directive 2001/83/EC on the Community Code Relating to Medicinal Products for Human Use. Available from: https://ec.europa.eu/health/sites/health/files/files/eudralex/vol-1/dir_2010_84/dir_2010_84_en.pdf.

European Commission (EC), 2010b. REGULATION (EU) No 1235/2010 of The European Parliament and of The Council of 15 December 2010 Amending, as Regards Pharmacovigilance of Medicinal Products for Human Use, Regulation (EC) No 726/2004 Laying Down Community Procedures for the Authorisation and Supervision of Medicinal Products for Human and Veterinary Use and Establishing a European Medicines Agency. Available from: https://ec.europa.eu/health/sites/health/files/files/eudralex/vol-1/reg_2010_1235/reg_2010_1235_en.pdf.

European Medicines Agency (EMA), 2006. Guideline on the Scientific Application and the Practical Arrangements Necessary to Implement Commission Regulation on The Conditional Marketing Authorization for Medicinal Products for Human Use Falling within the Scope of Regulation (EC) No. 726/2004. Available from: http://www.ema.europa.eu/docs/en_GB/document_library/Scientific_guideline/2009/10/WC500004908.pdf.

European Medicines Agency (EMA), 2011. CHMP Assessment Report EMA/CHMP/557664/2011. Available from: http://www.ema.europa.eu/docs/en_GB/document_library/EPAR_-_Public_assessment_report/human/002213/WC500109302.pdf.

European Medicines Agency (EMA), 2015. Scientific Guidance on Post-authorisation Efficacy Studies. EMA/PDCO/CAT/CMDh/PRAC/CHMP/261500/2015. Available from: http://www.ema.europa.eu/docs/en_GB/document_library/Scientific_guideline/2015/11/WC500196379.pdf.

Felis-Giemza, A., Moots, R.J., 2015. Measurement of anti-drug antibodies to biologic drugs. Rheumatology 54 (1), 1941−1943.

Food and Drug Administration (FDA), 2011. Guidance for Industry. Postmarketing Studies and Clinical Trials − Implementation of Section 505 (O)(3) of the Federal Food, Drug, and Cosmetic Act. Available from: https://www.fda.gov/downloads/Drugs/GuidanceComplianceRegulatoryInformation/Guidances/UCM172001.pdf.

Food and Drug Administration (FDA), 2015. Postmarketing Requirements and Commitments: Frequently Asked Questions. Available from: https://www.fda.gov/Drugs/GuidanceComplianceRegulatoryInformation/Post-marketingPhaseIVCommitments/ucm070766.htm#q14.

Food and Drug Administration (FDA), 2016. Postmarketing Requirements and Commitments: Introduction. Available from: https://www.fda.gov/drugs/guidancecomplianceregulatoryinformation/post-marketingphaseivcommitments/default.htm.

International Conference on Harmonisation (ICH), 2004. ICH of Technical Requirements for Registration of Pharmaceuticals for Human Use. ICH Harmonised Tripartite Guideline. Pharmacovigilance Planning E2E. Available from: https://www.ich.org/fileadmin/Public_Web_Site/ICH_Products/Guidelines/Efficacy/E2E/Step4/E2E_Guideline.pdf.

CHAPTER 7

PASS for Specialty Products

7.1 PASS for Biosimilars and Interchangeable Biologic Products..... 253
7.2 PASS for Medical Devices and Combination Products................. 277
7.3 PASS for Vaccines 293

Post-Authorization Safety Studies for Biosimilars and Interchangeable Biologic Products

Jaclyn L.F. Bosco[1], Nancy A. Dreyer[1], Ayad K. Ali[2]

[1]IQVIA, Durham, NC, United States; [2]Eli Lilly and Company, Indianapolis, IN, United States

INTRODUCTION

Biologic medicinal products are indicated for serious, chronic illnesses in the therapeutic areas of rheumatology, dermatology, oncology, immunology, neurology, nephrology, and endocrinology (Morrow and Felcone, 2004) and have had a profound impact on health care. Novel therapies such as trastuzumab and rituximab have demonstrated improved survival from HER2+ breast cancer (Duffy, 2013) and non-Hodgkin's lymphoma (Griffin and Morley, 2013), respectively; anti-tumor necrosis factor (TNF) alpha agents have revolutionized care for patients with Crohn's disease and ulcerative colitis by sustaining the duration of remission and reducing the need for surgery (Ferrante et al., 2009; Ahluwalia, 2012); and beta-interferons and targeted biologic therapies have led to fewer relapse and have slowed the disease progression in multiple sclerosis (Derwenskus, 2011) and rheumatoid arthritis patients (Horton and Emery, 2012), respectively. Biologics, such as insulin, red blood cell stimulation, and human growth hormone, have been around for decades, but novel research in genetic information and disease processes has greatly increased the number of targets that biologics affect (Morrow and Felcone, 2004).

Unlike medicinal products that are made from small molecules, biologic therapies are made from living organisms from humans, animals, plants, and microorganisms. Biologics require a complex manufacturing process and may have intricate requirements for processing, purification, storing, and testing; they often contain heterogeneous molecules and/or polypeptides, making their profiles dependent on the process used to produce and test each batch (Morrow and Felcone, 2004). By definition, biosimilars will never be exact copies of their reference product (Giezen et al., 2016).

CONTENTS

Introduction 253

Biologics and Biosimilars Regulation 255

Safety Concerns With Biologics and Biosimilars 256

Special Considerations for Biosimilars 258

Post-Authorization Safety Studies Designs for Biologics and Biosimilars 261
Interventional Post-Authorization Safety Studies............ 262
Noninterventional Post-Authorization Safety Studies............ 263

Methodological Considerations .. 265
Research Questions .. 265
Outcome Measurement 267
Exposure Measurement 268

253

Post-Authorization Safety Studies of Medicinal Products. https://doi.org/10.1016/B978-0-12-809217-0.00007-6

Comparator
Selection.................... 270
Validity
Considerations 270

References 273

Recent patent expirations have led to the introduction of biosimilars or copy biologics, terminology used to describe the generic versions of patented biologic therapies (see Table 7.1.1 for terms and synonyms). This terminology refers to products that contain a version of the active substance of an already authorized original biological medicinal product, the so-called "reference medicinal product" (EMA, 2006, 2015), which are similar or highly similar versions of an approved reference biologic.

Table 7.1.1 Biologics Terminology

Term	Definition
Biologic product	Virus, therapeutic serum, toxin, antitoxin, vaccine, blood, blood component or derivative, allergenic product, protein (except chemically synthesized polypeptides), or analogous product applicable to prevent, treat, or cure of a disease/condition in humans.
Originator, reference product, comparator, innovator, biologic product	Novel biologic product that has been patented.
Biosimilar, similar biotherapeutic product (WHO), similar biological medicinal product (EU), subsequent entry biologic (Canada), biotechnology follow-on biologic (Japan), biocomparable (Mexico)	Biologic product with identical primary amino acid sequence to an originator product; developed with intention to be as close to originator as possible; and demonstrated similarity in physiochemical characteristics, efficacy, and safety.
Biobetter, biosuperior	Biological product based on an originator product, but with improvements to increase efficacy, potency, marketability, safety (including immunogenicity), patient adherence, and/or ease of administration.
Copy biologic, Alternative biologic, B-NSRA	Copy of an originator product that has been approved in a country where no official biosimilar regulatory pathway exists or existed.
Follow-on biologic, Follow-on protein	Umbrella term encompassing biosimilars and copy biologics ("copy" of an off-patent originator biologic).
Me-too biologic	Targets same pathway as originator biologic but developed independently and is not compared to it.
Simple biologic, first-generation biologic	Biologic synthesized or made from living cells.
Complex biologic, second-generation biologic	Biologic produced in living cells.

B-NSRA, *biopharmaceutical not subject to regulatory approval;* EU, *European Union,* WHO, *World Health Organization.*

BIOLOGICS AND BIOSIMILARS REGULATION

Many countries, along with the World Health Organization (WHO), have based their guidance for biosimilars on the European Medicines Agency (EMA) guidelines or have fully adopted the EMA guidance as their own (WHO, 2009; Scheinberg and Kay, 2012). The chronological timeline of when biosimilar regulations and guidelines have been issued by the EMA and the FDA is illustrated in Fig. 7.1.1. Whether the government body is the EMA or the FDA, the premise of a biosimilar development program is to demonstrate similarity, not patient benefit—as patient benefit has already been established by the reference product. Biosimilars are authorized based on a reduced and less costly data package by building on the safety and efficacy experience of the reference product.

The regulatory pathway for approval for biosimilars is an abbreviated pathway since theoretically, if the mechanism of action is presumed to be the same across multiple indications, potentially none or only one head-to-head comparison trial may be needed. This trial is conducted in patients

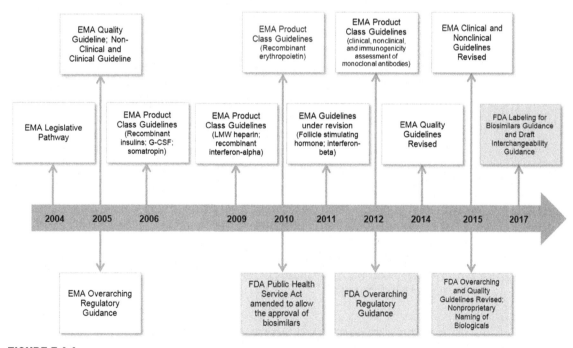

FIGURE 7.1.1
Timeline of overarching and product-specific biosimilar guidelines by the EMA and the FDA.

who are being treated for an indication that is determined, through discussions with regulators, to be the "most sensitive" indication. After demonstrating bioequivalence, it is highly likely that the biosimilar manufacturer will be granted extrapolation to many if not all other approved indications for the reference product without conducting clinical trials in these indications. Approval of extrapolation is based, in part, on scientific justification for the mechanism of action of each condition in which authorization is sought, e.g., target receptors for each relevant activity, the binding, or dose/concentration response, which is provided by the manufacturer (EMA, 2015; FDA, 2015b). This means that there is no clinical safety evidence available for each specific indication of the biosimilar for which it has authorization.

The indication that is deemed "most sensitive" may vary by regulatory agency and that scientific justification may be acceptable to some regulators in one region but not others. For example, the head-to-head comparison trial for the infliximab biosimilar was conducted in the rheumatoid arthritis indication (EMA, 2013). The EMA approved, through extrapolation, the authorization of several of the marketed indications for the reference product, which included other rheumatology diseases such as ankylosing spondylitis, psoriatic arthritis, and the gastroenterological indications of Crohn's disease and ulcerative colitis. The FDA authorized infliximab biosimilar with extrapolation to the adult indications of the reference product including the gastroenterological indications (FDA, 2016a). However, Health Canada did not approve extrapolation to the gastroenterological indications when it was initially approved in 2014 due to concerns with respect to the physicochemical and biological aspects of biosimilarity. Nevertheless, extrapolation to the gastroenterological indications was approved in 2016 following receipt of a supplemental application addressing the prior concerns (Health Canada, 2016).

The EMA has authorized 23 biosimilars since the introduction of their 2006 guidance (EMA, 2006, 2015), and as of October 2016, there were marketed 23 biosimilars for nine different reference products (EMA, 2016). As of the same date, four biosimilars have been authorized for four different reference products by the FDA under the 351(k) regulatory pathway (FDA, 2015b, 2016c), with the first approval in March 2015 and launch in September 2015 (Patel, 2015).

SAFETY CONCERNS WITH BIOLOGICS AND BIOSIMILARS

Unlike other pharmaceutical products, biologic therapies have special safety concerns given their complex manufacturing process and requirements for processing, purification, storing, and testing. Among these concerns are immunogenicity, manufacturing variability, product stability, product naming conventions, identification and traceability, and interchangeability and substitution of biosimilars. In addition to their safety consequences, these concerns also impart challenges during post-authorization safety studies (PASS) design and conduct for biologics and biosimilars.

Biologic products have the potential for immunogenic reactions by developing neutralizing antibody production. Immunogenicity is a concern for all biologic medicinal products and is an unwanted immune response that generally will not be of clinical significance, but in rare circumstances could result in serious and/or life-threatening events; thus considered "potentially clinically relevant" (EMA, 2016). Therefore, product-specific PASS may be required to determine if the identified risks are unrelated to or associated with the active substance or product class, or inactive ingredients (EMA, 2016).

A multitude of factors can affect immunogenicity. It can originate from one or more factors, including those related to product development, treatment administration or regimen, as well as the patient and disease profile in terms of genetic history, other concomitant medications, and underlying disease and immune status. The main concern is the introduction of neutralizing antibodies, which may lead to partial or complete loss of efficacy of the biologic product and can alter its pharmacokinetics.

Manufacturing variability refers to small and potentially insignificant changes to the manufacturing process (e.g., source materials, facilities, or regulatory requirements) that occur post-authorization (EMA, 2016). These changes are relevant within the same product (e.g., drift) and across products with the same international nonproprietary name (INN). These manufacturing changes can lead to different safety issues in terms of alteration of pharmacokinetics and immunogenicity. Both the reference product and biosimilar can independently undergo unique patterns of drift and evolution as the product evolves in the long-term post-authorization period (Ramanan and Grampp, 2014). Therefore, continuous life cycle implementation of PASS is important.

As with all biologic products, adherence to the appropriate storage and handling conditions, and good distribution practices are essential to maintain the stability of the product. Lack of such good practices can affect the stability and quality of the reference product or biosimilar, which then may introduce contamination or even immunogenicity. Therefore, maintaining pharmacovigilance at the level of the product and the batch number is important (EMA, 2016).

Both product and batch traceability are important considerations for updates to the risk management plan (EMA, 2016) because even small changes to the manufacturing process can alter the safety and immunogenicity profile, and product drift can occur over the post-authorization period. Products with the same INN must be distinguishable from one another to appropriately characterize the safety profile of a particular biologic product (reference or biosimilar), a particular challenge in the European Union (EU) where the biosimilar is authorized under the same INN as the reference product. Best practice for recording use of a reference product or biosimilar is for the health-care provider to record the trade name and batch number when different biologic products have the same INN, where the two products can be switched or substituted. Both of the identifiers should be available on the product packaging. However, there is no harmonization across health-care settings regarding the infrastructure for recording electronic health data and record linkage Moreover, most biologic medicinal products are administered in the hospital setting, so product identifiers may not be available in standard pharmacy databases.

SPECIAL CONSIDERATIONS FOR BIOSIMILARS

There are few special issues with biosimilars pharmacoepidemiologists need to consider, including interchangeability and substitution, naming conventions, and the context of use. The concept of interchangeability and substitution relates to the ability of a local pharmacy to provide a different product than what was requested by the prescriber. For biologics and biosimilars, this concept puts an extra burden on pharmacoepidemiologists for accurate exposure identification and understanding who is legally authorized to receive a biosimilar, whether the decision to substitute or switch a patient is made by the pharmacist or prescriber, and whether documentation of the switch or substitution will be available at the time of conducting PASS. Patients may not even be aware that they received a biosimilar as a substitute for the reference product.

The ability for a regulatory agency to determine interchangeability varies. For example, the decision regarding automatic substitution in the EU is up to the Member Countries, not the EMA (Thimmaraju et al., 2015). In the United States, the FDA can grant interchangeability of a biosimilar (FDA, 2015a), but the legislation about automatic substitution is the purview of each state (Cauchi, 2016).

The terms switching and substitution have been used synonymously, but they are actually distinctly different. Switching refers to when a prescriber makes the decision to exchange the one biologic for another with the same therapeutic intent in patients undergoing treatment (Ebbers and Chamberlain, 2014). Substitution on the other hand refers to when the pharmacist can dispense one product instead of another equivalent and interchangeable medicinal product without consulting the prescriber (Ebbers and Chamberlain, 2014). Table 7.1.2 summarizes the definitions for interchangeability, switching, and substitution. It is important to keep these terms straight to understand how interchangeability and substitution may impact PASS in terms of design, implementation, and interpretation of findings, particularly in relation to exposure classification.

In January 2017, the FDA issued its draft guidance for interchangeability, where it describes scientific considerations for demonstrating interchangeability (FDA, 2017a). The guidance outlines potential situations where post-authorization data of an already licensed biosimilar may support the demonstration of interchangeability; however, the specific type and amount of post-authorization data needed (e.g., surveillance data, PASS, or switching study) will depend on the residual uncertainty to establish interchangeability. In the United States as of July 2016, 23 states enacted laws allowing provisions of the pharmacist to substitute a biosimilar for a reference biologic. The legislation varies for each individual state, but common features include FDA approval, prescriber decision, "notification" versus "communication" to the prescriber, patient notification, retaining records, immunity, web lists, and cost or pricing.

As of October 2016, none of the four approved biosimilars in the United States have received interchangeable status. However, once FDA grants approval of interchangeability for a biosimilar, a prescriber may decide to prevent substitution by stating on the prescription "dispense as written" or "brand medically necessary." Some state legislation requires that the prescriber be notified of any substitution made by the pharmacist, but other legislation has modified the language to say that communication with

Table 7.1.2 Definitions of Interchangeability, Switching, and Substitution

Term	Definition
Interchangeability	Medical practice of changing one product for another that is expected to achieve the same clinical effect in a given clinical setting and in any patient on the initiative or with the agreement of the prescriber.
Switching	Decision by the treating physician to exchange one product for another with the same therapeutic intent in patients who are undergoing treatment.
Substitution	Practice of dispensing one product instead of another equivalent and interchangeable product at the pharmacy level without consulting the prescriber.

the prescriber via notation in the electronic medical record (EMR), pharmacy benefits management system record, or pharmacy record that can be electronically accessed by the prescriber is acceptable. In 12 states, the patient must be notified of the substitution or switch, and in some states the patient would be required to consent before any switch is made. The duration of how long a pharmacist and prescriber must retain records of the substitution is up to 5 years, but many states have not specified a duration. State legislation also varies in records to providing immunity for pharmacists who make a substitution that is in compliance with the biologics state law. Moreover, some states also mandate use of a public or web-based list of permissible interchangeable products. Finally, state legislation varies around the requirement for pharmacists to explain the cost or price of the biologic and interchangeable biosimilar, where in five states the substituted product must have the lowest cost. Specific details around the legislation in the United States by state can be found on the *State Laws and Legislation related to Biologic Medication and Substitution of Biosimilars* web page of the National Conference of State Legislatures (Cauchi, 2016).

There is some concern that in certain situations switching could be harmful to patients. The European Biopharmaceutical Enterprises, the European Federation of Pharmaceutical Industries and Associations, and the International Federation of Pharmaceutical Manufacturers and Associations have identified two situations in which they propose that switching from a reference product to a biosimilar (or between any products within a similar group of related products) should be avoided. Specifically, they caution against switching when the initial treatment choice (reference product or biosimilar) is no longer effective or the patient cannot tolerate the product because such switching may provoke the same lack of effectiveness and tolerability responses, and therefore, are unlikely to benefit the patient. They also expressed concern about the consequences of multiple exposures to the same group of related products and where such multiple exposures could affect the immunogenicity of future treatment with biologics, even though this appears to be speculation rather than based on real-world evidence. The groups also caution that a switch should be discouraged if the prescriber "feels that on balance a switch is likely to compromise future treatment options for the patient, e.g., with an alternate biological therapy." Thus, they advocate that prescribers should use their best clinical judgment to determine which product to prescribe (reference product or biosimilar) and that any decision to switch should be made in collaboration with, and with the full knowledge of the patient (EBE, 2017a,b).

The EMA uses identical INN for reference products and biosimilars and recommends that the trade name or brand name be used on prescribing to be able to distinguish between the products (EMA, 2015). However, in practice where prescribers will write down Remicade or Inflectra, for example, versus infliximab, may vary by prescriber, region, or country. Australia generally follows the EMA system for naming biosimilars (Australian Government, 2015); but in Japan, the INN is followed by "follow-on 1" (or 2, 3, etc., based on the order of approval) (Derbyshire, 2013), and South Korea uses only the proprietary (brand) name (Murphy, 2015).

In the United States, the FDA has used different naming practices for nonproprietary names from the first approved biosimilar to the second, third, and fourth approved biosimilar. The first biosimilar was named filgrastim-sndz with the 4-letter suffix representing the manufacturer name. Since the approval, the FDA revised their naming guidance for both biologics and biosimilars to carry a random 4-digit suffix (FDA, 2017b). The infliximab biosimilar was approved as infliximab-dyyb, the etanercept biosimilar was approved as etanercept-szzs, and the adalimumab biosimilar was approved as adalimumab-atto. The FDA has yet to grant interchangeability status to a biosimilar, and whether an interchangeable biosimilar will have a unique 4-letter suffix or the same suffix as the reference product is still to be determined (FDA, 2017b).

The WHO has proposed including a 4-letter suffix assigned at random as a biologic qualifier for naming purposes (WHO, 2015). For the time being, pharmacoepidemiologists should assume that naming conventions for biosimilars will vary by jurisdiction.

The context of use is important to consider when designing PASS for biosimilars. Reimbursement and health-care coverage can affect who receives a biologic or biosimilar. Many countries in Western Europe, such as the United Kingdom, have national health insurance schemes that will likely influence who receives the biologic or the biosimilar, especially for new users. In contrast, countries where patients bear much, if not all, the full cost of treatment, there could be fundamental differences in those who choose the biosimilar versus the reference product. Reimbursement for biologic products may also lead to selection bias in which patients can be recruited for prospective PASS. For example, identification and enrollment of an internal or contemporaneous comparator group receiving the reference product may not be possible once a health-care system supports the use of a biosimilar.

POST-AUTHORIZATION SAFETY STUDIES DESIGNS FOR BIOLOGICS AND BIOSIMILARS

Traditionally, randomized controlled trials (RCT) have been used to establish proof of efficacy and safety. Although such situations are elegant and widely accepted, trials are relatively expensive and by design, limit variability by controlling enrollment characteristics. For this reason, these studies will provide limited information about real-world product use where patients are likely to have comorbidities and other more heterogeneous clinical characteristics that may affect their treatment response. To address safety and effectiveness in these broader populations, real-world approaches are often used to provide more substance to regulatory submission packages and to provide evidence to clinicians and payers through presentations and publications.

PASS can help describe treatment patterns, demonstrate safety profile, and identify delayed risks related to biosimilars. The appropriate study design will depend on the research question and an understanding of the local regulations and clinical practice. Table 7.1.3 summarizes the key considerations for determining the appropriate PASS design for biologics and biosimilars.

The following are some of the study designs used in safety studies for biologics and biosimilars. More detail on each approach can be found in previous chapters.

Interventional Post-Authorization Safety Studies

Interventional designs, such as pragmatic clinical trials (PCT), may be the best option to answer questions about comparative safety when the patients of interest are not treated with the reference product or biosimilar of interest in routine clinical practice, or the use of the reference product or biosimilar is ubiquitous (i.e., no one is using the biologic product of interest, whether due to reimbursement decisions or prescriber adoption). The protocol-driven

Table 7.1.3 Key Considerations for Determining Appropriate Post-Authorization Safety Studies Design for Biologics and Biosimilars

PASS Design	Consideration
Interventional	<ul><li>Patients of interest are not being treated with the reference product or biosimilar of interest in routine clinical practice.</li><li>Use of the reference product or the biosimilar is ubiquitous.</li><li>Need for clinical data or assessments that are not performed in routine clinical practice.</li></ul>
Noninterventional prospective	<ul><li>Patients of interest are being treated with the reference product or biosimilar in routine clinical practice.</li><li>Clinical data captured from routine care and data collection is aligned with routine clinic visits.</li><li>Patient and/or physician reported information can be collected</li></ul>
Noninterventional retrospective	<ul><li>Patients of interest who are using the reference product or biosimilar can be identified from paper or electronic medical records or administrative databases.</li><li>Whether the patient is on the reference product versus the biosimilar can be distinguished without primary data collection.</li></ul>

aspect of PCT occurs at baseline, whether patients are randomized to treatment but are followed per routine clinical care.

Interventional PASS may be the best option when there is a need for clinical data or assessments to be collected that are not routinely performed in regular clinical practice on all patients. For example, if immunogenicity is of most concern, interventional PASS may be warranted to collect immunogenicity assays on all patients, not just those who experience a safety concern. Chapter 4.5 discusses PCT in detail.

Noninterventional Post-Authorization Safety Studies

Noninterventional PASS can be prospective, including primary data collection through patient registries, and retrospective, including chart reviews and existing databases (i.e., secondary use of data). A combination of retrospective and prospective approaches can be used in enriched studies. Chapter 4.5 discusses prospective designs, and Chapters 4.1—4.3 provide an overview of different retrospective designs commonly used for PASS. Enriched approaches are discussed with greater detail in Chapter 4.4.

Prospective designs may be the preferred approach when the patients of interest are being treated with the reference product or biosimilar in routine clinical practice. All of the data being collected are captured from routine care, and data collection is aligned with routine clinic visits (Glicklich and Dreyer, 2014). Careful design to minimize threats to validity must be taken into consideration when designing noninterventional PASS.

A patient registry in rheumatoid arthritis or ulcerative colitis, for example, can be conducted to enroll all patients diagnosed with the specific indication of interest. Alternatively a patient registry of all patients receiving a type of medicinal products (e.g., biologics) or specific product (e.g., infliximab) can also be conducted. An infliximab registry could be initiated to enroll all patients, regardless of indication, who receive the infliximab biologic of interest (reference or biosimilar). Both of these registry types would allow for contemporaneous comparator group information to be collected. Examples of existing biologic registries include the British Society for Rheumatology Biologics Register (Watson et al., 2005; Silman et al., 2003); Germany's Rheumatoide Arthritis: Beobachtung der Biologika-Therapie register (Deutsches Rheuma-Forschungszentrum, 2001); Antirheumatic Therapy in Sweden register (Neovius et al., 2011); and the British Association of Dermatologists' Biologic Interventions Register for patients with psoriasis treated with biologics (Burden et al., 2012). All of these country-specific registries are long-term observational registries of patients treated with biologic medicinal products.

Another patient registry option would be one of the biosimilar only or a "product registry" where patients are enrolled only if they are on a specific brand of infliximab biosimilar, for example. However, contemporaneous comparators would not be available in this approach and comparisons would need to be made to external or historical comparator groups. Chapter 3.3 provides an overview of registries as data sources for PASS.

On the other hand, retrospective PASS are best suited when the patients of interest are using the reference product or biosimilar of interest, and the product used by patients can be identified from EMR or other existing databases such as prescription databases and claims. Database studies can be used to determine feasibility and to develop hypotheses for prospective PASS. Discussions on claims and EMR as data sources for PASS are found in Chapters 3.1 and 3.2.

A retrospective PASS may be an ideal solution to provide descriptive information about the patient population receiving the biologic of interest, to quantify disease burden, evaluate treatment patterns, and compare across marketed products. Retrospective PASS are favorable when there is a need to look at extremely large populations or to identify rare events. However, the underlying information may not be collected in a systematic way and it can be difficult to interpret missing data; it is important to know why something is recorded and what its intended purpose is. With different modalities of data collection across health-care plans, regions, and countries, it is important to understand how data were coded and if a data dictionary exists. Other limitations of using existing data include the possibility of incomplete medical histories, nonuniform availability of data across countries of interest, and privacy issues that may create the need to use aggregated patient data. See Chapter 3.4 for an overview of big data.

It is important to remember that because biologic products are used to treat serious—and mostly chronic illnesses, dosing regimens may vary considerably depending on the type of biologic and the indication for which it is being administered. With serious illnesses come clinical complexity and the potential for substantial confounding, which may be intensified by missing data on prognostic indicators. Understanding the factors that influence initiation and discontinuation (switching vs. substitution) of a biologic product need to be carefully considered. Furthermore, clinical effectiveness measures are not typically reliably recorded in existing data, and the level of detail for most safety outcomes may lead to suboptimal sensitivity or specificity. In addition, careful attention must be paid to whether biological product prescriptions can be found in conventional pharmacy databases, which drug codes are used for the reference product and the biosimilar, and if the level of detail about the prescription and administration of the biologic are available.

As it was mentioned in Chapter 4.4, existing data can also be combined with prospective data capture resulting in "enriched" designs, which can be more cost-efficient than primary data collection alone. Integrated multisource data can provide a comprehensive view of the disease, care, and outcomes by using specific measures where needed, such as including patient-reported assessments and special clinical reported outcomes, and relying on existing data when sufficient.

As it is highly unlikely that any one database will include all data needed to describe full details on clinical characteristics, whether the prescribed biologic product was the one administered, or distinguish whether switching or substitution occurred. Prospective follow-up can be achieved through primary data collection, recording the brand of reference product or biosimilar administered and allowing for collection of patient- and prescriber-reported outcome data. Pharmacy and other data may be used to supplement prospectively collected data, depending on data availability and locality. Enriched PASS can be used for both prospective and PCT, where treatment assignment to a reference product or biosimilar is made by randomization and all follow-up is naturalistic.

METHODOLOGICAL CONSIDERATIONS

When designing PASS for biologics and biosimilars, pharmacoepidemiologists need to pay attention to key considerations for appropriate study design, implementation, and interpretation of findings. These include considerations related to the research questions, exposure and outcome measurements, comparator selection, and internal validity factors.

Research Questions

The best approach for generating reliable evidence for biologics will depend on the research question. Biologics-related research questions can be categorized into six broad types, which can contribute to understanding product risk: descriptive studies; treatment patterns and switching; safety and immunogenicity; clinical and comparative effectiveness; heterogeneity of exposure effect; and delayed risks and benefits.

Descriptive studies are those that describe the population with the indication of interest who are receiving the reference product or biosimilar of interest and clinical practice patterns. Studies of treatment patterns or drug utilization can be used to understand how the reference product was used for treatment before the launch of the biosimilar or can be used to understand switching patterns between the reference product and biosimilar. Depending on the data source, descriptive and drug utilization studies may be well suited for using existing or secondary data sources where it is possible to distinguish between the biosimilar and reference products. For example, in an Italian administrative claims database, the brand name of the product was available, making it an ideal data source to examine drug utilization and patterns of switching (Ingrasciotta et al., 2015). See Chapter 4.1 for a discussion about drug utilization studies and prescription-event monitoring studies.

To evaluate safety outcomes in secondary databases, it may be necessary to link the databases of prescription information with those that capture information on safety events, which should exist. However, the level of detail on a safety event may not be at the level of granularity needed for reporting purposes, and augmentation with prospective data collection may be required. For immunogenicity, unless there is a clinical concern, immunogenicity is not routinely performed in clinical practice, so obtaining immunogenicity in noninterventional PASS will be challenging. Therefore, if the objective is to study the immunogenicity profile of a specific biosimilar, RCT or minimally interventional studies would be the appropriate design to mandate the assessment of immunogenicity in all eligible patients, not just those with a concern.

Clinical effectiveness studies may be of particular interest for indications in which the biosimilar received authorization for through extrapolation for their indication (e.g., gastroenterological indications for infliximab). As with all biologics, clinical effectiveness measures may or may not be routinely recorded in secondary data sources. For renal anemia, hemoglobin is measured routinely and is available in some existing data sources to allow for the evaluation of the reference product or biosimilar in routine clinical practice. On the other hand, for reference products or biosimilars used to treat Crohn's disease, the Crohn's disease activity index (CDAI), or for psoriasis, the psoriasis area severity index (PASI) would not be routinely captured in existing databases. Primary data collection may be necessary to evaluate clinical effectiveness of a biosimilar.

Biosimilars PASS may require particular consideration regarding interchangeability, substitution and type of reimbursement, and coverage in the target countries of interest. If the study is being conducted in a country with a national health-care system where all patients receive the reference product or all patients receive the biosimilar, an internal comparator from the same site or country may be impossible to enroll contemporaneously, and PCT may be the only appropriate real-world evidence study design if comparative evidence is needed post-authorization. Depending on the reimbursement and health insurance coverage in the target countries of interest, there could be inherent differences in those who receive the reference product than those that are on the biosimilar. In particular, if a patient already has adequate reimbursement or coverage to receive the reference product, what would be the incentive to switch to the biosimilar? Examination of heterogeneity of exposure effect and other subgroup analyses will be important to understand which populations may have higher or lower benefits or risks. Ensuring enrollment of an adequate number of patients within the important subgroups of interest should be considered.

Information about exposure effect heterogeneity is important to patients, clinicians, and health-care systems, which could be addressed by focusing on some simple data that can be collected fairly easily by health-care providers, such as age, gender, race, ethnicity, disease severity, comorbidities, comedications, and previous treatments. Most, if not all of these "explanatory" variables are part of the health record and are easily recordable for every patient. Disease severity can be the most difficult to categorize, though for indications such as rheumatoid arthritis and non-Hodgkin's lymphoma, some relatively straight-forward measures can be used. Similarly, if the decision is made to record other product use, which can sometimes be the cause of a delayed safety event, it may be sufficient to collect only information about which products have been used and whether they are being used concurrently with the biologic or biosimilar of interest.

Depending on the length of observation affordable in any post-authorization study, it may also be beneficial to examine "delayed" risks and benefits because most RCT focus on the relatively short treatment duration and intermediate outcomes. Depending on the therapeutic indication and the labeled administration, there could be substantial clinical interest in systematic evaluation of longer-term effectiveness, especially when considering the use of concomitant medicinal products that are administered in combination with the reference product or biosimilar (e.g., chemotherapy). Delayed risks and benefits are also important to consider within the context of patients who switch from the reference product to the biosimilar. Considerations around whether the use of the reference product or biosimilar can be identified from the data source over the course of the study period will help determine whether any risks or benefits are simply delayed effects from use on the reference product or potentially due to the switch to the biosimilar.

Outcome Measurement

Effectiveness outcomes of interest may be difficult to identify from existing data sources alone. Typically, outcome measures that are used to establish the efficacy of a biologic product in pre-authorization RCT are generally not routinely or systematically collected in standard databases. Test results are sometimes captured as images in EMR, making it difficult to extract exact values. The exception being hemoglobin levels are captured in some databases. In contrast, for granulocyte-colony stimulating factors, the absolute neutrophil count is rarely captured and the temporal sequence may not be well established. For anti-TNF biologics, effectiveness measures for disease activity using particularly clinician- or patient-reported scales that are not generally available in existing records, despite their popularity, e.g., for Disease Activity Score (DAS28) for rheumatoid arthritis (NRAS, 2007); PASI (PASI Training, 2009); and CDAI (Best et al., 1976). Therefore, primary data collection may be needed to generate valid evidence on clinical effectiveness outcomes.

The completeness, accuracy, and level of detail for safety events of interest will vary by data source and recording practices in the countries or regions of interest. For example, although the FDA Sentinel System has developed validated algorithms for identifying safety outcomes with generally good operating characteristics, such as high specificity and positive predictive values, the algorithms for safety events of biologic products have had less desirable operating characteristics (FDA, 2008). In April 2015, a US initiative called the Biologic and Biosimilars Collective Intelligence Consortium, funded by managed care organizations, integrated delivery networks, pharmacy benefits managers, and Harvard Pilgrim Healthcare Institute, was initiated for the purpose of using the distributed data network (DDN) design of the Sentinel System to establish a data source for evaluating safety of reference and biosimilar products (AMCP Task Force on Biosimilar Collective Intelligence Systems, 2015). See Chapter 5.5 for more discussion on the Sentinel System.

Exposure Measurement

Exposure data may be more challenging to obtain using noninterventional PASS because many of biologic products, and hence biosimilars, can be administered by health-care providers in hospital settings. Population-based databases mainly include information from general practitioners and community pharmacies and will contain only limited information on patients who are exposed to biologic products. Biologics with multiple indications have different dosage regimens depending on the indication, which adds complexity to the ability to assess exposure and identifying the number of patients actually exposed from existing databases alone. Biologic medicinal products also have prolonged pharmacodynamics effects, which should be taken into consideration when defining the "at-risk window" or the period that a certain safety event could be attributed to the reference product or biosimilar.

Knowing how the biologic product is administered (e.g., self-administered injection or intravenous infusion) will help determine where to find the relevant data on treatment exposure, and in the United States, whether the biologic product is covered under the medical or pharmacy benefit. Chronic use of a reference product and/or biosimilar is also an important aspect to consider when defining exposure to treatment. Collection of start and stop dates, and dose escalations or reductions will be important to distinguish treatment "holidays" from discontinuation for the biosimilar versus the reference product. Switching and substitution should also be taken into account. Depending on reimbursement decisions and local substitution laws, switching may occur multiple times over the course of PASS and may occur in multiple ways between the reference product, biosimilar, or other biosimilars for the same reference product with or without prescriber's awareness. Being able to distinguish the biosimilar from its reference product is imperative to accurately attribute the benefits and risks to the correct product.

Coding of reference products and biosimilars may vary by country, region, or even specific data sources. Specifically in the United States, coding of biologic products for claims and reimbursement is based on the National Drug Code (NDC) and the Health Care Common Procedure Coding System (HCPCS) (CMS, 2016a; FDA, 2016b). The NDC identifies the product based on the dosage, manufacturer, and packaging and is required on a claim for pharmacy reimbursement under the pharmacy benefit (e.g., Medicare Part D). Although NDC can distinguish biosimilars from the reference products, even when the same INN is used, many of biologic products are not dispensed through outpatient pharmacies as they are typically intravenous infusions or injections.

Biologic products are typically administered by a health-care provider and reimbursed under the medical benefit (e.g., Medicare Part B). HCPCS was implemented by the Centers for Medicare and Medicaid Services (CMS) (CMS, 2016a), and they are required on medical claims for reimbursement of medicinal products administered by a health-care provider, but including the NDC on the claim is not required. Although an HCPCS code is unique, the unique code is assigned 1−2 years after market entry; thus the claims for newly authorized biosimilar products will be billed under a miscellaneous HCPCS code (J-codes) until a permanent HCPCS code is assigned. Although CMS will create different permanent HCPCS codes for biosimilars from their reference product, products that are considered therapeutic equivalents of a reference product or have similar clinical efficacy and indications often share the same HCPCS codes. Therefore, multiple biosimilars for the same reference product will likely have the same HCPCS code. CMS is mandating the use of a biosimilar-specific modifier on claims for biosimilars (CMS, 2016b). These modifiers are published on a quarterly basis on the *Part B Biosimilar Biological Product Payment and Required Modifiers* CMS web page. If an HCPCS code or corresponding modifier is not published, then the modifier is not required for the claim using the miscellaneous J-code.

Given how products are coded in the United States, the timing around the evaluation of existing electronic data sources for the number of patients exposed to a newly authorized biosimilar will be an important consideration during PASS design.

Comparator Selection

In the case of comparative PASS, naming conventions and interchangeability/ substitution practices may affect the feasibility of identifying and selecting appropriate comparators, and this will depend on the target market. The choice of comparator will depend on routine local clinical practice and product availability, and may be the reference product, other biosimilars of the same reference product, or other therapeutic options used to treat the condition. Because patients, prescribers, and payers are interested in current treatment choices, the collection of contemporaneous comparators can be useful for addressing the complex issue of having sufficiently detailed, clinically relevant, or timely data. Historical comparators are susceptible to bias due to changes over time in confounding risk factors that may contribute to potentially erroneous observed differences between the biosimilar and reference product in safety and effectiveness outcomes. Different patients may be treated now with different regimens and dosing, making it nearly impossible to address these issues using historical comparators. Thus, the validity of the comparison may be in question if other comparator choices are available. External comparators are useful for understanding the observed effects and to assess the generalizability of study findings. External comparator data are often generated from different methods and some data elements that are commonly used in RCT may be unavailable when real-world designs are used. Practical considerations and minimizing the potential for bias and confounding are critical aspects for selecting the appropriate comparator group in noninterventional settings. Table 7.1.4 summarizes key considerations regarding exposure classification.

Validity Considerations

Selection bias is likely in biologics and biosimilars PASS. It is essential to understand who prescribes biologics and biosimilars and if and how they differ. Different types of institutions or geographic locales may prescribe biosimilars. There may be differences in the type of patients who receive a biosimilar, such as economic differences in being able to afford the brand name biologic, which also will affect other health risks. For prospective PASS, there is also a potential for greater patient interest and high participation rates from regions with little to no reimbursement of biologics or inadequate insurance, especially when products may be available without charges for a study or be subsidized for the purpose of the study.

Table 7.1.4 Key Considerations for Exposure Measurement in Post-Authorization Safety Studies Design for Biologics and Biosimilars

Aspect	Consideration
Prescription	• Who and how is the biologic product administered? • Is the biologic product a monotherapy or a polytherapy? • For which indication and dosing regimen is the biologic being used for? • Is the product name or batch number recorded? • Is there health insurance coverage or reimbursement for the reference product or biosimilar of interest?
Long-term use	• Can start and stop dates be captured? • Is new biosimilar use distinguishable from prior reference product use? • Have there been changes in product availability over the study period?
Switching	• Is switching from a reference product to a biosimilar allowed in the countries of interest? • Is the physician deciding to switch a patient to a biosimilar from the reference product or is substitution occurring at the pharmacy level? • Are patients being "switched" multiple times over the study period?

There is a potential for exposure misclassification due to the ability or inability to identify whether a patient received the reference product or the biosimilar, and whether the necessary level of granularity is available (e.g., start and stop dates and identification over the duration of the study, not just at baseline). When using an existing data source, understanding how biosimilars are named and coded within the data source is critical. If a prescription is written, it is important to consider what was actually administered and where would that information be available. For self-administered biologics, was the original or biosimilar actually filled? For infusions, is the exposure information of which product was actually administered included in the patient's chart at the specialist office or only at the infusion center?

In addition to selection and information biases, confounding is a concern in all noninterventional PASS, and particularly so in real-world studies, where patients have chronic and severe conditions and may receive other concurrent therapies. As an example, patients with cancer receiving pegfilgrastim will also receive chemotherapy, making it challenging to tease apart the effects of the two treatments. Because biosimilars will be authorized for the same indications and at the same doses as the reference product, little to no confounding would be expected by patient-level factors or prognostic characteristics. However, there is a potential confounding by prescriber and patient preference, product supply, and insurance coverage; posing challenges to separate actual exposure effects from these extraneous factors.

Channeling bias, which occurs when therapies for similar indications are administered to subpopulations of patients with prognostic differences, can be a concern (Ali, 2013). Many biologics are second- or third-line therapies that are administered after failure of "standard therapy," which limits the patient population to those who tend to have more severe disease or poorer prognosis, which can lead to channeling bias. These patients may also have concomitant medicinal products that will need to be considered to tease out any safety outcomes of the biologic from the use of these other products. Physicians may prescribe new products more often to patients who have already failed an existing or first-line therapy. Preference for prescribing a biosimilar or not will be a challenge to consider when designing, implementing, and interpreting results of biosimilars PASS as it could obscure any differences between the biosimilar compared with the originator on long-term safety and effectiveness outcomes.

There is a possibility of confounding by severity where some countries or physician groups only allow patients who have not yet started a biologic for a specific indication to be on a biosimilar. Where a country's legislation only allow for patients who have been stable on a reference biologic to switch to a biosimilar. There would be obvious differences in disease status of the patients. Additionally, there may be an impact by the local legislations around switching and substation. Table 7.1.5 provides a summary of the

Table 7.1.5 Key Considerations for Internal Validity in Post-Authorization Safety Studies Design for Biologics and Biosimilars

Validity Threat	Consideration
Selection bias	• Different sites may prescribe the reference product than the biosimilar. • Patients on the biosimilar may be different than those on reference product. • Potential greater patient interest and higher participation rates from regions with little to no reimbursement of biologics or inadequate insurance.
Information bias	• Potential exposure misclassification due to the inability to identify whether a patient received the reference product or biosimilar with the necessary level of granularity. • Naming and coding considerations. • Recording of batch/lot number from the package in charts. • Potential exposure misclassification due to interchangeability and substitution laws and whether the physician and/or patient know which biologic (reference product or biosimilar) was administered.
Confounding	• Ability to distinguish whether outcomes are attributed to the reference product or biosimilar, or a concomitant medication. • Potential for confounding by severity due to local legislation around which patients can be switched to a biosimilar from a reference product or if only patients who are biologically naïve can receive the biosimilar.

considerations for the internal validity of the evidence from biologics and biosimilars PASS.

Depending on the study design, analytic methods such as exposure propensity scores should be considered to balance confounders at the initiation of the reference product or biosimilar (Rubin, 1997; Rassen and Schneeweiss, 2012). Most importantly, quantitative bias analysis can be used to examine the potential influence of missing confounding variables and misclassification on the findings from PASS (Lash et al., 2009). Chapters 5.1−5.3 discuss analytical approaches to account for bias and confounding in PASS.

PASS for biologics and biosimilars require careful design and implementation to generate quality evidence to support decision-making. The best approaches will consider the target countries and health-care systems of interest with regard to

- Clinical practice patterns and the acceptance of biosimilars among the specialty prescribers for the indications of interest
- Reimbursement and health-care coverage, particularly whether there is national health-care coverage, preferential reimbursements for biosimilars compared with the reference products, and the amount of copayment required from patients
- Naming and coding for reference products and biosimilars in the health-care system and data sources of interest, and whether biosimilars can be distinguished from reference biologics and from each other; and
- Whether pharmacists can automatically substitute a biosimilar for the reference product without notifying the prescribing physician, and whether product use can be linked to specific patients.

Understanding what to look out for and how these issues may impact PASS results is essential to achieve strong evidence and reliable interpretation to characterize the safety profile of biologics and biosimilars.

References

Ahluwalia, J.P., 2012. Immunotherapy in inflammatory bowel disease. Med. Clin. North Am. 96 (3), 525−544.

Ali, A.K., 2013. Methodological challenges in observational research: a pharmacoepidemiological perspective. Br. J. Pharmaceut. Res. 3 (2), 161−175.

AMCP Task Force on Biosimilar Collective Intelligence Systems, 2015. Utilizing data consortia to monitor safety and effectiveness of biosimilars and their innovator products. J. Manag. Care Spec. Pharm. 21 (1), 23−34.

Australian Government, 2015. Regulation of Biosimilar Medicines. Version 2.0, December 2015. Available from: https://www.tga.gov.au/publication/evaluation-biosimilars.

Best, W.R., Becktel, J.M., Singelton, J.W., Kern, F.J., 1976. Development of a Crohn's disease activity index. National cooperative Crohn's disease study. Gastroenterology 70 (3), 439−444.

Burden, A.D., Warren, R.B., Kleyn, C.E., McElhone, K., Smith, C.H., Reynolds, N.J., on behalf of the BSG, 2012. The British Association of Dermatologists' Biologic Interventions Register (BADBIR): design, methodology and objectives. Br. J. Dermatol. 166 (3), 545–554.

Cauchi, R., 2016. State Laws and Legislation Related to Biologic Medications and Substitution of Biosimilars. National Conference of State Legislatures. Updated June 1, 2016. Available from: http://www.ncsl.org/documents/health/Biologics_BiosimilarsNCSLReport2015.pdf.

Centers for Medicare & Medicaid Services (CMS), 2016a. HCPCS- General Information. Available from: https://www.cms.gov/Medicare/Coding/MedHCPCSGenInfo/index.html?redirect=/medhcpcsgeninfo/.

Centers for Medicare & Medicaid Services (CMS), 2016b. Part B Biosimilar Biological Product Payment and Required Modifiers. Baltimore, MD. Available from: https://www.cms.gov/Medicare/Medicare-Fee-for-Service-Part-B-Drugs/McrPartBDrugAvgSalesPrice/Part-B-Biosimilar-Biological-Product-Payment.html.

Derbyshire, M., 2013. Biosimilar development and regulation in Japan. GaBI J. 2 (4), 207–208.

Derwenskus, J., 2011. Current disease-modifying treatment of multiple sclerosis. Mt. Sinai J. Med. 78 (2), 161–175.

Deutsches Rheuma-Forschungszentrum, 2001. RABBIT - Rheumatoide Arthritis: Beobachtung der Biolgoika-Therapie. Available from: http://www.biologika-register.de/en/home/.

Duffy, M.J., 2013. The war on cancer: are we winning? Tumor Biol. 34 (3), 1275–1284.

Ebbers, H.C., Chamberlain, P., 2014. Interchangeability. An insurmountable fifth hurdle? GaBI J. 3 (2), 88–93.

European Biopharmaceutical Enterprises (EBE), European Federation of Pharmaceutical Industries and Associations (EFPIA), International Federation of Pharmaceutical Manufacturers and Associations (IFPMA), 2017a. Considerations for Physicians on Switching Decisions Regarding Biosimilars. Available from: http://www.efpia.eu/uploads/Modules/Documents/annex-1–-considerations-for-switching-decisions_biosimilars-and-rbps-final.pdf.

European Biopharmaceutical Enterprises (EBE), European Federation of Pharmaceutical Industries and Associations (EFPIA), International Federation of Pharmaceutical Manufacturers and Associations (IFPMA), 2017b. EBE, EFPIA and IFPMA Have Today Launched a Position Paper Entitled "Considerations for Physicians on Switching Decisions Regarding Biosimilars" [Press Release]. Available from: http://www.efpia.eu/mediaroom/384/43/EBE-EFPIA-and-IFPMA-have-today-launched-a-position-paper-entitled-Considerations-for-physicians-on-switching-decisions-regarding-biosimilars.

European Medicines Agency (EMA), 2016. European Public Assessments Reports. Available from: http://www.ema.europa.eu/ema/index.jsp?curl=pages/medicines/landing/epar_search.jsp&mid=WC0b01ac058001d124&searchTab=searchByAuthType&keyword=Enter%20keywords&searchType=name&alreadyLoaded=true&status=Authorised&status=Withdrawn&status=Suspended&status=Refused&jsenabled=false&searchGenericType=biosimilars&orderBy=authDate&pageNo=1.

European Medicines Agency (EMA) (CHMP/437/04 Rev 1), 2015. Guideline on Similar Biological Medicinal Products. (CHMP/437/04 Rev 1). European Medicines Agency. Available from: http://www.ema.europa.eu/docs/en_GB/document_library/Scientific_guideline/2014/10/WC500176768.pdf.

European Medicines Agency (EMA) (CHMP/437/04), 2006. Guidelines on Similar Biological Medinical Products. European Medicines Agency. Available from: http://www.ema.europa.eu/docs/en_GB/document_library/Scientific_guideline/2009/09/WC500003517.pdf.

European Medicines Agency (EMA) (EMA/168402/2014), 2016. Guideline on Good Pharmacovigilance Practices (GVP). Product- or Population-specific Considerations II: Biological Medicinal Products (EMA/168402/2014). Available from: http://www.ema.europa.eu/docs/en_GB/document_library/Scientific_guideline/2016/08/WC500211728.pdf.

European Medicines Agency (EMA) (EMA/CHMP/589422/2013), 2013. Inflectra Assessment Report. Available from: http://www.ema.europa.eu/docs/en_GB/document_library/EPAR_-_Public_assessment_report/human/002778/WC500151490.pdf.

Food and Drug Administration (FDA), 2008. The Sentinel Initiative: National Strategy for Monitoring Medical Product Safety. FDA. Available from: http://www.fda.gov/downloads/Safety/FDAsSentinelInitiative/UCM124701.pdf.

Food and Drug Administration (FDA), 2015a. Biosimilars: Additional Questionss and Answers Regarding Implementation of the Biologics Price Competition and Innovation Act of 2009. Guidance for Industry. (Revision 1). Available from: http://www.fda.gov/downloads/Drugs/.../Guidances/UCM273001.pdf.

Food and Drug Administration (FDA), 2015b. Scientific Considerations in Demonstrating Biosimilarity to a Reference Product. U.S. Food and Drug Administration. Available from: http://www.fda.gov/downloads/drugs/guidancecomplianceregulatoryinformation/guidances/ucm291128.pdf.

Food and Drug Administration (FDA), 2016a. Inflectra Prescribing Information. (Reference No. 3912620). Available from: http://www.accessdata.fda.gov/drugsatfda_docs/label/2016/125544s000lbl.pdf.

Food and Drug Administration (FDA), 2016b. National Drug Code Directory. Available from: https://www.fda.gov/Drugs/InformationOnDrugs/ucm142438.htm.

Food and Drug Administration (FDA), 2016c, CDER 23 October 2016, CBER 30 August 2016. Puple Book. Available from: http://www.fda.gov/Drugs/DevelopmentApprovalProcess/HowDrugsareDevelopedandApproved/ApprovalApplications/TherapeuticBiologicApplications/Biosimilars/ucm411418.htm.

Food and Drug Administration (FDA), 2017a. Considerations for Demonstrating Interchangeability With a Reference Product: Guidance for Industry (Draft Guidance). Available from: http://www.fda.gov/ucm/groups/fdagov-public/@fdagov-drugs-gen/documents/document/ucm537135.pdf.

Food and Drug Administration (FDA), 2017b. Nonproprietary Naming of Biological Products: Guidance for Industry. Available from: http://www.fda.gov/downloads/drugs/guidances/ucm459987.pdf.

Ferrante, M., D'Haens, G., Rutgeerts, P., Vermerire, S., Van Assche, G., 2009. Optimizing biologic therapies for inflammatory bowel disease (ulcerative colitis and Crohn's disease). Curr. Gastroenterol. Reb. 11 (6), 504–508.

Giezen, T.J., Avendaño-Solá, C., Wolff-Holz, E., Weise, M., Ekman, N., Laslop, A., Annese, V., 2016. Roundtable on biosimilars with European regulators and medical societies, Brussels, Belgium, 12 January 2016. GaBI J. 5 (2), 74–83.

Glicklich, R.E., Dreyer, N.A., 2014. In: Leavy, M.B. (Ed.), Registries for Evaluation Patient Outcomes: A User's Guide, third ed. Agency for Healthcare Research and Quality. Available from: https://ahrq-ehc-application.s3.amazonaws.com/media/files/registries-guide-3rd-edition-vol-2-140430.pdf.

Griffin, M.M., Morley, N., 2013. Rituximab in the treatment of non-Hodgkin's lymphoma – a critical evaluation of randomized controlled trials. Expet Opin. Biol. Ther. 13 (5), 803–811.

Health Canada, 2016. Inflectra: Summary Basis of Decision (SBD). Available from: http://www.hc-sc.gc.ca/dhp-mps/prodpharma/sbd-smd/drug-med/sbd_smd_2014_inflectra_159493-eng.php.

Horton, S.C., Emery, P., 2012. Biological therapy for rheumatoid arthritis: where are we now? Br. J. Hosp. Med. 73 (1), 12–18.

Ingrasciotta, Y., Giorgianni, F., Bolcato, J., Chinellato, A., Pirolo, R., Tari, D.U., Trifirò, G., 2015. How much are biosimilars used in clinical practice? A retrospective Italian population-based study of erythropoiesis-stimulating agents in the years 2009–2013. BioDrugs 29 (4), 275–284.

Lash, T.L., Fox, M.P., Fink, A.K., 2009. Applying Quantitative Bias Analysis to Epidemiologic Data. Springer, Springer Dordrecht Heidelberg London New York.

Morrow, T., Felcone, L.H., 2004. Defining the difference. What makes biologics unique. Biotechnol. Healthc. 1 (4), 24-26, 29-29.

Murphy, B., 2015. Debate over naming of biosimilars intensifies ahead of WHO meeting. Pharmaceut. J. 294. Available from: http://www.pharmaceutical-journal.com/news-and-analysis/news/debate-over-naming-of-biosimilars-intensifies-ahead-of-who-meeting/20068663.article.

National Rheumatoid Arthritis Society (NRAS), 2007. The DAS28 Score. Available from: http://www.nras.org.uk/the-das28-score.

Neovius, M., Simard, J., Sundström, A., Jacobsson, L., Geborek, P., Saxne, T., Group ftAS, 2011. Generalisability of clinical registers used for drug safety and comparative effectiveness research: coverage of the Swedish Biologics Register. Ann. Rheum. Dis. 70 (3), 516–519.

PASI Training, 2009. Psoriasis Area and Severity Index (PASI). Available from: http://www.pasitraining.com/.

Patel, N., 2015. Novartis Launches First Biosimilar Zarxio in the US. Available from: http://www.pmlive.com/pharma_news/novartis_launches_first_biosimilar_zarxio_in_the_us_812623.

Ramanan, S., Grampp, G., 2014. Drift, evolution, and divergence in biologics and biosimilars manufacturing. BioDrugs 28 (4), 363–372.

Rassen, J.A., Schneeweiss, S., 2012. Using high-dimensional propensity scores to automate confounding control in a distributed medical product safety surveillance system. Pharmacoepidemiol. Drug Saf. 21, 41–49.

Rubin, D.B., 1997. Estimating causal effects from large data sets using propensity scores. Ann. Intern. Med. 127 (8 Pt 2), 757–763.

Scheinberg, M.A., Kay, J., 2012. The advent of biosimilar therapies in rheumatology—"O Brave New World". Nat. Rev. Rheumatol. 8 (7), 430–436.

Silman, A., Symmons, D., Scott, D.G.I., Griffiths, I., 2003. British society for rheumatology biologics register. Ann. Rheum. Dis. 62 (Suppl. 2), ii28–ii29.

Thimmaraju, P.K., Rakshambikai, R., Farista, R., Juluru, K., 2015. Legislations on Biosimilar Interchangeability in the US and EU - Developments Far from Visibility. GaBI Online - Generics and Biosimilars Initiative. Available from: http://www.gabionline.net/Sponsored-Articles/Legislations-on-biosimilar-interchangeability-in-the-US-and-EU-developments-far-from-visibility.

Watson, K., Symmons, D., Griffiths, I., Silman, A., 2005. The British Society for Rheumatology biologics register. Ann. Rheum. Dis. 64 (Suppl. 4), iv42–iv43.

World Health Organization (WHO), 2009. Annex 2. Guidelines on Evaluation of Similar Biotherapeutic Products (SBPs) (Sixteenth). WHO Press, Geneva, Switzerland. Available from: http://apps.who.int/medicinedocs/documents/s21091en/s21091en.pdf.

World Health Organization (WHO), 2015. Biological Qualifier an INN Proposal: Program on International Nonproprietary Names (INN) (INN Working Doc. 14.342 Rev. Final October 2015). WHO, Geneva, Switzerland. Available from: http://www.who.int/medicines/services/inn/WHO_INN_BQ_proposal_2015.pdf?ua=1.

Post-Authorization Safety Studies for Medical Devices and Combination Products

Jessica J. Jalbert[1], Theodore C. Lystig[2], Mary E. Ritchey[3], Ayad K. Ali[4]

[1]LASER Analytica, New York, NY, United States; [2]Medtronic, Minneapolis, MN, United States; [3]RTI Health Solutions, Durham, NC, United States; [4]Eli Lilly and Company, Indianapolis, IN, United States

INTRODUCTION

A medical device is any "instrument, apparatus, appliance, software, material, or other article," including combinations and accessories, which are used in humans for the "diagnosis, prevention, monitoring, treatment, or alleviation" of disease, injury, handicap, or replacement of an anatomical part or physiological process (EEC, 1993). In addition, a medical device must not "achieve its principal intended action by pharmacological, immunological, or metabolic means" (EEC, 1993). In other words, a medical device is a product other than a medicinal product, which is used to maintain or improve human health.

Dependent on the potential risk of the product, medical devices can be classified into four classes. *Class I* devices are those with the lowest risk, e.g., syringes without needles, corrective glasses and frames, and adhesive bandages. *Class IIa* generally includes devices, which are intended for short-term use in body orifices, transient surgical use, or to administer, exchange, or remove substances to and/or from the body, e.g., vaginal pessaries, single use scalpels, infusion pumps, and cryosurgery equipment. *Class IIb* devices are generally those, which are intended for long-term use in body orifices, supply energy/ionizing radiation, or administer medicine in short term, e.g., tracheal cannula, vascular closure devices, therapeutic X-ray, and blood warmers. *Class III* devices are those with the highest potential risk, e.g., implanted neurostimulators (EC, 2010a).

Regulatory review of medical devices occurs within a distributed system, which differs from the centralized assessment provided by the EMA for medicinal products and may be at increased risk of variability in regulation interpretation

CONTENTS

Introduction 277

Safety Concerns With Medical Devices 278

Methodological Considerations .. 279
Device Exposure Measurement 279
Data Sources 281
Registries 281
Administrative Claims .. 282
Electronic Medical Record 283
Validity Considerations 284
Provider-Level Factors. 284
Healthy-User Bias 285
Immortal-Time Bias 286
Confounding 287
Analytical Considerations 288

References 290

and enforcement (Sorenson and Drummond, 2014). The "CE marking" indicates that applicable pre-authorization requirements for the device have been completed. Unlike medicinal products, devices need to provide evidence of effectiveness or "performance" for regulatory approval, with no specific mention of safety (Sorenson and Drummond, 2014).

There are products that have both medicinal and device attributes. These "combination" products, including drug-delivery products, may be regulated as medical devices or as medicinal products, depending on their primary function (EC, 2010b). For example, prefilled syringes or pens, patches for transdermal drug delivery, or polymer matrices intended for drug release after implantation are all regulated as medicinal products. However, port systems, drug-eluting stents, and bone cements containing antibiotic agents are regulated as medical devices. Products determined to be primarily medicinal are subject to the regulations of medicinal products, and products determined to be primarily devices are subject to the regulations of medical devices (EC, 2010b).

On June 27, 2016, the European Union (EU) declared that an agreement has been reached toward improving surveillance and traceability of medical devices, which included "the reinforced requirement for manufacturers to collect data about the real-world use of their devices" and is based on proposed legislation from 2012. New regulations in 2017 apply for most medical devices within 3 years and for in vitro devices within 5 years after regulations are published (EC, 2016). Additionally, postmarket clinical follow-up (PMCF) studies might be required, which are the medical device version of PASS for medicinal products. Based on draft regulations, a European Commission expert panel or other independent scientific body may review the PMCF study plans and reports—similar to the Pharmacovigilance Risk Assessment Committee for medicinal products (CEU, 2015). Moreover, there may be expectation that the PMCF report be updated annually, along with the summary of safety and clinical performance of medical devices (CEU, 2015).

SAFETY CONCERNS WITH MEDICAL DEVICES

Reporting of adverse events for medical devices is expected for all classes of devices. In some cases, the manufacturer is expected to obtain specific data after obtaining the CE marking, which is accomplished through PMCF studies that are planned and conducted to address specific, outstanding questions regarding the safety or performance of the device at time of CE marking achievement. However, as opposed to PASS for medicinal products, there is no requirement for protocols or results from PMCF studies be shared publicly. Thus, it is difficult to determine whether real-world studies conducted within the EU are conducted under the PMCF requirements as it may not be mentioned in the methods, if the study is published at all.

PMCF studies may be required to assess risks that were not fully understood during the pre-authorization phase, whether this be quantifying known risks or identifying possible residual risks from pre-authorization phase. Limitations of pre-authorization data may include limited length of follow-up, small number of device users, relative homogeneity of patients or clinical settings, and limited data for the full range of patient conditions and comorbidities in the real-world. PMCF studies might be desirable for devices that are innovative, of high risk (based on design, target population, or challenges of treatment), with unanswered questions of long-term safety or performance (where subpopulations are unstudied, if risks are identified for similar marketed devices, or if CE marking was based on equivalence to other marketed devices) (EC, 2012).

The PMCF study should include the approach to collecting or obtaining data sufficient to address the acceptability of known performance or safety attributes of the device or to detect emerging risks. The collection of clinical data for PMCF studies is subject to the same standards as pre-authorization studies, with the exception that PMCF studies are not considered interventional in nature.

METHODOLOGICAL CONSIDERATIONS

In addition to the required PMCF studies, additional safety and performance data may also be requested by regulators. Post-authorization safety data for medical devices are also often needed for formulary and other health technology assessments. Clinical data collected within the EU may also be used in submissions to the FDA or other national regulatory agencies. Irrespective of the motivation for assessing the real-world safety of devices, the following considerations for study design and methodologies are applicable to all types of medical device safety studies.

Device Exposure Measurement

Pharmacoepidemiologists should consider factors related to device life cycle, device system types, and unique device identifiers (UDIs) for exposure definition in device PASS. Medical devices can be marketed as individual, separate components, or as full systems. For example, hip arthroplasty systems can include femoral stems, femoral heads, articular interfaces, and acetabular shells. When a device system is implanted, it cannot be assumed that all components of the same system are implanted, as physicians may choose to mix and match components from different systems. Each component within a system may have a different life cycle, and minor design or material differences in components within a system may result in different safety profiles. One study estimated that ~25% of patients undergoing total hip replacements between 2003 and 2013 in England and Wales received femoral stems, femoral heads, or acetabular shells from more than one company (Tucker et al., 2015). Depending on which components are mixed, revision rates could be higher, similar, or lower compared to hip replacement procedures where all components from one system are used.

The product life cycle of medical devices tends to be much shorter than those of medicinal products (1.5-2 years compared to ≥10 years) depending on the remainder of the patent duration and plans for extension (MedTech Europe, 2014). Although any change in the chemical structure, formulation, dose, and mode of administration of an authorized medicinal product requires a new regulatory submission based on randomized controlled trials (RCT), a new CE marking may not be required if a minor modification of a marketed device is not expected to affect the safety and performance of the deice. If the modification is considered to be major, a submission for the CE marking will likely be required, but the evidence for such submissions is more likely to be from laboratory testing, literature reviews, or a small study, rather than from full-scale RCT (FDA, 2012). In this regulatory environment, manufacturers tend to modify the design of marketed device frequently, with the intent of improving performance or to overcome shortcomings. Devices may therefore be on the market for only a short time before being discontinued and replaced by newer versions or innovative alternatives.

The short life cycles of devices may complicate safety assessments because patients in a given population may have been exposed to multiple versions of the same device. If the performance of device iterations differs but a uniform safety profile is assumed, this could lead to a biased assessment of the device and could overlook any safety problems with specific versions of the device. Stratification can be applied to assess the possibility that the safety of a device may differ by lot and version, as well as by model and manufacturer.

The regulatory landscape for medical devices in the EU is not centralized, and each country has its own regulatory agency overseeing products sold within its borders. As a consequence of this structure, different national approaches to device identification currently exist. The lack of a single UDI system harmonized across Europe (and beyond) can hinder the conduct of studies needing to combine multiple data sources, as the capture and specificity of device information may vary by data source and by country. The report by the UDI working group at the International Medical Device Regulators Forum, indicated that an international UDI system would provide a "single, globally harmonized system for positive identification of medical devices," which could be used to "increase safety and optimize patient care" (IMDRF, 2013). In addition, the UDI could also be used to link various data sources together to perform PASS. The UDI could provide a key to perform exact matching of patients across various data sets (e.g., linking registries to administrative claims or linking electronic medical record [EMR] across health-care providers), when other unique identifiers—such as social security numbers, are not available. Ultimately, the usefulness of the UDI system for device PASS will depend on how UDI systems will be integrated into existing data sources, such as claims. The timeline for implementation of UDI will vary across countries.

Data Sources

Data sources for medical device PASS ranges from primary data collection with interventional, de novo studies and registries, to secondary use of available data, such as EMR and claims. The cost of interventional PASS for medical devices tends to be much higher than noninterventional PASS, and delivery of care in participating centers might be altered as a result. Therefore, noninterventional designs are frequently used in PMCF studies. Data sources most commonly used for PASS are discussed in Chapters 3.1–3.5.

Registries

Registries can be created to identify cohorts of patients exposed to particular devices. In 2013, there were an estimated 101 registries for implantable medical devices in Europe, with more than 66% of the registries in the field of cardiac implants or arthroplasty (Niederlander et al., 2013). There is some type of implanted device registry in almost every European country, with some countries running more than one type of registry, and others running multiple registries in the same field. As mentioned in Chapter 3.3, registries may differ substantially in objective, structure, quality, and accessibility for research.

There are two main population-level approaches to enrolling patients into a device registry. The first consists of enrolling all patients exposed to the device, e.g., the National Joint Registry in the United Kingdom, which collects data on all hip, knee, ankle, elbow, and shoulder joint replacements across the National Health Service and the independent health-care sector (NJR, 2014). The other more common approach is to sample the population, usually by enrolling a maximum number of patients from a preselected subset of sites where the device is used. This is frequently performed by self-selection rather than by random sampling, as participation by the site and patient is often voluntary. As such, while sampling may be more resource-efficient than enrolling all patients exposed to the device, consideration must be given to the likelihood of selection bias, and impact on representativeness of the sampled population to the source population.

Although most registries collect device-specific information (such as UDI, manufacturer, catalog number, and individual components), their usefulness for device PASS will depend on availability and length of follow-up, their size, and data quality (Sedrakyan et al., 2011). The ability of device registries to evaluate long-term safety will be limited if data are only collected when the device is either implanted or used, or if there is considerable attrition after the encounter. For PASS of long-term risks, it may be necessary to link device registries to secondary data sources where the outcomes may be validly identified (Lalmohamed et al., 2013). Multiple registries may also need to be combined to have an adequate powered PASS, depending on the incidence rate of the outcome of interest, and the type and scale of use of device or device combinations of interest. For example, initiatives such as the International Consortium of Orthopaedic Registries and the International Consortium of Cardiovascular Registries have sought to leverage data from registries across multiple countries for post-authorization evaluation of the benefits and risks of medical devices, including for safety surveillance (Sedrakyan et al., 2011, 2013). Lastly, the value of device registry for PASS depends on data content and quality, which is a function of the design (e.g., registry objective, site and patient participation, stakeholder involvement, and site burden), as well as data collection and quality control procedures. Data quality, in terms of completeness, validity, breadth, and timeliness, can be heterogeneous across registries and within sites of a given registry, which limits the utility of data from certain registries or sites for device PASS. See Chapter 3.3 for an overview of registries.

Administrative Claims

Health insurance administrative claims are derived from billable interactions between patients and health-care systems, mediated by physicians, pharmacies, hospitals, and other health-care providers. Claims data tend to fall into four general categories: enrollment, inpatient, outpatient, and pharmacy. Depending on the country and how the health-care system is organized, the source of administrative claims can be from a single payer (e.g., the Danish Nationwide Registers) (Thygesen et al., 2011), or from multipayer health-care systems (e.g., the German sickness funds) (RatSWD, 2009). Claims data are useful sources for conducting device PASS due to their scale, which can contain longitudinal data on millions of patients.

In some claims databases, it may be possible to identify patients receiving durable medical equipment. In Germany, for example, UDI such as the *Hilfsmittelpositionsnummer* can be used to identify patients receiving devices such as wheelchairs, walkers, and nebulizers. For other types of devices, procedure codes are generally needed to capture device exposures. Procedure codes may include country-specific versions of the International Classification of

Diseases codes and/or other types of codes, e.g., *SKS-klassifikationerne* in Denmark and *Operationen und Prozedurenschlüssel*, or *Einheitlicher Bewertungsmaßstab* codes in Germany. However, procedure codes tend to convey more information about the procedure than the device and can only identify devices for which a procedure is billed. As such, the use of claims data for device PASS will tend to be limited to implantable devices (e.g., carotid stents or cerebral aneurysm coils), device-specific procedures (e.g., dialysis or extracorporeal membrane oxygenation), or durable medical equipment (e.g., insulin pumps or motility assistive equipment). In certain cases, additional information about the device or procedure can be obtained by supplementing claims data with procedure-specific registries (e.g., Western Denmark Heart Registry and Nordic Arthroplasty Register Association) (Schmidt et al., 2010; Havelin et al., 2011).

Specificity regarding device identification is not the only limitation to consider when using claims data for PASS of devices that are not durable medical equipment. Although procedure dates are generally available, diagnoses are reported for the hospitalization and dates are not generally provided; thus, temporality of the association between the device and the event of interest cannot be determined. For example, in PASS investigating the link between coronary stent and cardiovascular risks, for a patient with a claim for myocardial infarction who received a coronary stent during a hospitalization, it will be challenging to determine whether the patient was admitted with an infarction and then received a stent; the patient was admitted with an infarction, received a stent, and had an infarction as a complication; or the patient received a stent and then had an infarction.

Moreover, depending on the procedure, determining the exact anatomical location where the device was implanted may not be possible as the location specified in the procedure code and modifiers may be too general or not specified at all. If it is unclear whether the procedure is a revision or a new procedure because the device can be implanted in multiple parts of an organ or body part (e.g., cardiac coronary stents) or on either side of the body (e.g., knee arthroplasty), it may not be possible to use claims data to assess certain device failures or revisions without additional information. Nonetheless, the linkage of claims and procedure-specific registries may be useful in identifying certain outcomes with greater specificity than would be possible using either data source in isolation. Chapter 3.1 discusses claims data with greater detail.

Electronic Medical Record

In 2012, the European Commission expressed its commitment to develop a centralized European health record system by 2020 (Milieu Ltd. and Time.lex., 2014). Currently, EMR are in use in all member countries, but not all countries have infrastructures allowing health-care providers from different institutions to access and update patient data. As of January 2017, shared EMR systems are fully implemented in eight countries (Bulgaria, Denmark, Estonia, Finland, Hungary, Malta, the Netherlands, Sweden, and the United Kingdom), with other countries either developing, piloting, or deploying such systems. For systems that are not fully shared, patient care provided outside of a clinic, hospital, or network within a country will not be captured. In the context of device PASS, this means that it may not be possible to identify all patients with the device and that follow-up may be incomplete.

One advantage that EMR have over claims is that information about the device, disease severity, and outcomes may be more granular. Some of this granularity might be found in free-text fields in the EMR such that, tools like natural language processing might be needed to extract the relevant information into more standard data fields. Perhaps the most challenging aspect of EMR use for device PASS is the lack of widespread standardization of data fields. Although data standardization has become more prevalent in clinical research through the work of organizations such as the Clinical Data Interchange Standards Consortium (CDISC, 2016), adoption of such standards has been less swift across EMR systems. These can be site-specific coding values for anything from the device itself, to family history of disease, to functional assessments, and to laboratory values. Consequently, working with data generated from separate EMR systems can be very challenging because a considerable amount of work may be needed to extract and standardize data across institutions to perform PASS for medical devices and combination products. Chapter 3.2 provides an overview of EMR as a data source for PASS.

Validity Considerations

Pharmacoepidemiologists should consider multiple factors that might affect the validity of device PASS, including biases and confounding, in addition to provider-level and health-care system factors.

Provider-Level Factors

Many devices are part of a medical procedure, which may require that the physician has a certain set of skills. For instance, robotic-assisted surgery, which offers an alternative to laparoscopic or open surgery, requires that physicians undergo training to use the device. The more technically complex the medical procedure is to use or to implant the device, the more likely that the device will be associated with a learning curve. As the physician becomes more familiar with the device and procedure, patient outcomes are likely to improve because of increased proficiency and improved ability to identify patients who are likely to benefit from the procedure. In the presence of a learning curve, device performance may change over time and not taking into account provider's proficiency could lead to erroneous conclusions regarding the safety of a device. For example, an analysis of coronary stent implantation performed between 2003 and 2004 using the Swedish Coronary Angiography and Angioplasty Registry found a higher risk of mortality among patients receiving drug-eluting stents compared with bare metal stents (Lagerqvist et al., 2007). A subsequent study using the same registry with data from 2006 to 2010 found that drug-eluting stents was associated with lower rates of restenosis, stent thrombosis, and mortality (Sarno et al., 2012). The difference in the findings between the two studies was explained by diffusion in use of the drug-eluting stents, better patient selection, and the introduction of improved stent technology.

The clinic, center, or hospital in which the device is used or implanted can affect device performance. An institution's experience with the device may allow it to tailor the aftercare of patients. For example, if a certain complication commonly arises with the use or implantation of a device, the center may choose to make refinements to the procedure or take other measures to avert complications. Teaching affiliation, staffing, ownership (public vs. private), center size, and bed occupancy can also influence device performance insofar as it can impact quality and availability of training resources, clinical team makeup, and nature of pre- and postprocedural care.

Exploring the relationship between device performance and provider characteristics is essential to making appropriate conclusions regarding the safety of a device. In comparative PASS where the device is compared to another treatment, provider characteristics should be evaluated as potential confounders or effect measure modifiers. In PASS without comparators, stratification by provider characteristics will be helpful in understanding the overall risk profile of the device in the context of provider case-mix. Measures of the learning curve and proficiency may include lifetime or recent procedural volume, complication rates, and length of operation. Other proxies may include physician specialty and board certification, specialty center status, or caseload complexity. Center characteristics potentially associated with facility organization, financial means, and quality of care should also be considered. From a statistical perspective, accounting for clustering of patients within providers (physicians or hospitals) is recommended as the independence of patient outcomes within provider clusters is unlikely to hold.

Healthy-User Bias

Healthy-user (or healthy-adherer) bias may arise when patients who receive a therapy tend to more actively to seek out preventative care and engage in other healthy behaviors than patients who do not receive therapy. Health-seeking behaviors may include eating a healthy diet, exercising regularly, and wearing a seat belt. Incomplete adjustment for such behaviors can lead to spurious inferences regarding the safety of the device of interest because healthy behaviors are associated with a reduced risk of a number of poor health outcomes. For example, a study comparing insulin pumps with real-time continuous glucose monitoring to self-injecting insulin regimens may overstate the effect of insulin pumps on outcomes such as mortality, stroke, or myocardial infarction if the patients receiving insulin pumps sought out this treatment with the aim of obtaining tighter glucose control. Controlling for healthy-user bias in PASS tends to be quite challenging when using secondary data sources, as healthy behaviors and personality traits they represent are difficult to measure in such data sources. Proxies may include evidence of health screening such as yearly physicals, mammography, or colonoscopy; or the receipt of preventative therapies such as influenza vaccine.

Additionally, patients who adhere to their treatment are more likely to engage in healthier behaviors than nonadherent patients. This source of bias may be of concern in PASS where a device may be preferentially used to treat patients with difficulty adhering to their treatments. In the earlier example, if insulin pumps are reserved for patients with poor adherence to their self-injecting insulin regimens, estimates may be biased against the pumps because nonadherent patients may be engaging in more risk-taking and less health-seeking behaviors than patients remaining on the self-injecting insulin regimens. Failing to account for the behaviors that correlate with treatment adherence could lead to erroneous conclusions regarding the safety of a device.

Immortal-Time Bias

Immortal person-time can be introduced in a study when cohort definition is dependent on everyone having survived up to a certain point (Ali, 2013). For example, in PASS assessing the long-term safety of implantable cardioverter defibrillator (CD), a cohort may be defined as all patients that have had a CD implanted for ≥ 3 years. Because all patients in the cohort must survive for at least 3 years after having received the implantable CD or they would not be eligible for inclusion in the study, the time is "immortal." Including the time during which the patient could, by definition, not have died will result in rates that are biased downward because the denominator is artificially inflated by the inclusion of immortal person-time. This holds true even if the outcome of interest is not death or an event that can be fatal, e.g., stroke. The correct approach to dealing with immortal-time bias is to remove the immortal person-time from the denominator by starting PASS follow-up once all inclusion criteria have been met.

Additionally, immortal-time bias may also be introduced when two treatments are compared and the ways their follow-up periods are defined are different, as treatment is not yet selected by the time that the observation of patients begins

(Ali, 2013). When comparing the safety of implantable CD to medications for heart failure, the time prior to CD implantation among patients who received the implantable CD is "immortal" because patients must survive from the beginning of follow-up up to CD implantation. This comparison will introduce immortal-time bias if the time prior to CD implantation is not appropriately allocated or statistically handled.

Confounding

In device safety studies, confounding by indication would arise when patients exposed to a device are different than those not receiving the device because they do not have the indication for treatment. This may occur if diseases are managed in a stepwise approach such that a device may be used to treat the disease when other alternatives have failed (or vice versa) (Ali, 2013). For instance, obese patients who undergo gastric banding are likely to have higher body mass index values and have a greater obesity-related comorbidity burden than obese patients who are treated with medications or lifestyle interventions. A common way of dealing with this type of confounding would be to restrict the analysis to patients with the indication. In this example, the analysis should be restricted to obese patients who are eligible to receive the gastric lap band rather than all obese patients (some of whom would not be covered by the indication for the device).

Even when a comparison group consists of patients who have the same disease and indication for the device, differences in disease severity and other risk factors may still exist between people treated with the device and those not treated with the device. In the case of implanted devices, there is usually a short-term risk associated with the implantation, and the least invasive treatment may be reserved for the healthiest patients (or the sickest if used as last-line therapy). If such differences are not adequately accounted for, confounding by disease severity may be introduced (Ali, 2013). In the above example, although the analysis may be restricted to obese patients with the indication for gastric lap banding, there will likely still be differences in the distributions of body mass index, diabetes severity, and level of hypertension among patients receiving and not receiving a gastric lap band.

Channeling patients to a treatment when other alternatives for the same indication exist may result in bias if patients channeled to that treatment have differences in factors affecting prognosis (Ali, 2013). Channeling bias can occur at any point during the life cycle of medical devices, but it tends to be of particular concern when the device is newly launched. This type of confounding by indication may occur if a device is perceived to be more effective and is reserved for patients with more severe disease, or for those patients who are not appropriately managed using other alternatives due to effectiveness or tolerance issues.

Newer devices may initially be reserved for patients with more severe disease or those who have failed on first-line therapies. For example, transcatheter aortic valve replacement (TAVR) is a more recent and less invasive alternative to open-heart surgical aortic valve replacement (SAVR). It was initially approved in Europe for patients considered inoperable due to unacceptably high-surgical risk. As a result, unadjusted comparisons of outcomes following TAVR and SAVR could favor the latter, not necessarily because TAVR was less safe, but because the population to whom the device was channeled had a higher risk of poor outcomes. As the indication for TAVR was expanded to high-surgical risk patients, the imbalance in risk profiles will lessen. Such channeling could persist indefinitely or not, depending on approved indications, speed of uptake, and perceptions in the medical community regarding the safety and effectiveness profile of the device.

Analytical Considerations

With sufficiently detailed information on disease severity and risk factors or their proxies, confounding and bias may be handled through analytical approaches, such as exposure propensity scores (EPS) or instrumental variables (IV) analyses (D'Agostino and D'Agostino, 2007; Ali, 2013). In addition to these approaches, pharmacoepidemiologists should consider factors related to generalization and extrapolation of PASS findings, systems for device surveillance, and establishing frameworks for continuous updates to the benefit—risk profile of medical devices and combination products. Chapters 5.1—5.3 discuss the application of EPS, disease risk scores, and IV as means for confounding control in PASS.

Extrapolation of data from one population to support indications in other populations may provide a potential solution to the issue of scarcity of data for certain populations. This scarcity may be driven by limits in the size of the target population or by the number of subjects willing to take part in clinical research studies. Because of data scarcity, the enrollment time for interventional PASS or time needed to have enough patients exposed to perform meaningful analyses for noninterventional PASS could exceed length of time that a device version is available on the market. Rather than allowing off-label use to continue without any realistic means of assessing device performance, information may be borrowed from a related population in which safety and performance has previously been demonstrated, and for which, it could be argued that the results for this related population might be similar to that of the as-of-yet unknown results in the population. This process of leveraging data from a related population to support inference in another population is known as data extrapolation.

Examples of where extrapolation might be useful include leveraging data from adult to pediatric populations or from one European country to another.

In these cases, leveraging the related information, possibly through the use of a Bayesian hierarchical model, could yield a desirable level of confidence in the distribution of the parameter of interest that would not ordinarily be obtainable where leveraging techniques are not available. Use of Bayesian hierarchical models to perform such extrapolation for devices in pediatric populations is explicitly discussed in FDA's guidance document (FDA, 2016).

Furthermore, patients and physicians in PASS may not be representative of the likely future population of recipients or operators of medical devices. For example, younger and healthier patients and high-volume centers with expert practitioners may be overrepresented in interventional PASS. When the study population is a random sample exhibiting proportionality between the sample and the parent population, and all relevant subgroups have been captured, it is relatively straightforward to calibrate estimates of component subgroups of a populations. For the purpose of calibration, the relevant subgroups are those patients with differential performance of the device, which may be specific to the therapy area or type of device. Although the question of generalizability becomes moot if a complete census-type registry approach is used for device PASS, it will remain for any other study that does not include the entire population.

As mentioned in Chapter 5.5 (proactive safety surveillance), distributed data networks (DDNs) such as the Sentinel System have been used to perform proactive safety surveillance of medicinal products in the United States, and the feasibility using European databases in such networks has been demonstrated (Schuemie et al., 2013: Gagne et al., 2018). DDN operate by using similar instructions on separate data sets to perform the analyses, the results of which are then synthesized into a coherent whole. The system can work well when each data source is sufficiently large such that outputs obtained by running the analysis instructions are stable. For example, survival estimates can be reliably obtained when the number of patients at risk is as small as 100,000. Although this number may be easily attained for analyses of products on a population scale, the number of patients exposed to a specific device may be 100 or less in a given data set. It may therefore be necessary to restrict the type of analyses performed to those that will be stable given population sizes or seek other alternatives to the DDN framework. For example, a sufficient subset of data elements from multiple coordinated research networks could be sent to a single repository where analyses could be executed.

PASS of medical devices are generally geared toward updating our understanding about the safety of a device but rarely also provide updated information about the effectiveness and performance of the same device. Device PASS (in form of PMCF studies) have traditionally been used to learn about safety, but there are minimal structural hurdles against using similar approaches to learn about performance as well, particularly when many effectiveness metrics are simply the mirror image of safety metrics. Establishing a framework where both safety and effectiveness information are updated would provide greater context and direction around how to handle potential safety signals. If the overall benefit–risk profile of the device is not materially impacted by the new safety information, then the impetus to take action is greatly diminished. A worthwhile objective would be to agree on transparent means to define and update the benefit–risk profile and indicate how it could be calibrated to reflect different weights for components of safety and effectiveness. This would allow for the incorporation of patient preferences or potentially personalization of the benefit–risk ratio to incorporate key factors for individual patients.

PASS for medical devices and combination products require special considerations in terms of data source and design approach, especially with factors related to exposure measurement, including single device versus system of devices, life cycles, and unique identifiers. Understanding potential threats to the validity and how they can be minimized is essential to allow for proper interpretation of PASS findings and better characterization of the benefit–risk profile of medical devices.

References

Ali, A.K., 2013. Methodological challenges in observational research: a pharmacoepidemiological perspective. Br. J. Pharmaceut. Res. 3 (2), 161–175.

Clinical Data Interchange Standards Consortium (CDISC), 2016. Available from: www.cdisc.org/.

Council of the European Union (CEU), 2015. Proposal for a Regulation of the European Parliament and of the Council on Medical Devices, and Amending Directive 2001/83/EC, Regulation (EC) No 178/2002 and Regulation (EC) No 1223/2009 2015. Available from: http://data.consilium.europa.eu/doc/document/ST-12040-2015-ADD-1/en/pdf.

D'Agostino Jr., R.B., D'Agostino Sr., R.B., 2007. Estimating treatment effects using observational data. J. Am. Med. Assoc. 297 (3), 314–316.

European Commission (EC), 2010a. Classification of Medical Devices. Available from: http://ec.europa.eu/DocsRoom/documents/10337/attachments/1/translations/en/renditions/native.

European Commission (EC), DG Enterprise and Industry, 2010b. Borderline Products, Drug-delivery Products and Medical Devices Incorporating, as an Integral Part, an Ancillary Medicinal Substance or an Ancillary Human Blood Derivative. Available from: http://ec.europa.eu/DocsRoom/documents/10328/attachments/1/translations/en/renditions/native.

European Commission (EC), Directorate General for Health and Consumers, 2012. Post Market Clinical Follow-up Studies: A Guide for Manufacturers and Notified Bodies. Available from: http://ec.europa.eu/DocsRoom/documents/10334/attachments/1/translations/en/renditions/native.

European Commission (EC), 2016. Commission Welcomes New Agreement for Safer Use of Medical Devices. Available from: http://ec.europa.eu/growth/tools-databases/newsroom/cf/itemdetail.cfm?item_id=8863&lang=en&tpa_id=1061&title=Commission-welcomes-new-agreement-for-safer-use-of-medical-devices.

European Economic Community (EEC), 1993. Council Directive 93/42/EEC of 14 June 1993 Concerning Medical Devices. Available from: http://eur-lex.europa.eu/legal-content/EN/TXT/PDF/?uri=CELEX:31993L0042&from=EN.

Food and Drug Administration (FDA), 2012. Unsafe and Ineffective Devices Approved in the EU that Were Not Approved in the US. US Food and Drug Administration. Available from: http://www.elsevierbi.com/~/media/Supporting%20Documents/The%20Gray%20Sheet/38/20/FDA_EU_Devices_Report.pdf.

Food and Drug Administration (FDA), 2016. Leveraging Exisiting Clinical Data for Extrapolation to Pediatric Uses of Medical Devices: Guidance for Industry and Food and Drug Administration Staff. Available from: http://www.fda.gov/downloads/medicaldevices/deviceregulationandguidance/guidancedocuments/ucm444591.pdf.

Gagne, J.J., Houstoun, M., Reichman, M.E., Hampp, C., Marshall, J.H., Toh, S., 2018. Safety assessment of niacin in the US Food and drug Administration's mini-sentinel system. Pharmacoepidemiol. Drug Saf. 27, 30–37.

German Council for Social and Economic Data (RatSWD), 2009. Administrative Data from Germany's Statutory Health Insurances for Social, Economic, and Medical Research. Available from: http://www.ratswd.de/download/RatSWD_WP_2009/RatSWD_WP_122.pdf.

Havelin, L.I., Robertsson, O., Fenstad, A.M., Overgaard, S., Garellick, G., Furnes, O., 2011. A scandinavian experience of register collaboration: the nordic arthroplasty register association (NARA). J. Bone Joint Surg. Am. 93 (Suppl 3), 13–19.

International Medical Device Regulators Forum (IMDRF), 2013. UDI Guidance: Unique Device Identification (UDI) of Medical Devices. Available from: http://www.imdrf.org/docs/imdrf/final/technical/imdrf-tech-131209-udi-guidance-140901.pdf.

Lagerqvist, B., James, S.K., Stenestrand, U., Lindback, J., Nilsson, T., et al., 2007. Long-term outcomes with drug-eluting stents versus bare-metal stents in Sweden. N. Engl. J. Med. 356 (10), 1009–1019.

Lalmohamed, A., MacGregor, A.J., de Vries, F., Leufkens, H.G., van Staa, T.P., 2013. Patterns of risk of cancer in patients with metal-on-metal hip replacements versus other bearing surface types: a record linkage study between a prospective joint registry and general practice electronic health records in England. PLoS One 8 (7), e65891.

MedTech Europe, 2014. The European Medical Technology Industry in Figures. Available from: http://www.ub.edu/medicina/grauEB/2014%20The%20European%20medical%20technology%20industry%20in%20figures.pdf.

Milieu Ltd and Time.lex., 2014. Overview of the National Laws on Electronic Health Records in the EU Member States and Their Interaction with the Provision of Cross-border EHealth Services: Final Report and Recommendations. Available from: http://ec.europa.eu/health/ehealth/docs/laws_report_recommendations_en.pdf.

National Joint Registry (NJR), 2014. About the NJR. Available from: http://www.njrcentre.org.uk/njrcentre/default.aspx.

Niederlander, C., Wahlster, P., Kriza, C., Kolominsky-Rabas, P., 2013. Registries of implantable medical devices in Europe. Health Pol. 113 (1–2), 20–37.

Sarno, G., Lagerqvist, B., Frobert, O., Nilsson, J., et al., 2012. Lower risk of stent thrombosis and restenosis with unrestricted use of 'new-generation' drug-eluting stents: a report from the nationwide Swedish Coronary Angiography and Angioplasty Registry (SCAAR). Eur. Heart J. 33 (5), 606–613.

Schmidt, M., Maeng, M., Jakobsen, C.J., Madsen, M., Thuesen, L., et al., 2010. Existing data sources for clinical epidemiology: the Western Denmark Heart Registry. Clin. Epidemiol. 2, 137–144.

Schuemie, M.J., Gini, R., Coloma, P.M., Straatman, H., et al., 2013. Replication of the OMOP experiment in Europe: evaluating methods for risk identification in electronic health record databases. Drug Saf. 36 (Suppl 1), S159–S169.

Sedrakyan, A., Paxton, E.W., Phillips, C., Namba, R., Funahashi, T., Barber, T., Sculco, T., et al., 2011. The international consortium of orthopaedic registries: overview and summary. J. Bone Joint Surg. Am. 93 (Suppl 3), 1–12.

Sedrakyan, A., Marinac-Dabic, D., Holmes, D.R., 2013. The international registry infrastructure for cardiovascular device evaluation and surveillance. J. Am. Med. Assoc. 310 (3), 257–259.

Sorenson, C., Drummond, M., 2014. Improving medical device regulation: the United States and Europe in perspective. Milbank Q. 92 (1), 114–150.

Thygesen, L.C., Daasnes, C., Thaulow, I., Bronnum-Hansen, H., 2011. Introduction to Danish (nationwide) registers on health and social issues: structure, access, legislation, and archiving. Scand. J. Publ. Health 39 (7 Suppl), 12–16.

Tucker, K., Pickford, M., Newell, C., Howard, P., Hunt, L.P., Blom, A.W., 2015. Mixing of components from different manufacturers in total hip arthroplasty: prevalence and comparative outcomes. Acta Orthop. 86 (6), 671–677.

Post-Authorization Safety Studies for Vaccines

Priscilla Velentgas[1], Roger Baxter[2], Philip Bryan[3], Mendel Haag[4], Lorna Hazell[5], Rachel Jablonski[1], Alena Khromova[6], Ombretta Palucci[1], Saad Shakir[5], Walter Straus[7], Robert P. Wise[8], Ayad K. Ali[9]

[1]IQVIA, Cambridge, MA, United States; [2]Kaiser Permanente, Oakland, CA, United States; [3]Medicines and Healthcare Products Regulatory Agency, London, United Kingdom; [4]Seqirus, Amsterdam, The Netherlands; [5]Drug Safety Research Unit, Southampton, United Kingdom; [6]Sanofi Pasteur, Toronto, Canada; [7]Merck and Co., Inc., Kenilworth, NJ, United States; [8]AstraZeneca, Gaithersburg, MD, United States; [9]Eli Lilly and Company, Indianapolis, IN, United States

DISCLAIMER/ACKNOWLEDGMENTS

The authors of this chapter and the editors of the book would like to recognize with great respect, fondness, and appreciation, the contributions of Dr. Roger Baxter, previously codirector of the Kaiser Permanente Vaccine Study Center, to this chapter prior to his death in late 2016. His contributions to vaccine safety research will be lasting and he will be missed.

INTRODUCTION

Particular challenges for evaluating the safety of vaccines include their widespread use in healthy populations, administration in settings different from routine care, leading to challenges for exposure and outcome assessment; and for influenza vaccine, the need for rapid assessment of safety and effectiveness in each flu season, i.e., near real-time analyses. In addition to other guidance for development of post-authorization safety studies (PASS), a draft European Medicines Agency (EMA) guideline requires annual surveillance of seasonal influenza vaccine safety and effectiveness encompassing PASS and enhanced passive surveillance activities.

Unlike other medicinal products, there are specific challenges of PASS and safety surveillance for vaccines, including public health and public perception of vaccines. Immunization programs are a fundamental pillar of public health protection, and on a global level, substantially reduce morbidity and help to prevent millions of deaths every year. Along with access to clean water and

CONTENTS

Disclaimer/
Acknowledg
ments 293

Introduction 293

Special
Considerations for
Vaccine Post-
Authorization
Safety Studies ... 295

Vaccine Safety
Surveillance
Programs 297

Regulatory
Requirements for
Vaccine Post-
Authorization
Safety Studies ... 298

Enhanced Passive
Safety Surveillance
for Vaccines 300

Utility of Enhanced
Passive Safety
Surveillance in
Seasonal Campaigns 302

Designs for Vaccine
  Post-Authorization
  Safety Studies ... 304
Signal
Detection.................... 305
Signal
Evaluation 307
Cohort and
Case–Control
Designs 308
Vaccinee-Only
Designs 310
Data Sources
for Vaccine Post-
Authorization
Safety Studies............ 312
Claims and Electronic
Medical Record 312
Vaccination
Registries 313
Primary Data
Collection................... 313
Considerations for
Vaccine Exposure
Measurement 314
Vaccine Indication......... 314
Vaccine Formulation 315
Vaccine
Recommendations 316
Vaccine Dosing
Schedule 316
Vaccine Route, Lot, and
Expiration Date............. 317
Vaccine Administration
Setting.......................... 317

Methodological
  Considerations .. 318
Seasonal and Regional
Considerations 318
Site Selection 319
Patient Enrollment ... 320
Patient Retention 320
Data Collection
Methods 321
Case Definition 322

adequate nutrition, vaccines contribute more to public health than any other intervention. Near universal access to childhood vaccines has 86% of infants worldwide receiving three doses of diphtheria–tetanus–pertussis (DTP or DTaP), and 83% receiving three doses of Hepatitis B vaccine in 2015 (WHO, 2016). Adults and adolescents are now also routinely protected against a range of diseases. Immunization programs are continuously evolving and expanding as manufacturers develop new and improved vaccines, and more infectious diseases are becoming vaccine-preventable.

From a pharmacovigilance perspective, the basic requirements and principles of PASS and other forms of safety surveillance are not different for vaccines than other medicinal products. We need to detect and refine safety signals, and where possible, to test the resulting hypotheses. In addition, we need to quantify risks (and to balance these against benefits), and to ensure these processes are continued for the life cycle of the product. There are several features of vaccines and their use, though, which create particular postlicensure challenges and expectations. In contrast to most medicinal products, which are usually administered to individual patients on a discretionary basis (i.e., to treat an existing condition), recommendations for vaccine use to prevent diseases typically arise from medical professional associations and/or national or international governmental agencies or advisory committees. Vaccines are generally administered on a population level with an expectation that—barring known contraindications—an entire population will receive a vaccine. High vaccine coverage provides direct protection to vaccinated individuals, as well as for most vaccines, societal benefits from herd protection. Some recommendations for vaccination are also mandatory at national or regional levels, for instance, requirements prior to entry into school or for certain professions. Additionally, most vaccines are administered to healthy children, who typically do not (in comparison to older populations) concurrently receive many other medicinal products but can receive multiple concomitant vaccinations during childhood immunization. These factors greatly increase expectations of product safety. The tolerance for risks or uncertainty about them is much lower for vaccines than for most medicinal products.

The role of governments in establishing recommendations for requirements for vaccination may also raise concerns over individual freedoms that do not exist in most therapeutically oriented patient–provider interactions.

A further factor in public trust is the dynamic nature and public perception of benefit–risk balances for vaccines. For rare diseases, including those that have become rare through successful immunization programs, the public perception of benefit from vaccinations can decline. When used as intended, a vaccine will, over time, reduce the burden of disease from the target infection; societal concern about that infection then wanes, raising concerns about the value of the vaccine and an associated lower tolerance of actual and potential risks (Ellenberg and Chen, 1997). Another challenge to public perception of benefit–risk balance of vaccines may arise for a disease with long latency between infection and disease onset (and accordingly, need for immunization at an early age relative to the overt disease risk), human papillomavirus (HPV) infection being an example.

Background Event
Rates 322
Confounding 322

References 324

A consequence of mass immunization is an inevitably large number of suspected adverse event reports in the early postlicensure period and arguably more so than for other medicinal products (Weber, 1984; Hartnell and Wilson, 2004; Moro et al., 2015). Certain latent pediatric illnesses (e.g., autism and autoimmune conditions) become manifest throughout childhood, creating fertile ground for parents to attribute them to an external cause, such as a recent vaccination (the post hoc ergo propter hoc fallacy). Although confirmation and characterization of new risks is paramount for any vaccine or medicinal product, unfounded vaccine safety fears can significantly degrade vaccine coverage in the wider population, leading to reemergence of disease. To counter this threat, it is of the utmost importance for public health communities (governmental, industrial, and academic) to develop and sustain capabilities for rapid assessment of safety concerns. With good safety surveillance systems, the fragility of hypotheses posed by anecdotal reports of adverse events can be lucidly described to the public, and invalid concerns can be refuted as objective data emerge. The recent experience in the United Kingdom, when unfounded links between measles, mumps, and rubella (MMR) vaccine and development of autism led to a significant fall in vaccine uptake, demonstrates that public confidence in vaccines with very high uptake can erode rapidly (Friederichs et al., 2006). In risk management planning for vaccines, there is therefore a requirement to anticipate that such concerns or unconfirmed signals may arise, and for there to be proactive plans in place to rapidly evaluate and respond to them.

Collectively, these factors create societal expectations for product safety (and benefit) that are particularly high for vaccines. PASS are an important means to evaluate vaccine safety after licensure and to provide the public reassurance essential to develop and sustain high levels of vaccine coverage.

SPECIAL CONSIDERATIONS FOR VACCINE POST-AUTHORIZATION SAFETY STUDIES

Structural considerations bear on vaccine PASS designs and implementation. Although the scale of vaccine clinical development is generally large (Phase III randomized controlled trial [RCT] usually involve thousands–ten thousands of participants) and these studies are designed to address vaccine efficacy and general safety, they are typically not powered to detect rare safety events. An exception was the development of the second generation rotavirus vaccines, which were specifically powered to rule out an elevated risk of intestinal intussusception (which had led to withdrawal of the first rotavirus vaccine) (Patel et al., 2009). Consequently, vaccine PASS can augment the spontaneous reporting systems (with capacity to identify rare adverse events) by providing a mechanism to explore a specific safety signal and broader safety monitoring of new or seasonally updated vaccines.

In terms of PASS, a significant practical challenge is that very high uptake of a vaccine results in a low proportion of unvaccinated individuals, which can affect the ability to identify suitable controls for a noninterventional study. The pool of unvaccinated subjects may be relatively small, and they may not be representative of the target population because seasons for nonvaccination may influence risk for the outcome of interest (e.g., health status and/or socioeconomic factors), resulting in confounding by indication or "healthy-vaccinee bias" (Remschmidt et al., 2015). Self-controlled designs are usually required to overcome these factors. Another challenge for vaccine PASS is short-term use of new vaccines (either a novel vaccine strain or a new vaccine construct) in a campaign or to control a disease outbreak. A notable example is pandemic influenza, when novel vaccines are used in mass immunization over a period of only a few months. Such situations require very specific planning and unique design for near real-time surveillance and PASS.

Many vaccinations occur in settings outside of the traditional health-care environment in which medicinal products are usually prescribed and dispensed. For example, adolescent immunizations may be administered via school-based programs, whereas influenza vaccines are increasingly available through community pharmacies and places of employment, as well as primary care institutions. Particularly for vaccine PASS based on routinely collected electronic medical record (EMR), it is important to fully understand vaccine exposures and to record them at national and local levels to minimize risks of underascertainment (which could be severely biased, as when the working well might be more likely to receive vaccinations in different settings) and misclassification of exposure. Another difference between vaccines and most medicinal products other than biologicals is that different formulations of a particular vaccine type (e.g., target disease) and the same vaccine may be used simultaneously in a given population. This factor can affect PASS and other forms of safety surveillance by requiring attention to the product variables of manufacturer, vaccine type, and lot identification codes (lot IDs). Vaccines are biological products, unlike most small molecule products, so that differences may emerge among safety profiles of multiple brands of a single vaccine type and among lots of a single vaccine brand. Close surveillance of safety in these dimensions provides the critically important opportunity to detect product quality issues at the earliest possible point. Threats, including inadvertent contamination, loss of a shipment refrigeration, counterfeiting, and tampering, are among the potential mechanisms that could increase reactogenicity of a vaccine dose.

VACCINE SAFETY SURVEILLANCE PROGRAMS

In discussing approaches to vaccine PASS, it is necessary to describe various programs that have been developed in the European Union (EU) and United States specifically to provide ongoing safety surveillance of vaccines, and research infrastructure that may be leveraged to conduct PASS. Other countries, including Canada and Taiwan, also have developed programs with similar objectives (Huang et al., 2010; Canadian Vaccine Network, 2017). Vaccine PASS may also be initiated outside of such programs, usually through the sponsorship of the marketing authorization holder.

The European Centre of Disease Prevention and Control supported the Vaccine Adverse Event Surveillance and Communication consortium (VAESCO), a collaborative network of agencies responsible to collect and collate information on adverse events following immunization in Europe (VAESCO, 2017) The consortium developed guidelines for vaccine safety surveillance, and built infrastructure to support vaccine safety research, including studies conducted between 2009 and 2011.

In 2013m the Innovative Medicines Initiative established the Accelerated Development of Vaccine Benefit-Risk Collaboration in Europe as a platform for rapid conduct of studies on vaccine benefit—risk assessments in Europe. Description of the program's recent activities, including profiling of potential data sources and technical requirements for data sources that may be used to assess vaccine benefit—risk balance in the EU, are available on the program website (IMI, 2017).

The US Centers for Disease Control and Prevention (CDC) Immunization Safety Office and the Food and Drug Administration (FDA) Center for Biologics Evaluation and Research have four major projects, involving vaccine safety, which conduct ongoing surveillance and research studies addressing specific hypotheses. These systems are the Vaccine Adverse Event Reporting System (VAERS); the Clinical Immunization Safety Assessment (CISA) network; the Vaccine Safety Datalink (VSD); and the Postlicensure Rapid Immunization Safety Monitoring (PRISM) program.

The VAERS is a collaborative effort of CDC and FDA as a passive surveillance system, designed similarly to the FDA Adverse Event Reporting System for medicinal products and therapeutic biological products (FDA, 2016) to which medical providers and vaccinated persons can report any suspected vaccine reaction. It has proven helpful to find new safety information related to vaccines, but because of the passive nature with typically extensive underreporting and vulnerability to multiple biases, such as effects of publicity on reporting patterns, VAERS is generally not useful for causality assessments or hypothesis testing PASS (HHS, 2016).

The CISA network is a collaboration between the CDC and a number of academic and health-care organizations, which gives expert consultations on unusual adverse events following immunizations and provides causality assessments and guidance on revaccinations. Supporting these consultations, retrospective noninterventional analyses on adverse events are sometimes performed using data from the Kaiser Permanente Northern California health plan (CDC, 2016).

The VSD is a group of vaccine researchers forming a voluntary network of integrated health delivery organizations throughout the United States has collaborated since 1991 on the conduct of vaccine safety studies, primarily utilizing administrative claims and EMR data (McNeil et al., 2014). The VSD has pioneered various methodologies, including Rapid Cycle Analysis, in which data files are updated weekly at sites and adverse events following immunizations monitored over time to look for indications of increases associated with vaccines. One issue with monitoring and analyzing adverse events over time is the effect of multiple comparisons on statistical significance. Over time, the risk of false positive results will continually increase unless there is an adjustment for each observation. However, methods have been developed to limit false positive findings. The VSD data structure and governance are discussed with greater detail in Chapter 5.5.

The PRISM program was created in 2009 as a response to the challenge of the 2009−2010 H1N1 influenza epidemic and need for monitoring of influenza vaccine safety (Nguyen et al., 2012). It has subsequently been incorporated as part of the FDA Sentinel System for post-authorization safety monitoring of medicinal products and vaccines. Through use of the Sentinel DDN, it allows greater ability to detect rare adverse events, such as Guillain−Barré syndrome (GBS), and to support stratified analyses in key subpopulations.

REGULATORY REQUIREMENTS FOR VACCINE POST-AUTHORIZATION SAFETY STUDIES

At the time licensure of a vaccine (and assuming a marketing authorization is approvable based on an acceptable balance of benefits and risks), the available safety data should allow the general reactogenicity of a vaccine to be established (i.e., solicited local and systemic adverse events) and should usually allow reliable characterization in terms of frequency and severity of other common adverse events. However, because of the size of RCT and as in the development of any new medicinal product, it may neither be possible to assess causality of isolated serious adverse events reported in the RCT nor to identify and characterize very rare risks. Similarly, it may not be possible to evaluate safety in populations or subgroups excluded from RCT (e.g., those with certain clinical risk factors, pregnant women, and particular age groups) who may nonetheless be recommended to receive a vaccine in routine clinical practice.

Aside from the standard requirement for routine pharmacovigilance to monitor safety in the postlicensure period, regulators may request or require a particular PASS at the time of licensure to evaluate specific areas of uncertainty, potential risks, or missing information arising from the clinical development program, but which did not preclude a marketing authorization. PASS may also be requested to evaluate the outcome of specific risk minimization measures (e.g., to evaluate compliance with an important contraindication or restricted access condition). Such PASS or surveillance may be a specific obligation or condition that must be fulfilled in a given period for a marketing authorization to remain valid. Other PASS may be voluntary, undertaken by the manufacturer to further characterize potential risks or father new information (which could still affect the status of the authorization if the studies should yield significant new safety concerns). Similarly, regulators may request or require specific PASS at any time during the post-authorization life cycle of a product to evaluate a new safety concern that has arisen during routine clinical use.

At the time of licensure of a vaccine and at any time during the postlicensure life cycle, regulators may request additional safety surveillance (i.e., in addition to routine pharmacovigilance activities) other than (or in addition to) PASS. Such forms of additional pharmacovigilance activities may include proactive surveillance methods or enhanced passive surveillance methods using observed versus expected approaches.

Regulators may themselves undertake or commission vaccine PASS or other surveillance activities, independent from the manufacturer, to inform regulatory decision-making at any point in the life cycle of a particular vaccine.

The need for vaccine PASS or other additional surveillance is not just a consideration for regulators or for manufacturers as part of their vaccine development program. Immunization programs have many stakeholders, including national public health authorities who purchase vaccines and implement immunization programs. Public health authorities may therefore undertake or commission vaccine PASS to inform national decision-making at any point of the life cycle of a particular vaccine. Similarly, academic institutions, often in partnership with public health authorities, may undertake vaccine PASS that is independent from any regulatory or manufacturer-sponsored studies. Public health authorities may require PASS in advance of an immunization program to establish incidence rates of prespecified events, with prospective PASS to timely compare them to rates in immunized cohorts.

Increasingly, novel vaccines are being developed to prevent diseases that are endemic to certain low- and middle-income countries, but not present in the countries where clinical research is most commonly conducted. Many of these vaccines will be introduced into countries that lack robust spontaneous reporting systems (Gates Foundation, 2011). In these settings, enhanced surveillance systems or targeted PASS may provide a mechanism to address postlicensure safety assessment (WHO, 2012a).

A risk management plan (RMP) is required in the EU as part of marketing authorization application for new medicinal products and vaccines, and many countries have adopted guidelines similar to those of the EU. The RMP is regularly refined following licensure. For older products introduced prior to this requirement, an RMP may also be requested by regulators at any point in the life cycle in response to an emerging safety concern. The structure of RMP is discussed with greater detail in Chapter 2.1. Among the components of the RMP, a pharmacovigilance plan describes the requirements for routine and additional pharmacovigilance activities, including risk minimization measures. These plans may include PASS and other forms of surveillance to further characterize important identified risks, or to actively evaluate (or refute) important potential risks, or to gather missing information and PAES (see Chapter 6.2 for more information about PAES and their utility in benefit–risk evaluations). The RMP remains in place throughout the product life cycle, during which time-specific commitments may be removed (e.g., as PASS is completed) or they may be added to address new areas of concern arising from the emerging postlicensure experience. PASS and other forms of surveillance may also be required to evaluate the effectiveness and impact of risk minimization measures, such as compliance with important contraindications and warnings (Chapter 2.2 discusses risk minimization with detail).

ENHANCED PASSIVE SAFETY SURVEILLANCE FOR VACCINES

Although the passive surveillance approaches described in this section do not rise to the level of PASS, the EU draft guidance of 2014 on influenza vaccine safety surveillance provides vaccine manufacturers with the options of conducting either PASS or enhanced passive safety surveillance (EPSS) to fulfill the requirement for enhanced safety surveillance of seasonal influenza vaccines and are thus described below (EMA, 2014).

Routine safety surveillance for vaccines is based on conventional spontaneous reporting systems, such as the UK Yellow Card Scheme and the US VAERS. These systems comprise collections of case reports of suspected adverse reactions submitted by health-care professionals, consumers, and other sources. The purpose of these systems is to detect safety signals in the early postlicensure period. They often cover entire populations and provide a means of monitoring vaccines throughout their life cycle. However, they have limitations, including a general underreporting, selective reporting, and the lack of a true denominator to measure the population at risk.

To minimize the limitations of conventional passive surveillance, various EPSS methods have been developed to encourage or stimulate reporting of adverse events that may occur following vaccination. Their goal is to increase reporting overall, to identify safety signals more rapidly, and improve data quality. EPSS can be used as an open-ended surveillance, with no restriction on the types of adverse events reported or on the time frame of interest, or to focus on specific outcomes of interest.

EPSS can be implemented in different ways. Posters can be displayed in vaccination clinics to raise awareness of reporting, or vaccine recipients may be given awareness materials such as instruction leaflets on how to report adverse reactions. A more direct option is to issue a Safety Report Card (SRC) on which vaccinees report any suspected reactions. The SRC can be pre-populated with key information, such as the vaccine lot number and contact information to be used to report suspected reactions. Electronic devices have also been used to facilitate timely reporting, whereby vaccinees are contacted within days of vaccination through message or email. This allows simple "yes/no" responses to be given to basic questions but can be expanded should follow-on questions be needed, by providing links to more detailed web-based questionnaires.

EPSS can also be used to characterize the safety of live attenuated vaccines to detect symptoms of infection following vaccination. An example is the Varicella Zoster Virus Identification Program, an EPSS focused on viral characterization of virus isolates collected from varicella vaccine recipients with manifestations of zoster to characterize the isolates as wild-type or vaccine-type strains (Goulleret et al., 2010).

Another enhancement of conventional passive surveillance is to collect exposure denominator information, for example, by recording the number of vaccinees given the reporting material (e.g., the SRC) or the number contacted by messages or emails. These denominators allow calculation of reporting rates (for passive surveillance) or incidence rates (when ascertainment has been consistent) for detected adverse events.

Regardless of the method, care needs to be taken in the timing and communication to vaccinees of information regarding safety surveillance so as not to alarm patients or discourage uptake of vaccination.

Utility of Enhanced Passive Safety Surveillance in Seasonal Campaigns

A particular challenge arises when monitoring vaccines that may change in composition on a seasonal basis, such as influenza vaccines with virus strains that may vary from year to year. In addition, the target population comprises large numbers of relatively healthy individuals vaccinated in a short period in each successive season. Conventional passive surveillance methods could be modified to improve detection of safety signals in a timely manner. The EMA recommends that all seasonal influenza vaccines undergo EPSS with emphasis on rapid detection of typically common and minor "reactogenicity events" in the early flu season, particularly monitoring by age group and lot number (EMA, 2014). Marketing authorization holders and research providers have adopted a variety of approaches in response. Vaccine Working Party, the EMA's Pharmacovigilance Risk Assessment Committee (PRAC), emphasized that the key element is timeliness of the results, i.e., the aim of PASS or EPSS is to inform real-time regulatory actions during the ongoing season. Vaccines Europe, an organization representing vaccine manufacturers proposed that a model based on EPSS would provide an option to achieve near real-time surveillance that could be integrated into routine pharmacovigilance systems (Vaccine Europe, 2016).

An example of how EPSS has been used in this context is demonstrated by the UK experience for the children's flu vaccine. Public Health England recommended that children in selected age groups should be offered the intranasal vaccine as part of the national immunization campaign in general practices and in schools. A pilot EPSS program was designed and implemented in England in the 2015−16 flu season. Vaccinees or their representative were given an SRC at the time of vaccination with instructions to return the card to the marketing authorization holder if the child experienced a suspected adverse reaction. Surveillance was open-ended with no restriction on time window of reporting or the type of suspected adverse reactions. By simultaneously collecting data from participating immunization providers on the number of SRC handed out (n = 8753), it was possible to calculate a crude reporting rate for each reported suspected adverse reaction overall, and by lot and age group. The majority of reported suspected reactions were nonserious, and no safety signal was identified in the pilot program.

A key principle of the EPSS required by the EMA is to monitor, from year to year, the frequency and severity of commonly reported suspected adverse reactions after vaccination, with the focus on early detection of any increase in the expected frequency or severity of such suspected reactions in each flu season (EMA, 2014). EPSS is a feasible option in this respect by comparing reporting rates in a given season with the respective rates in the preceding seasons. In the example above, patients were instructed to return the SRC only in case of a suspected reaction, and the numbers of SRC returned with adverse events was relatively small (n = 165), representing about 2% of all SRC issued. Thus, the capacity to detect important differences between age groups or vaccine lots was limited. Despite the small numbers, the method appears to be a feasible means of increasing the overall reporting rate, as this was $\sim$200-folds higher than that expected from routine passive surveillance during the same period. Nevertheless, experience to date highlights a number of factors that must be considered in designing a successful EPSS program to select a representative and adequate sample of vaccinees and to ensure communication strategies are designed to encourage reporting without causing alarm or safety concerns (Box 7.3.1).

The most recent review of EPSS by PRAC encourages the marketing authorization holder to collect data on available lots per site at the end of the data collection period. In addition, potential signals arising from EPSS and

---

BOX 7.3.1 FACTORS TO CONSIDER IN ENHANCED PASSIVE SAFETY SURVEILLANCE IN SEASONAL FLU CAMPAIGNS

- Identify a key market to conduct EPSS in preparation of the new season (tenders may change on annual or biannual basis)
- Requirements for ethics committee and other approvals
- Target sample size and required number of vaccination sites
- Representativeness of population in selection of vaccination sites
- Projected vaccine uptake at selected sites
- Timeliness of vaccination clinics to ensure early seasonal data capture
- Options for reporting modalities and preferences of respondents
- Provision of surveillance materials in multiple languages
- Targeted events of interest or open-ended surveillance
- Facility to follow-up with health-care professionals
- Promotion of surveillance to vaccinees
- Methods to capture vaccine lot identification information
- Integration with routine pharmacovigilance to ensure timely processing of safety reports

conventional reporting systems should be investigated and communicated to the competent authorities using applicable established procedures. In the long term, the expectation is that reference rates for adverse event reporting will be established over time as data from the passive approach accumulate across multiple seasons.

As new vaccine products become available to prevent additional diseases in various parts of the world, the demand for effective pharmacovigilance systems in low- and middle-income countries is increasing. To help establish such systems in all countries, the World Health Organization (WHO) developed the Global Vaccine Safety Blueprint (WHO, 2012b). The development of further important vaccines, such as those against dengue, HIV, malaria, and tuberculosis—of primary interest for use in low-income countries—will make the challenge even more acute because these vaccines have never previously been used anywhere. Because of the limitations of spontaneous reporting systems, improved systems are used to monitor newly available vaccines in a timely fashion. For example, CYD tetravalent dengue vaccine has been licensed in several countries to date. It has been introduced to the public vaccination program in the first country, the Philippines, in April 2016. The vaccine was administered as part of a school-based program targeting fourth grade children (aged 9–10 years) in three highly endemic regions. Approximately 248,000 children were immunized. In this cohort, adverse events following immunization were monitored through EPSS. All serious events were investigated promptly and reviewed by an independent expert committee. Thus far, 518 adverse events have been reported, including 21 serious with 2 deaths, an example of how EPSS worked well in a mass immunization campaign with a reporting rate of 0.2% in a resource limited setting.

DESIGNS FOR VACCINE POST-AUTHORIZATION SAFETY STUDIES

PASS for vaccines might be conducted for multiple reasons, but in general, manufacturers and regulators are aiming to evaluate the safety of a product in the real-world (i.e., as given in clinical practice rather than the controlled context of RCT). Many of these studies are noninterventional rather than interventional in approach because once a vaccine is licensed and recommended for a particular group, it may no longer be ethical to randomize subjects in this group to potentially not receive the vaccine. Although there are instances of RCT for licensed products, such as comparisons of a newer vaccine formulation to a licensed older one.

Noninterventional studies can assess product safety in typical real-world settings, where patients may be more heterogeneous, and medical treatment follows usual care rather than a study protocol, and where cold chains and other factors may not be as meticulous as in clinical trials. Additionally, these studies can be much larger, offering power to detect infrequent and rare risks that could otherwise escape recognition during clinical development programs. Real-world study populations may also include those excluded from clinical development, e.g., pregnant women. Programs such as the VSD are described previously in this chapter, but differentiated from PASS, which are designed to evaluate the safety of a specific product and/or assess a specific hypothesis, although VSD may serve as a data source for PASS. Objectives for vaccine PASS may include routine surveillance and signal detection, as well as targeted hypothesis testing. A range of study designs might be used to address these objectives, as described below.

Signal Detection

As part of routine pharmacovigilance activities conducted by the manufacturer, PASS may be designed in whole or in part to provide additional safety surveillance for potential adverse events of newly licensed or seasonally modified vaccine products. Following licensure of the adolescent and adult formulation of the tetanus, diphtheria, and acellular pertussis (Tdap) vaccine in the United States, a safety study with a risk interval and historic cohort design was conducted within a large integrated health-care organization and subsequently monitored over 120,000 vaccinees for potential adverse events (Baxter et al., 2016).

The EMA called for influenza vaccine manufacturers to conduct EPSS of each year's formulation, with a primary objective to detect a potential increase in reactogenicity and allergic events intrinsic to the product (not due to specific lot deviations or local programmatic issues) in near real-time in the earliest vaccinated cohorts (EMA, 2014). It is noted that the guidance is evolving since its initial implementation and has been modified by the Vaccines Working Party in discussion with Vaccines Europe (de Lusignan et al., 2017). In 2014, a pilot cohort study was conducted to evaluate the safety and reactogenicity of the intranasal live attenuated influenza vaccine, in which vaccinees were recruited from the mass vaccination program in the United Kingdom (McNaughton et al., 2016).

Cohort studies, whether designed primarily for safety surveillance or hypothesis testing, allow for the direct estimation of risk of an event or events of interest stated as a cumulative incidence (number of events over the specified follow-up period of interest divided by number vaccinated) or incidence rate (number of events divided by sum of person-time for the period of interest) with associated confidence intervals. In this manner, both a point estimate of absolute risk of an event of interest, which may be used in benefit–risk assessments, and estimation of attributable risk, as well as upper and lower bounds for the true risk in a similar population, are obtained. The estimation of these incidence measures and confidence intervals is straightforward (Rothman et al., 2008).

A retrospective cohort study was conducted using a distributed research network approach among a number of large US health insurers to address concerns regarding VAERS reports of GBS following meningococcal conjugate vaccination (MCV4) in the year after licensure among adolescents in the United States (Velentgas et al., 2012). In this study, incidence rates were calculated for categories of person-time defined in relation to timing of MCV4 exposure, i.e., the day of and 42 days after vaccination, days more than 42 days after MCV4, and days unexposed to MCV4, and reported as number of GBS cases per 100,000 person-years, with exact 95% confidence intervals.

The attack rate (risk) or cumulative incidence of GBS per million vaccinations was calculated by dividing the number of observed GBS cases by the number of total vaccinations for each vaccine type. An estimate of the attributable risk of GBS was obtained by subtracting the expected number of vaccine-exposed cases of GBS per million vaccinations from the risk or the upper bound of the confidence interval for risk of GBS per million vaccinations, with one-sided 95% confidence intervals (upper bounds) for the attack rate and attributable risk of GBS per million vaccinations calculated using exact binomial confidence intervals.

Between the passive surveillance and broad signal detection approaches such as VAERS and Sentinel have evolved the area of near real-time safety surveillance for vaccines and other medicinal products. With near real-time surveillance approaches, prespecified adverse events of interest are investigated in the period shortly after launch of a new vaccine or seasonal update of a previous vaccine formulation (i.e., targeted surveillance), usually based in EMR data from a single health-care system or a distributed research network such as the VSD (Chen et al., 1997). To allow for ongoing evaluation of vaccine safety with reevaluation of the risk of an adverse event of interest compared with a historical or other background rate, methods allow for continuous testing of a hypothesis or multiple hypotheses as new events accrue. The method most frequently used is the maximized sequential probability ratio test, which can evaluate the observed data against a composite alternative hypothesis such as relative risk >1, thus representing an evolution of the original sequential probability ratio test (SPRT) method (Leite et al., 2016). It has been suggested that proactive surveillance using the SPRT method in VSD would have detected an increased risk of intussusception following rotavirus vaccine after about 2600 doses of vaccine, at about the same time as the first VAERS reports were received (Davis et al., 2005).

Signal Evaluation

PASS may address specific safety hypotheses to evaluate safety signals, which provide evidence to confirm or refute possible safety signals following introduction of new or seasonally updated vaccines. Spontaneous reports to the VAERS describing intussusception among recipients of the first approved rotavirus vaccine began to accumulate during the months after licensure. A positive but statistically insignificant association has been evaluated from Phase 3 RCT. Urgently conducted PASS confirmed a very strong statistical association, leading initially to withdrawal of the vaccine from the marketplace and reinforcing the need for stronger (larger) Phase 3 studies of subsequent rotavirus vaccines to assure a positive benefit–risk balance prior to licensure (CDC, 2004).

In another example, although methodologic questions persist, multiple studies with diverse designs appeared to confirm an association between narcolepsy and an H1N1 influenza vaccine in multiple countries after initial recognition of spontaneously reported cases among Scandinavian recipients of the adjuvant pandemic influenza vaccine in 2010 (Verstraeten et al., 2016).

Table 7.3.1 presents the range of usual study design choices for vaccine PASS, along with some of the key drivers for selection of one design over another. Refer to Chapters 4.1–4.5 for more discussion on specific designs.

Table 7.3.1 Study Design Options for Vaccine Post-Authorization Safety Studies

Design	Objective	Consideration for Selection
Single-arm cohort (Chapter 4.1)	• Characterize vaccinated population • Estimate risk of adverse events following vaccination, including upper/lower bounds for confidence intervals	• Multiple or all adverse events are of interest • Interest in putting upper bound on risk of specific events.
Two-arm cohort (Chapter 4.3)	• Characterize vaccinated population • Estimate risk of adverse events • Compare vaccinated with unvaccinated persons within defined source population • Identify potential causal associations of vaccine and risk of events (hypothesis testing)	• Multiple or all adverse events are of interest • Interest in putting upper bound on specific event • Comparison to unvaccinated is of interest • Estimate attributable risk (risk difference) and relative risk
Case–control (Chapter 4.3)	• Hypothesis testing	• Very rare events • Comparison to unvaccinated is of interest • Unvaccinated persons can be identified
Vaccinee-only (Chapter 4.2)	• Hypothesis testing • Mainly acute adverse events with defined risk window.	• High coverage vaccines with less exposure variation, e.g., childhood vaccines • Not for delayed onset events • Vaccinated persons with events, e.g., SCCS • Estimate risk difference and relative risk

When the link between a specific adverse event of interest and vaccination is in question and a prespecified hypothesis is being evaluated, observed-to-expected comparisons in the form of risk differences, relative risks, odds ratios, and other measures developed for use in vaccine safety studies may be estimated. An example of estimation of relative risks in a cohort study of vaccinated and unvaccinated children can be seen in a retrospective cohort of all children born in Denmark between 1991 and 1998 to evaluate a possible association between MMR vaccine and autism. Adjusted relative risks (incidence rate ratios) were calculated using log-linear Poisson regression with vaccination as a time-dependent covariate. Overall, no association was seen between vaccination and autism or other autism-spectrum disorders (Madsen et al., 2002).

A study of intussusception following second-generation rotavirus vaccine administrations in the United States utilized a self-controlled risk interval (SCRI) and cohort designs to estimate attributable risks and relative risks of intussusception after rotavirus vaccine exposures (Yih et al., 2014). The SCRI approach had the potential to better control for confounding as values for important measured and unmeasured confounders are the same within individuals, and the cohort analysis had greater statistical power, due to the greater amount of historical and concurrent unexposed person-time included in the analysis. In the SCRI analysis, the number of cases in the risk intervals (1–7 days and 1–21 days after vaccination) and control intervals (22–42 days after vaccination) was compared using logistic regression with an offset term to adjust for differential risk of intussusception by age in the risk and control intervals. In the cohort analysis, rates of the outcome during exposed and unexposed person-time were compared using Poisson regression, with adjustment for age, sex, and health plan. Both analyses showed an increased risk of intussusception in the risk interval of 1–21 days following a first dose of vaccine.

Cohort and Case–Control Designs

Cohort PASS may include patients vaccinated with the product of interest only (single-arm designs), e.g., cohort event monitoring studies (Chapter 4.1) designed to estimate incidence rates for a range of predefined adverse events of special interest or events reported in a given time frame following vaccination. Without an internal or designated external comparison group, there is no adjustment for confounding. But study aims may be to quantify risks associated with the vaccine with sufficient precision to contribute to the manufacturer ongoing pharmacovigilance efforts; detection of unexpected adverse reactions; and—depending on study size—to identify rare adverse events associated with the vaccine. A postlicensure cohort study of the safety of MF59 adjuvant cell culture–derived influenza vaccine in the 2009–2010 H1N1 influenza pandemic enrolled about 4000 individuals from four EU and South American countries (Reynales et al., 2012). Basic health information was collected at the immunization clinic on the day of vaccination, and patients were contacted 7 days following vaccination, and monthly thereafter for 6 months to collect information on all adverse events for which patients sought medical attention and for adverse events of special interest, including neuritis, seizure, anaphylaxis, encephalitis, vasculitis, GBS, demyelinating conditions, Bell's palsy, and laboratory-confirmed vaccination failure. Counts of adverse events that occurred within the prespecified risk window were compared against expected rates using sequential testing methods (Lieu et al., 2007). Only two seizure cases occurring outside the 7-day risk window were reported, and other adverse events were consistent with the known safety profile of MF59 adjuvant influenza vaccine.

Alternative to single-arm designs, vaccine PASS can be comparative cohorts. In one such study, the CDC and clinicians at participating hospitals enrolled a cohort of over 5000 pregnant women with confirmed vaccination histories at the time of presentation at the hospital for live birth or miscarriage, to examine the association of influenza vaccination with risk of small for gestational age and preterm births. The investigators found that influenza vaccination was associated with a significantly lower adjusted risk for preterm birth, and no effect on small for gestational age or birth weight (Olsen et al., 2016).

In contrast to cohort PASS, which compare the occurrence of adverse events in vaccinated and unvaccinated individuals, case–control PASS might begin by identifying all persons with a specific rare event within a defined population, and then measuring the frequency of immunization in those with (cases) and without (controls) the outcome. The VAESCO-GBS case–control study group conducted a case–control study of GBS following the 2009–10 H1N1 pandemic influenza vaccination campaign, using EMR, vaccination registries, and other data from five EU countries (Dieleman et al., 2011). About 100 GPS cases that met the Brighton case definition or were confirmed by a neurologist were identified from a source population of over 50 million individuals and matched with one or more controls. Data on medical history, including influenza-like illness, upper respiratory infections, pandemic and seasonal influenza vaccination in the prior 6 weeks, and past history of GBS and other conditions were collected to adjust for potential confounding. The results helped to put an upper bound on the expected increase in cases of GBS of 3 per million vaccinated cases. Chapter 4.3 discusses cohort and nested case–control designs with details.

Vaccinee-Only Designs

The challenges of identifying suitable unvaccinated comparison groups has led to the development of designs that avoid the need for selection of comparable unvaccinated patients by comparing vaccinated individuals to themselves or to other vaccinated individuals, some of which were developed specifically for vaccine safety evaluation (Farrington, 1995; Whitaker et al., 2006; Fireman et al., 2009). Examples of these vaccinee-only designs include the *risk interval designs*, such as the SCRI and the self-controlled case series (SCCS); and *case-centered designs*. More details on self-controlled study designs can be found in Chapter 4.2.

These designs generally define a risk interval, a biologically plausible window of time following a vaccine when an adverse event could be due to the vaccine (Rowhani-Rahbar et al., 2012). If a vaccine is causing the adverse event (with a sufficiently high attributable risk for detection in the sample studied), we would expect clustering of the events shortly after immunization. Clustering in time alone may suggest, but does not always confirm, an inference of causality. In one VSD experience, a preliminary finding of clustering for hair loss after vaccinations appeared to confirm a hypothesis from several reports to VAERS. However, examination of case records by the investigators disclosed a misclassification of diagnosis dates. Young children had been seen for "well baby" or other medical visits, during which they received routine vaccinations. But during these visits their parents had also described hair loss, which preceded the vaccinations but prompted referrals to dermatologists. When the children saw the dermatologists days or weeks later, the diagnoses of alopecia were entered into their medical records, providing an appearance that the hair loss followed vaccinations. This experience highlights the importance of ascertaining the correct dates of vaccination and adverse event onset in any study using a risk interval.

The basic risk interval method is depicted in Fig. 7.3.1A. Risk interval study designs have been used in numerous PASS. Examples of vaccine PASS include studies on HPV vaccine (HPV4) (Klein et al., 2012); live attenuated nasal influenza vaccine (Baxter et al., 2012a,b); live attenuated zoster vaccine (Baxter et al., 2012c); tetanus toxoid; reduced diphtheria toxoid; acellular pertussis vaccine (Baxter et al., 2016); and DTaP-inactivated poliovirus-hemophilus B conjugate vaccine (Hansen et al., 2016).

Conditioning on the individual in a risk interval cohort study distinguishes an SCRI design. The SCCS design utilizes only individuals that have a particular adverse event under study and uses the timing of vaccination in relation to the adverse event to assess possible causality. Both of these self-controlled methods effectively control for time-stable confounders, e.g., date of birth, sex, and other genetic variables (Whitaker et al., 2006).

(A)   Risk Interval Design

Research Question: Do adverse events cluster in the risk interval after vaccination compared with the comparison interval?

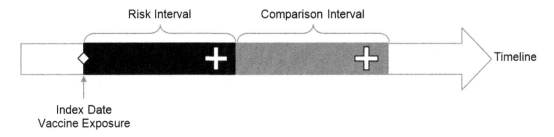

(B)   Case-Centered Design

Research Question: Do vaccines cluster in the exposure interval prior to the adverse event compared with the comparison interval?

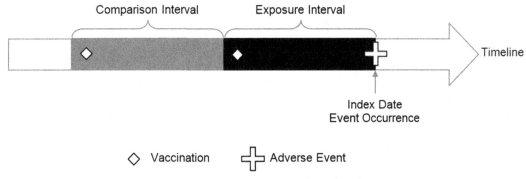

FIGURE 7.3.1
Illustration of vaccine-only designs commonly used in vaccine PASS.

Fig. 7.3.1B depicts the basic case-centered design. The case-centered method is equivalent to a case–control study but has some advantages for vaccines (Fireman et al., 2009). In this design, expected rates of immunization may be calculated from the entire general population, stratified by age and sex. This method has the advantages of adjusting for seasonality and making use of population-based immunization patterns, allowing calculation of the risk difference and attributable risk, which is not possible when only the vaccination of cases is known.

Data Sources for Vaccine Post-Authorization Safety Studies

Vaccine PASS utilize standard epidemiologic approaches and data sources, including those described in detail in Chapters 3.1–3.5, with basic requirements for collection of information about vaccine exposure of interest and consistent ascertainment of the outcomes, i.e., disease, syndrome, or other potential adverse events of interest independent of vaccination status. For immunizations, common data sources include administrative claims, EMR, immunization or disease registries, and prospectively collected data from patients and health-care professionals across a range of settings (either supplemental detail beyond what is typically recorded in the patient record or clinical outcomes assessments). Selection of the optimal data source for a given study depends on strategic exploitation of information resources for the particular study objectives and research questions.

Claims and Electronic Medical Record

In addition to serving as the underlying source data for research infrastructure such as the VSD, PRISM, and other projects, secondary data sources such as claims and EMR are frequently used for vaccine PASS. They are considered relatively complete and accurate sources for information on the type (indication) of vaccine administered, date of administration for vaccines administered in a clinic for EMR, or for which payment was processed by insurance provider with respect to claims. Lot identifications and sometimes the manufacturer or specific product/brand of vaccine for which there are multiple manufacturers may not always be available in secondary data sources. Particularly for higher cost vaccines, such as meningitis and HPV vaccines, these sources are likely to be quite complete for populations seen within a defined health-care system and/or covered by a specific health insurer. For vaccines that are commonly delivered in multiple care settings and may be paid for out-of-pocket, such as seasonal influenza vaccine, these data sources require careful evaluation as to their suitability for the population of interest.

For some safety events of interest, claims and/or EMR data may be appropriate for outcome data, bearing in mind whether patients are likely to seek medical care for the event of interest. Milder injection site reactions and other reactogenicity may be difficult or impossible to study in such data sources and may require de novo data collection (EMA, 2014). These data allow for access to extremely large populations for PASS of rare adverse events following vaccination, e.g., GBS. However, because algorithms for identifying adverse events based on diagnostic coding systems may yield a mix of confirmed and "rule-out" diagnoses, potential outcomes identified through claims or EMR data require further direct confirmation through medical record abstraction, chart review, or contact with the treating physician for adequate rigor. More discussion can be found in Chapter 3.1 for claims and Chapter 3.2 for EMR data.

Vaccination Registries

Vaccination or immunization registries are data source that attempts to record vaccinations for all persons of interest within a geographic region, such as a city, state, or country. Although vaccination registries provide valuable information on vaccination exposure for a population, they do not typically include any information on adverse events following vaccination and may not be easily linked to other data sources to be able to identify associations between vaccine exposures and outcomes of interest. Registries as data source for PASS are discussed with detail in Chapter 3.3.

Primary Data Collection

Information commonly collected from health-care providers and vaccination clinics include medical history, specific details of vaccines administered, and adverse events that may be observed shortly after vaccination, e.g., injection site reactions and events following vaccination for which patients may seek medical care. Chapter 4.5 provides an overview of prospective study designs, including primary data collection approaches.

Vaccination and adverse event information collected directly from the vaccinee can supplement study data elements and capture information not reported to health-care providers or vaccination sites. These approaches are particularly beneficial to assess adverse events for which medical attention may not be sought, including many reactogenicity events, as well as cases where the vaccinee does not return to the vaccination site following immunization, and it is known which health-care provider would be consulted should have an adverse event following immunization occur to collect or verify the necessary safety data, e.g., through SRC in EPSS. Limited knowledge of vaccine exposure detail may be expected from parents or patients through direct patient data collection, with vaccine indication and dates of administration being likely more easily and accurately recalled than the brand or lot of the vaccine. Chapter 4.4 discusses enriched study design where secondary data and primary data sources can be linked to serve objectives of PASS.

Providing alternative modes of data collection and use of fit-for-purpose technology may increase the likelihood of high response rates across multiple age groups, income levels, and geographic regions. Electronic data capture (EDC) systems, commonly used in prospective noninterventional studies, now often provide electronic patient-reported outcomes (PRO) capabilities that give patients access to online questionnaires through a link sent by email or to their smartphones or tablets, as well as facilitating electronic reminders to complete questionnaires as scheduled by text messaging or email.

Electronic questionnaires may be difficult to older generations with less technological literacy and/or may be less accessible to lower income or resource-poor populations. Paper questionnaires are an alternative that should be considered for these populations and interactive voice response speech recognition. Irrespective of format, translation of questionnaires into local languages must also be incorporated into study planning and costs.

An example of direct patient data collection methods is the previously described study conducted in 2009 to assess postlicensure safety of MF59 adjuvant influenza vaccine used during a global pandemic (Reynales et al., 2012). Despite challenges surrounding patient follow-up with a large cohort in relatively short time frame, the overall response rate at 6 months was about 97%, with only 59 patients lost to follow-up, 5 patients who withdrew from the study, and 3 deaths. Several follow-up methods were used in this study contributing to this high response rate, including electronic (internet-based) and paper (via mailing) PRO questionnaires available depending on preference or need, as well as telephone surveys, which were the most common method employed.

Considerations for Vaccine Exposure Measurement

Countries have different vaccination systems, recommendations, and schedule of vaccine administration. All these factors, together with the selected setting and population, determine which data sources are appropriate for collecting vaccine exposure data. Here we summarize specifics of vaccine exposure characteristics and general considerations for sources of data on vaccine exposure, the availability of which are ideally confirmed through a feasibility assessment of the potential data sources prior to implementing a study.

Table 7.3.2 lists specific characteristics of vaccine exposure to consider when selecting an exposure data source and defining the exposure status, not all of which may be needed, depending on the research question. Some of these characteristics can be inferred from the applicable vaccine recommendations or from distribution or manufacturing data.

Vaccine Indication

A licensed indication is a legally valid reason for using a vaccine product. In contrast to curative medicinal products, vaccines are used for disease prevention, and hence, their use is not limited to persons only after they have become ill or injured. A vaccine indication is defined by the disease it aims to prevent, except for therapeutic vaccines (e.g., cancer treatment) and

Table 7.3.2 Vaccine Exposure Characteristics to Consider in Vaccine Post-Authorization Safety Studies

Characteristic	Example
License holder or manufacturer	Licensed, in-licensed products
Indication	Infectious disease, age group, and preventive postexposure prophylaxis
Formulation	Live attenuated, killed, nonadjuvant, cell culture, x-valent, combination vaccine, and proprietary vaccine name
Vaccine recommendations and schedule	Routine vaccination as per recommendations (e.g., childhood, seasonal, risk groups, and pregnant women), outbreak, travel, professional (e.g., health-care workers), voluntary, reimbursed, and out-of-pocket paid
Dosing schedule	Single vaccination, dose series (e.g., priming, booster, and revaccination)
Production	Lot identification and expiry date
Presentation	Vial (e.g., monodose, multidose, and prefilled syringe), and application device (e.g., needle, needle-free, and spray)
Route of administration	Oral, intranasal, injectable, injection site (e.g., intradermal, intramuscular, and subcutaneous), and other application devices
Setting of administration	General practitioner, hospital, vaccination center, pediatric clinic, travel clinic, school program, employer program, pharmacy, commercial available vaccine, and community based child care
Concomitant vaccination	Vaccines given concomitantly with the vaccine of interest

postexposure prophylaxis (e.g., rabies, varicella, and tetanus). Approved vaccine indications generally also vary by age group and sometimes sex.

As for medicinal products, use of the vaccine in the routine practice may differ from the licensed indication. An example of use of vaccine outside its licensed sex indication (i.e., off-label use) is the HPV vaccine. Initially licensed in the United States for use in the female population from age 9 to 26 years, the vaccine was used off-label in the high-risk male population for prevention of genital warts until 2009 and anal cancer until 2010, when both indications were added to the label as the completed trial data become available.

Vaccine Formulation

The specific composition of a vaccine determines its safety, efficacy, stability, and storage methods. The fundamental structural consideration for a vaccine is inclusion of one or more epitopes that will induce an appropriate immune response. These epitopes may be presented in one or more forms: vaccines may contain live viruses that have been attenuated (i.e., weakened or altered so as not to cause illness); inactivated or killed viruses; inactivated bacterial toxins (for bacterial diseases where toxins generated by the bacteria cause illness); or components of the pathogen (e.g., polysaccharides in subunit and conjugate vaccines). A specific challenge is posed by combination vaccines that contain antigens targeting different pathogens. These combination vaccines are intended to minimize the number of vaccinations administered to a child but may lead to difficulty in interpreting vaccination exposure data if records do not capture brand and manufacturer, or if this information is not recorded in prospective PASS. As an example, one vaccine product covers diphtheria, tetanus, pertussis, poliovirus, and hepatitis B (FDA, 2002); whereas another vaccine product covers hemophilus influenza type B in addition to above illnesses (FDA, 2008). In addition, the formulation may include excipients, adjuvants, preservatives, stabilizers, surfactants, emulsifiers, animal products (e.g., egg), or DNA in various compositions.

Vaccine Recommendations

For vaccines, national and local public health recommendations play a major role in determining who receives the vaccine, and these recommendations in turn inform the selection of data sources and health-care settings that are likely to reflect immunizations administered to the target population regarding age, high-risk groups, immunocompromised patients, children, or pregnant women, and certain professions such as health-care workers and whether the vaccine is reimbursed by insurance.

Vaccine Dosing Schedule

The number of doses to be provided of a particular vaccine depends on several factors, including the type of vaccine, age, and other factors, impacting the status of the immune system. Some vaccines, such as tetanus and pertussis, require periodic booster doses after initial immunization.

Live attenuated vaccines can result in lifelong immunity with just one or two doses. In contrast, primarily inactivated vaccines are not based on replication and will result in a less robust and less diverse memory response. Some vaccines protect against agents that change often enough that older versions would not offer protection. The influenza vaccine is a key example, requiring new versions virtually every season.

Age is an important determinant for the immune response. Younger persons have more robust immune responses to vaccines than do older persons. Dose schedules generally differ according to age. For example, the shingles vaccine given to adults contains about 14 times more vaccine virus than the chickenpox vaccine given to children, even though both vaccines are prepared using the same Oka strain of the varicella virus. Similarly, the adult version of the hepatitis A vaccine contains higher doses than the one for children. In contrast, the Tdap vaccine used in adolescents, teens, and adults contains lesser quantities of the antigens to reduce the chance for swelling of the arm than was common in older children and adults. Immune senescence, or aging-related changes in the immune system, also may lead to reactivation of chronic infections such as herpes zoster, with implications for vaccination later in life.

Finally, persons with altered immunocompetence may require an alternative dosing schedule (or even different types of vaccines) than healthy subjects.

Vaccine Route, Lot, and Expiration Date

In some situations, it can be important to identify exposure to one particular formulation or production lot, specifically for investigations of production-related issues, or when the effectiveness of the vaccine may depend on whether the vaccine was properly administered. Lot identifications and particularly expiration dates are characteristics that may not be commonly recorded as part of routine care, limiting the usefulness of secondary data for PASS needing these details.

Different routes of administration may influence the nature of local reactions experienced by vaccine recipients. Route of administration often differs by age group and settings. For example, intranasal vaccine for very young children may be challenging for the recipient to inhale as instructed. Contraindications may also differ by the route and formulation of a vaccine. Deviation from the recommended route of administration might reduce vaccine effectiveness or increase the risk for local adverse reactions.

Vaccine Administration Setting

An ideal data source for estimating individual exposure or population coverage with a vaccine would capture vaccinations by all service providers, including public and private hospitals, health centers, and physicians. For PASS, identification of data sources or populations through which information on vaccination exposure and outcome can be systematically obtained is more important, as long as sufficient numbers of vaccinated patients, including key groups of interest (e.g., children, adults, elderly, or pregnant women) are encompassed within the data sources or can be enrolled through the health-care sites. For example, enrollment of patients through multiple general practitioner sites up to a target sample size may be an appropriate approach for prospective PASS looking at the safety of seasonal influenza vaccines.

The study of vaccination programs implemented outside the care of health-care professionals may require data collection beyond these settings, e.g., school-based programs for vaccination against HPV may require working with the cooperation and approval of school-based clinics.

Persons who do not belong to the recommended target groups for vaccination may also more likely receive vaccines outside the care of their general practitioner. This is the case with influenza vaccines, which are available without prescription in a wide range of settings, such as through public health campaigns, company vaccination programs, and pharmacies. Information derived from these sources may be more limited than those provided through healthcare professionals, which have access to additional patient information beyond vaccine administration. Different settings may thus capture exposure status of different types of recipients. Recording practices of vaccine characteristics may also differ between settings.

METHODOLOGICAL CONSIDERATIONS

Vaccine PASS pose challenges for successful implementation and reporting, and some specific challenges arise in prospective studies in which data are collected directly from health-care professionals or clinical sites, patients, or a mix. Strategies surrounding efficient study start-up, timing, and representativeness of patient enrollment, data collection methods, and other factors should be considered (Palucci, 2016).

Seasonal and Regional Considerations

Efficient implementation of study start-up activities is critical for successful PASS implementation to ensure the appropriate patients can be enrolled into the study in time for vaccine receipt and at sites suitable for study needs. This is particularly true when undertaking vaccine PASS for seasonal diseases (e.g., dengue, influenza, and Zika), in which a peak vaccination time window exists at the beginning of the disease season during which nearly all vaccinations occur. Failure to successfully complete study start-up activities in time for enrollment during these peak vaccination time frames could result in an inability to identify and enroll patients at or shortly following vaccination, as they would likely have already received the vaccine for the season and past the acceptable time frame for collection of adverse event information. Additionally, the length of these peak vaccination time frames varies by disease, climate, country, and vaccine availability. Therefore, it is important to understand well in advance when these time frames will occur, and plan so as to ensure all necessary tasks to screen and initiate sites and potential patients can be completed before the majority of the season vaccinations occur.

For many vaccine PASS, geographic region is also an important consideration when selecting sites and navigating processes for study start-up. Several factors critical for successful study start-up may vary by region or country and present obstacles to patient enrollment and timely study conduct if not preemptively anticipated. For example, peak vaccination time frames may differ by temperate versus tropical climates. Patterns of uptake and availability of vaccines may differ according to country or health-care system, overall and for specific age groups. Vaccinations administered outside of typical care settings, such as schools and vaccination centers in mass campaigns, may require partnering with investigators and administrators of these clinics/sites to capture the desired population. It is necessary to plan for these variations when designing and implementing PASS to be able to set realistic patient enrollment targets by country and to select appropriate sites to carry out the study and fulfill regulatory requirements.

Understanding the epidemiology of the disease under study is necessary for this planning, as well as determining more broadly, which regions or countries make sense to be included in the study, in conjunction with any country-specific requirements for PASS specified by regulatory authorities. The geographic distribution of the disease influences seasonality, as well as disease incidence, and in turn, likely numbers of individuals seeking vaccine, both adults and children, within that area. Selecting sites in countries or regions with earlier vaccine availability, peak vaccination time frames similar to necessary study start dates, and high expected vaccination usage among the patient population in question will improve likelihood of meeting enrollment targets in a timely manner and collecting useful data to meet PASS reporting requirements.

In evaluating the geographic burden of disease for site and patient selection, it is also important to consider how differences in development stage of the countries to be included would affect the study, and specifically study start-up activities. These challenges may include availability of resources for study conduct such as technology or health-care centers and challenges of working in remote locations, such as patient travel distances to vaccination centers and vaccine availability at sites. Strategic decisions must be made regarding whether to include sites in these areas, and if so, how to overcome several of these barriers in a productive manner so as to ensure a smooth and efficient study start-up process.

Site Selection

Site selection is one of the most important factors in ensuring the successful conduct of a prospective vaccine PASS, both from the perspective of achieving enrollment targets and ensuring representation of key subgroups in the study. Contrary to conduct of RCT where vaccine administration and distribution is typically centralized to one or several specific locations, in the postlicensure context, vaccinations are administered from many different locations and types of sites, all of which could fall within different cities, villages, or towns.

A strategy for site selection must thus ensure that the final set of chosen sites will capture the targeted patient population, including key subgroups such as pediatric patients, if relevant, while also having a high likelihood of reaching the overall target sample size for the study.

Understanding vaccine distribution and where the targeted patient population chooses to receive vaccines is necessary to ensure sites are reflective of community vaccine preferences and behavior patterns. For example, receipt of vaccinations from pharmacies may be common for elderly patients in the United States, whereas pediatric patients may typically receive vaccines at pediatric outpatient clinics. Where possible, existing vaccination networks may be leveraged to address these site identification challenges.

Patient Enrollment

Study enrollment of patients within specific age categories to meet regulatory guidance requires thorough understanding of country-specific regulations for patient consent, particularly as they relate to enrollment of vulnerable populations into the study, including pediatric and geriatric patients who are typically at high risk for adverse events. Such requirements include use of parental informed consent forms for pediatric patients, customization of child consent forms for younger versus older pediatric patients, and customization of material for parental or legal guardian involvement.

Predetermined enrollment targets by age group are also important to consider during implementation of PASS for assessment of rare adverse events. Large sample sizes within each age category are required to be able to detect rare or very rare events (occurring in rates <0.1%). These enrollment targets can be challenging to meet if patient enrollment windows are short (e.g., seasonal influenza PASS). If detection of rare events is within the objectives of the study, prior considerations should be made during site selection processes that will deliver approximately the number of required patients within each age category of interest (e.g., ensure pediatric clinics are included as study sites if ascertainment of rare events in children is desired or necessary for regulatory requirements).

Patient Retention

Translation of all patient study material into local languages and making any follow-up calls or other direct-to-patient contacts in the local language of the patients should be incorporated into the study conduct when multiple countries or regions are involved, so as to reach out to patients in a language and/or dialect familiar to them to reduce the work required for the patient to report requested information, and to increase the likelihood that the information will be provided completely and accurately.

Providing modest incentives for completion of patient questionnaires such as small credit with patient's mobile phone provider if follow-up is done by telephone is another useful tool to improve data completeness, and patient follow-up and engagement throughout the study time frame. This is a well-accepted practice and if done with approval through appropriate regulatory channels, e.g., institutional review board or ethics committee approval, consistent with regional requirements, and described clearly in patient consent materials, no ethical concerns exist.

Data Collection Methods

Issues common to noninterventional studies in general, such as patient engagement and outreach, loss to follow-up, and the potential for missing data also exist for PASS. Vaccine PASS also face challenges relating to the need for rapid follow-up with the patient postvaccination for assessment of adverse events.

As vaccinees are in general a healthy population that is not necessarily expected to be seen again by the health-care professional or vaccination center during the follow-up period of interest, as discussed earlier in this chapter, direct patient data collection methods for reporting adverse events of particular value can be used. If used, EDC systems also permit real-time data queries and edit checks with study sites to increase the likelihood that data are entered properly the first time and to limit subsequent data issues when reporting results. Risk-based monitoring can be applied remotely in these study settings through use of the EDC; these efforts are most effective when implemented as a collaboration between clinical and data management study personnel to review data collected through the system (Box 7.3.2).

BOX 7.3.2 STRATEGIES TO AID IN DATA COLLECTION AND PATIENT FOLLOW-UP IN PROSPECTIVE VACCINE POST-AUTHORIZATION SAFETY STUDIES

- Utilize direct-to-patient data collection methods with multiple modalities for questionnaire completion to accommodate differing patient populations
- Employ remote risk-based monitoring of data entry through electronic data capture systems
- Provide study-related materials in local languages to increase patient engagement and improve retention rates
- Actively follow-up with nonresponders to reduce missing data
- Provide patients nonmonetary incentives where possible to increase rates of retention and completion of patient questionnaires

Case Definition

In 1999, the Brighton Collaboration was established to further methods for studying vaccine safety, engages in a wide range of research and standards development in support of methodologically sound vaccine safety research (Brighton Collaboration, 2016). In addition to conducting research studies and support of the VAESCO research infrastructure for vaccine research in the EU, the Brighton Collaboration has made a substantial contribution in the development of standard case definitions for outcomes of interest to vaccine safety. Its library of case definitions currently includes over 28 definitions, ranging from local reactions and seizures to GBS and Fisher syndrome. Use of standard case definitions should increase comparability across studies and help fill gaps in availability of specialists such as neurologists in many parts of the developing world.

Background Event Rates

Although to some extent the development and broad use of vaccinees-only designs for vaccine PASS has made the need for background incidence rates of adverse events somewhat less pressing, it remains important to contextualize incidence rates observed in a single study to broader population rates, especially in studies of rare events where the background rate of events may be based on a small number of events within a given study population. Additionally, near real-time safety surveillance methods require an expected number of events of interest from the same or similar population for comparison to the observed counts of events of interest (Belongia et al., 2010). When available, as in the case of claims and EMR data, historical rates estimated from similar patients using the same data source may be ideal (Burwen et al., 2012); however, in the case of prospective PASS, an external source of information on expected incidence of rare events, such as GBS, anaphylaxis, seizure, autoimmune, and other conditions, may be needed to ensure a stable comparator to a small number of observed cases (Black et al., 2009).

Confounding

In general, noninterventional PASS are vulnerable to confounding—differences between vaccinated and unvaccinated individuals that could influence the analytic results for reasons other than direct effects of the vaccine. Confounding can often be controlled in the study design (e.g., by matching cases with controls on a variable of concern or use of self-controlled designs) and/or in the analysis (e.g., by stratification or multivariable regression).

Vaccinated persons can be very different from unvaccinated persons, and often these differences are difficult to measure, so that they cannot be fully controlled through statistical analyses (Jackson et al., 2006, 2013; Fireman et al., 2009;

Baxter et al., 2010;). For example, people who choose not to be vaccinated or who do not allow their children to be vaccinated may have very different health-care utilization patterns from people who do receive routine vaccines. The former may make more extensive use of "alternative" providers or may have less trust in conventional medical providers, or have religious, political, or other beliefs that keep them from seeking medical care.

Vaccine recommendations and reimbursement are also essential to understand and take into account when studying vaccine exposure patterns, especially if they involve comparisons with other vaccines. Recommendations and reimbursement factors can help researchers to identify important confounding factors, choose the appropriate comparator vaccines or comparison risk windows, and select appropriate study populations. Age and immune status are two main drivers for vaccine recommendations. Standards for vaccination practices are very common and often vary by age group. Recommendations for the age at which vaccines should be administered are influenced by age-specific risks for disease, risks for complications, and capacity to respond to a vaccine.

Priority groups for vaccination may include those at higher risk of infection with the target disease (which the vaccine is intended to prevent) or complications from it, such as immunocompromised patients, children, elderly, and pregnant women. As a result, those who are vaccine-exposed may include a higher proportion of persons with more severe comorbidity than an unexposed group. Crude estimates of the association between exposure to vaccine and outcomes in such studies may therefore be biased, with various effects depending on the outcome of interest. For estimation of vaccine safety, more adverse events may be observed in the exposed compared to unvaccinated individuals. The reverse may happen when choice of vaccination is less dependent on vaccine indication and is associated with good functional status or healthy lifestyle and has been described as the *healthy-vaccinee effect* in the context of obtaining influenza vaccinations per recommendation (Remschmidt et al., 2015). In this case, crude estimates of vaccine safety underestimate the true effects.

In some populations, particularly among infants, immunization rate can be very high ($\geq 95\%$), making the unvaccinated a highly selected group that is unlikely to be similar in all ways to the vaccinated group, so that relatively few suitable controls are available, and those that can be found may differ substantially from vaccinated patients. For example, unvaccinated persons may more often have contraindications to vaccination, such as immune deficits.

Seasonality of vaccine-preventable illnesses such as influenza, pneumococcal pneumonia, and rotavirus represents an additional potential confounding factor. Confounding by indication may also occur if the presence of temporary acute illness would result in deferred or delayed vaccination and introduce differences between vaccinees and nonvaccinees. Specific attention must be paid to this potential issue in designs that use prevaccination periods as comparison windows.

References

Baxter, R., Lee, J., Fireman, B., 2010. Evidence of bias in studies of influenza vaccine effectiveness in elderly patients. J. Infect. Dis. 201, 186–189.

Baxter, R., Toback, S.L., Sifakis, F., et al., 2012a. A postmarketing evaluation of the safety of Ann Arbor strain live attenuated influenza vaccine in adults 18-49 years of age. Vaccine 2012 (30), 3053–3060.

Baxter, R., Toback, S.L., Sifakis, F., et al., 2012b. A postmarketing evaluation of the safety of Ann Arbor strain live attenuated influenza vaccine in children 5 through 17 years of age. Vaccine 2012 (30), 2989–2998.

Baxter, R., Tran, T.N., Hansen, J., et al., 2012c. Safety of Zostavax—a cohort study in a managed care organization. Vaccine 2012 (30), 6636–6641.

Baxter, R., Hansen, J., Timbol, J., et al., 2016. Post-licensure safety surveillance study of routine use of tetanus toxoid, reduced diphtheria toxoid and 5-component acellular pertussis vaccine. Hum. Vacc. Immunother. 12 (11), 2742–2748.

Belongia, E.A., Irving, S.A., Shui, I.M., Kulldorff, M., Lewis, E., Yin, R., Lieu, T.A., et al., 2010. Real-time surveillance to assess risk of intussusception and other adverse events after pentavalent, bovine-derived rotavirus vaccine. Pediatr. Infect. Dis. J. 29 (1), 1–5.

Black, S., Eskola, J., Siegrist, C.A., Halsey, N., Macdonald, N., Law, B., Miller, E., Andrews, N., et al., 2009. Importance of background rates of disease in assessment of vaccine safety during mass immunisation with pandemic H1N1 influenza vaccines. Lancet 374 (9707), 2115–2122.

Brighton Collaboration, 2016. Who We Are. Available from: https://brightoncollaboration.org/public/who-we-are.html.

Burwen, D.R., Sandhu, S.K., MaCurdy, T.E., Kelman, J.A., Gibbs, J.M., Garcia, B., et al., 2012. Surveillance for Guillain–Barré syndrome after influenza vaccination among the Medicare population, 2009–2010. Am. J. Publ. Health 102 (10), 1921–1927.

Canadian Vaccine Network, 2017. Available from: http://cirnetwork.ca/network/national-ambulatory-network/.

Centers for Disease Control and Prevention (CDC), September 13, 2004. Suspension of rotavirus vaccine after reports of intussusception – United States, 1999. Mort. Morb. Weekly Rep. 53 (34), 786–789. Available from: https://www.cdc.gov/mmwr/preview/mmwrhtml/mm5334a3.htm.

Centers for Disease Control and Prevention (CDC), 2016. Clinical Immunization Safety Assessment Project (CISA). Available from: http://www.cdc.gov/vaccinesafety/ensuringsafety/monitoring/cisa/.

Chen, R.T., Glasser, J.W., Rhodes, P.H., Davis, R.L., Barlow, W.E., Thompson, R.S., 1997. Vaccine Safety Datalink project: a new tool for improving vaccine safety monitoring in the United States. Pediatrics 99 (6), 765–773.

Davis, R.L., Kolczak, M., Lewis, E., Nordin, J., Goodman, M., Shay, D.K., Platt, R., Black, S., et al., 2005. Active surveillance of vaccine safety: a system to detect early signs of adverse events. Epidemiology 16 (3), 336–341.

de Lusignan, S., Dos Santos, G., Correa, A., Haguinet, F., Yonova, I., Lair, F., Byford, R., Ferreira, F., Stuttard, K., Chan, T., 2017. Post-authorization passive enhanced safety surveillance of seasonal influenza vaccines: protocol of a pilot study in England. BMJ Open 7 (5), e015469.

Dieleman, J., Romio, S., Johansen, K., Weibel, D., Bonhoeffer, J., et al., 2011. Guillain-Barré syndrome and adjuvanted pandemic influenza A (H1N1) 2009 vaccine: multinational case-control study in Europe. BMJ 343, d3908.

Ellenberg, S.S., Chen, R.T., 1997. The complicated task of monitoring vaccine safety. Publ. Health Rep. 112 (1), 10–20 discussion 21.

European Medicines Agency (EMA), 2014. Interim Guidance on Enhanced Safety Surveillance for Seasonal Influenza Vaccines in the EU. EMA/PRAC/222346/2014. Available from: http://www.ema.europa.eu/docs/en_GB/document_library/Scientific_guideline/2014/04/WC500165492.pdf.

Farrington, C.P., 1995. Relative incidence estimation from case series for vaccine safety evaluation. Biometrics 511, 228–235.

Fireman, B., Lee, J., Lewis, N., Bembom, O., van der Laan, M., Baxter, R., 2009. Influenza vaccination and mortality: differentiating vaccine effects from bias. Am. J. Epidemiol. 170, 650–656.

Food and Drug Administration (FDA), 2002. Pediarix Product Insert. Available from: http://www.fda.gov/downloads/BiologicsBloodVaccines/Vaccines/ApprovedProducts/UCM241874.pdf.

Food and Drug Administration (FDA), 2008. Pediacel Product Insert. Available from: http://www.fda.gov/downloads/BiologicsBloodVaccines/Vaccines/ApprovedProducts/UCM109810.pdf.

Food and Drug Administration (FDA), 2016. FDA Adverse Event Reporting System (FAERS). Available from: http://www.fda.gov/Drugs/GuidanceComplianceRegulatoryInformation/Surveillance/AdverseDrugEffects/.

Friederichs, V., Cameron, J.C., Robertson, C., 2006. Impact of adverse publicity on MMR vaccine uptake: a population based analysis of vaccine uptake records for one million children, born 1987–2004. Arch. Dis. Child. 91 (6), 465–468.

Gates Foundation, 2011. A Report of the Post-market Safety and Surveillance Working Group. Available from: https://docs.gatesfoundation.org/documents/SSWG%20Final%20Report%2011%2019%2013_designed.pdf.

Goulleret, N., Mauvisseau, E., Essevaz-Roulet, M., Quinlivan, M., Breuer, J., 2010. Safety profile of live varicella virus vaccine (Oka/Merck): five-year results of the European Varicella Zoster Virus Identification Program (EU VZVIP). Vaccine 28 (36), 5878–5882.

Hansen, J., Timbol, J., Lewis, N., et al., 2016. Safety of DTaP-IPV/Hib vaccine administered routinely to infants and toddlers. Vaccine 34, 4172–4179.

Hartnell, N.R., Wilson, J.P., 2004. Replication of the Weber effect using postmarketing adverse event reports voluntarily submitted to the United States Food and Drug Administration. Pharmacotherapy 24, 743–749.

Health and Human Services (HHS), 2016. Vaccine Adverse Event Reporting System (VAERS): About the VAERS Program. Available from: https://vaers.hhs.gov/about/index.

Huang, W.T., Chen, W.W., Yang, H.W., Chen, W.C., Chao, Y.N., Huang, Y.W., et al., 2010. Design of a robust infrastructure to monitor the safety of the pandemic A(H1N1) 2009 vaccination program in Taiwan. Vaccine 28, 7161–7166.

Innovative Medicines Initiative (IMI), 2017. ADVANCE Project: About ADVANCE. Available from: http://www.advance-vaccines.eu/?page=home.

Jackson, L.A., Jackson, M.L., Nelson, J.C., Neuzil, K.M., Weiss, N.S., 2006. Evidence of bias in estimates of influenza vaccine effectiveness in seniors. Int. J. Epidemiol. 35, 337–344.

Jackson, M.L., Yu, O., Nelson, J.C., et al., 2013. Further evidence for bias in observational studies of influenza vaccine effectiveness: the 2009 influenza A(H1N1) pandemic. Am. J. Epidemiol. 178, 1327–1336.

Klein, N.P., Hansen, J., Chao, C., et al., 2012. Safety of quadrivalent human papillomavirus vaccine administered routinely to females. Arch. Pediatr. Adolesc. Med. 166, 1140–1148.

Leite, A., Andrews, N.J., Thomas, S.L., 2016. Near real-time vaccine safety surveillance using electronic health records—a systematic review of the application of statistical methods. Pharmacoepidemiol. Drug Saf. 25, 225–237.

Lieu, T.A., Kulldorff, M., Davis, R.L., Lewis, E.M., Weintraub, E., Yih, K., et al., 2007. Real-time vaccine safety surveillance for the early detection of adverse events. Med. Care 45, S89–S95.

Madsen, K.M., Hviid, A., Vestergaard, M., Schendel, D., Wohlfahrt, J., etal, 2002. A population-based study of measles, mumps, and rubella vaccination and autism. N. Engl. J. Med. 347, 1477–1482.

McNaughton, R., Lynn, E., Osborne, V., Coughtrie, A., Layton, D., Shakir, S., 2016. Safety of intranasal quadrivalent live attenuated influenza vaccine (QLAIV) in children and adolescents: a pilot prospective cohort study in England. Drug Saf. 39 (4), 323–333.

McNeil, M.M., Gee, J., Weintraub, E.S., et al., 2014. The Vaccine Safety Datalink: successes and challenges monitoring vaccine safety. Vaccine 32, 5390–5398.

Nguyen, M., et al., 2012. The Food and drug Administration's post-licensure rapid immunization safety monitoring program: strengthening the federal vaccine safety enterprise. Pharmacoepidemiol. Drug Saf. 21 (S1), 291–297.

Olsen, S.J., Mirza, S.A., Vonglokham, P., Khanthamaly, V., Chitry, B., Pholsena, V., Chitranonh, V., et al., 2016. The effect of influenza vaccination on birth outcomes in a cohort of pregnant women in Lao PDR, 2014–2015. Clin. Infect. Dis. 63 (4), 487–494.

Palucci, O. Operational experience and lessons learned on influenza vaccination post authorization safety studies. In: Vaccines & Vaccination Global Summit and Expo. 16–18 June, 2016. Available from: http://vaccines.global-summit.com/europe/ppt/2016/operational-experience-and-lessons-learned-on-influenza-vaccination-post-authorization-safety-studies.

Patel, M.M., Haber, P., Baggs, J., Zuber, P., Bines, J.E., Parashar, U.D., 2009. Intussusception and rotavirus vaccination: a review of the available evidence. Exp. Rev. Vaccines 8 (11), 1555–1564.

Moro, P.L., Arana, J., Cano, M., Lewis, P., Shimabukuro, T.T., 2015. Deaths reported to the vaccine adverse event reporting system, United States, 1997–2013. Clin. Infect. Dis. 61 (6), 980–987.

Remschmidt, C., Wichmann, O., Harder, T., 2015. Frequency and impact of confounding by indication and healthy vaccinee bias in observational studies assessing influenza vaccine effectiveness: a systematic review. BMC Infect. Dis. 15, 429.

Reynales, H., Astudillo, P., de Valliere, S., Hatz, C., Schlagenhauf, P., Rath, B., et al., 2012. A prospective observational safety study on MF59® adjuvanted cell culture-derived vaccine, Celtura® during the A/H1N1 (2009) influenza pandemic. Vaccine 30 (45), 6436–6443.

Rothman, K.J., Greenland, S., Lash, T.L. (Eds.), 2008. Modern Epidemiology, third ed. Wolters Kluwer, Phildelphia.

Rowhani-Rahbar, A., Klein, N.P., Dekker, C.L., et al., 2012. Biologically plausible and evidence-based risk intervals in immunization safety research. Vaccine 31, 271–277.

Vaccine Adverse Event Surveillance and Communication consortium (VAESCO), 2017. Who We Are. Available from: http://vaesco.net/vaesco/about-us.html.

Vaccines Europe, 2016. Who We Are. Available from: http://www.vaccineseurope.eu/about-vaccines-europe/who-we-are/.

Velentgas, P., Amato, A.A., Bohn, R.L., et al., 2012. Risk of Guillain-Barré syndrome after meningococcal conjugate vaccination. Pharmacoepidemiol. Drug Saf. 21 (12), 1350–1358.

Verstraeten, T., Cohet, C., Dos Santos, G., Ferreira, G.L., Bollaerts, K., Bauchau, V., Shinde, V., 2016. Pandemrix™ and narcolepsy: a critical appraisal of the observational studies. Hum. Vacc. Immunother. 12 (1), 187–193.

Weber, J.C.P., 1984. Epidemiology of adverse reactions to nonsteroidal antiinflammatory drugs. In: Rainsford, K.D., Velo, G.P. (Eds.), Advances in Inflammation Research, vol. 6. Raven Press, New York, pp. 1–6.

Whitaker, H.J., Farrington, C.P., Spiessens, B., Musonda, P., 2006. Tutorial in biostatistics: the self-controlled case series method. Stat. Med. 25, 1768–1797.

World Health Organization (WHO), 2012a. Report of WHO/CIOMS Working Group. Definition and Application of Terms for Vaccine Pharmacovigilance. Available from: http://www.who.int/vaccine_safety/initiative/tools/CIOMS_report_WG_vaccine.pdf.

World Health Organization (WHO), 2012b. Global Vaccine Safety Blueprint. Available from: http://apps.who.int/iris/bitstream/10665/70919/1/WHO_IVB_12.07_eng.pdf.

World Health Organization (WHO), WHO Imnunization Fact Sheet Updated September 2016. Available from: http://www.who.int/mediacentre/factsheets/fs378/en/.

Yih, W.I., Lieu, T.A., Kulldorff, M., Martin, D., McMahill-Walraven, C.N., Platt, R., et al., 2014. Intussusception risk after rotavirus vaccination in U.S. Infants. N. Engl. J. Med. 370 (6), 503–512.

CHAPTER 8

The European Union Post-Authorization Study Register

Thomas Goedcke, Xavier Kurz

European Medicines Agency, London, United Kingdom

DISCLAIMER/ACKNOWLEDGMENTS

The views expressed in this article are the personal views of the authors and may not be understood or quoted as being made on behalf of or reflecting the position of the European Medicines Agency or one of its committees or working parties.

INTRODUCTION

The 2010 European Union (EU) pharmacovigilance legislation has significantly changed the landscape of pharmacovigilance and post-authorization supervision of medicinal products with a strong legal basis for regulators to request and oversee post-authorization studies (PAS). PAS are aimed at addressing safety (i.e., PASS) and effectiveness (i.e., PAES) questions that could not been answered at the time of authorization, and they became an important regulatory tool to assess whether benefits outweigh risks once a new medicinal product has been approved. In 2012, the mandate of the Pharmacovigilance Risk Assessment Committee explicitly includes the regulatory supervision of PASS, including protocol approval for studies imposed as a condition of marketing authorization and to monitor the safe and effective use of products in normal clinical practice. An important success factor of pharmacovigilance activities and the surveillance of medicinal products are transparency and public awareness about the regulatory measures, the applied methodologies, and the results of important PAS. A number of EU initiatives such as the establishment of the European medicines web portal and the European Union post-authorization study (EU PAS) Register underpin this transparency initiative.

The EU PAS Register is a web-based resource that provides patients, health-care professionals, researchers, and the general public with easy access to information on publicly and privately funded PAS. The Register is maintained by the

CONTENTS

Disclaimer/
Acknowledg
ments 329

Introduction 329
Regulatory
Requirements for
Post-Authorization
Safety Studies............ 331
Registering Studies... 332
Searching the European
Union Post-Authorization
Study Register........... 332
Monitoring
Compliance................ 333

References 335

Post-Authorization Safety Studies of Medicinal Products. https://doi.org/10.1016/B978-0-12-809217-0.00008-8

European Medicines Agency (EMA) and currently hosted on the European Network of Centers for Pharmacoepidemiology and Pharmacovigilance (ENCePP) website, and it is a unique publicly accessible resource for the registration of noninterventional PAS, building on the 2010 initiative of ENCePP to establish the same transparency standards provided for interventional clinical trials since the launch of the US FDA clinical trials website (www.clinicaltrials.gov) in February 2000.

Both PASS and PAES may be submitted to the EU PAS Register. As mentioned in earlier chapters, the EU legislation defines PASS as studies relating to an authorized medicinal product conducted with the aim of identifying, characterizing, or quantifying a safety hazard, confirming the safety profile of the product or of measuring the effectiveness of risk minimization measures (EU, 2001). PASS may be interventional or noninterventional. The majority of records in the EU PAS Register provide information on noninterventional studies, which require the following (EMA, 2016a,b):

- the medicinal product is prescribed in the usual manner in accordance with the terms of the marketing authorization;
- the assignment of the patient to a particular therapeutic strategy is not decided in advance by a trial protocol but falls within current practice, and the prescription of the product is clearly separated from the decision to include the patient in the study; and
- no additional diagnostic or monitoring procedures are applied to the patients, and epidemiological methods are used for the analyses of collected data.

In the EU, the clinical trials regulation defines a noninterventional study as any clinical study other than a clinical trial (EU, 2014); however, PASS can have either designs, and therefore, the EU PAS Register may also include information on clinical trials.

Registering a study, including protocol and study results in the EU PAS Register, facilitates sharing of analytical and methodological "know how" among investigators, regulators, and the wider general public across borders. It also promotes peer review to determine the validity of pharmacoepidemiological research with its vast variety of study designs and analytical methods. High levels of public scrutiny of registered study protocols help to increase trust in pharmacoepidemiological study designs and reduce the chance for manipulation of predefined endpoints (Schneeweiss and Avorn, 2011), increasing the value of noninterventional/observational research for regulatory decision-making.

The EU PAS Register has emerged as a key tool developed by ENCePP to strengthen post-authorization monitoring of medicinal products by facilitating the conduct of transparent, independent, and methodologically robust noninterventional studies, which regulators increasingly rely on to support decision-making on the safety and effectiveness of products authorized inside and outside the EU. The EU PAS Register not only supports EU pharmacovigilance activities but also important ENCePP initiatives on best practice for the conduct of PAS, including the ENCePP Code of Conduct (ENCePP, 2016) and the ENCePP Guide on Methodological Standards in Pharmacoepidemiology (ENCePP, 2010), providing a set of rules and principles at all steps of study planning, design, conduct, analysis, and reporting. Although the launch of the EU PAS Register has been a key step to promote transparency and collaboration in noninterventional research, the quality of a study and the validity of the results will ultimately depend on how the study design controls for bias and confounding.

Regulatory Requirements for Post-Authorization Safety Studies

The EU PAS Register is reflected in the guideline on Good Pharmacovigilance Practices (GVP) module VIII on PASS (EMA, 2016a), which includes specific provisions for imposed noninterventional studies. By means of the EU PAS Register, the EMA and marketing authorization holders (MAH) comply with their EU pharmacovigilance legislation requirements to make public the protocols and abstracts of results of noninterventional PASS imposed as an obligation of marketing authorization by a competent authority (EU, 2001, 2004). In particular, Annex III of the Commission Implementing Regulation, which aims at facilitating these legal provisions, specifies that the date of study registration in the EU PAS Register shall be included as a milestone in the final study report (EU, 2012). It is important to emphasize that, as a general recommendation, all noninterventional PASS and PAES should be registered—regardless whether they are initiated, managed, or financed by MAH, or whether they are conducted by a research institution, including from outside the EU.

The GVP specifically recommend that PASS initiated, managed, or financed voluntarily by an MAH, and which are required in the risk management plan (RMP) to further investigate safety concerns or to evaluate the effectiveness of risk minimization activities, and any other relevant PASS should also be entered in the EU PAS Register to support the same level of transparency, scientific, and quality standards as required by law for imposed noninterventional PASS.

PASS that fall under the definition of a clinical trial in accordance with the clinical trials regulation may also be registered in the EU PAS Register, including a reference to registration in other databases such as the US clinical trials website. MAH should register PAES in the EU PAS Register.

Registering Studies

A study may be submitted to the EU PAS Register by the lead investigator or any staff member of an academic research center, public, or private study sponsor. The lead investigator identified in the study protocol has to ensure that the provided information is correct and kept up to date at all times. This includes the provision of contact details, which allow anybody with an interest in the study to contact the lead investigator or a designated contact person to verify the study information. A user-friendly step-by-step guide on how to access the EU PAS Register and to register a new study, to update existing study records, or to search for study information can be downloaded from www.encepp.eu.

The disclosure of study information in the EU PAS Register at an early stage is encouraged, preferably before the study has actually started (i.e., a priori registration). The study start date is usually the date when the primary data collection starts, and the first subject is recorded in the data set in prospective studies or registries where data is collected during routine clinical practice. In case of secondary use of data, the start date is the date when data extraction starts (e.g., from claims and electronic medical record [EMR]). An advantage of a priori study registration is the comparison of initial and final protocol once the study has been completed. Early study registration may also benefit collaboration within the scientific community, allowing for best use of resources and preventing unnecessary duplication of research (Goedecke and Arlett, 2014). Table 8.1 provides an overview of study information held in the EU PAS Register.

The study protocol should be uploaded once finalized and prior to the start of data collection. Any substantial protocol amendments, progress reports, and the final study report should also be made public in the register preferably within 2 weeks after finalization. A redacted protocol may be made public where publication of the full protocol may jeopardize the validity of the study due to information bias, or there is a need to protect intellectual rights. For imposed noninterventional PASS, the GVP require that the final study report is submitted within 12 months after the end of data collection, and this timeline is also recommended for PASS included in the RMP of a medicinal product or conducted voluntarily in the EU.

Searching the European Union Post-Authorization Study Register

Searching the EU PAS Register is entirely free of charge and there is no registration or personal identification required. The search function allows browsing noninterventional study records based on a number of criteria, which can also be combined for advanced searches. All study information fields marked with an asterisk in Table 8.1 are searchable, either by means of predefined

Table 8.1 Overview of Study Information Held in the European Union Post-Authorization Study (EU PAS) Register. Searchable Information is Highlighted by *

Administrative Information	Targets of the Study
Study identification:*	Information of study medicinal product:*
• EU PAS Register number	• Substance class
• Status of study	• Substance generic name
• Title of study/acronym	• Brand product name
• Study type	Medical conditions to be studied*
• Study requested by a regulator	Population under study (age groups)*
• Risk management plan study category	Number of patients
• Other registration number	Source of data
Research centers and investigator details:*	Scope of the study*
• Coordinating study entity	Main objectives
• Research network	Study design
Study timelines:	Follow-up of patients
• Initial administrative steps	Data analysis plan
• Progress reports	ENCePP seal*
• Final report	Full protocol
Source of funding	Study results
Contact details for inquiries	Other relevant information

values from dropdown lists or as free-text field. Studies can also be searched via the unique study identifier.

The EU PAS Register has become an important resource for research in regulatory science. The role and objectives of drug utilization studies in measuring the effectiveness of risk minimization measures are described in a review based of 18 protocols that could be retrieved for a total of 36 drug utilization studies registered by the end of 2013 (Kurz and Blake, 2016). Acknowledging that study registration is encouraged by regulators for those studies requested in RMP, and that the EU PAS Register does not represent the entirety of drug utilization research conducted in the EU, the authors could demonstrate that multinational drug utilization research is feasible, with more than 50% of registered studies conducted in more than one country. The EU PAS Register has also been the source to provide perspectives and trends for PASS requested by regulators (Engel, 2016).

Monitoring Compliance

The introduction of a unique study identifier with the latest release of the EU PAS Register in 2016 was a significant step toward the EU PAS Register being a valid reference for publicly funded noninterventional PASS. Other study registration identification numbers, such as the EUDRACT number and links to URL may be provided as applicable, which is especially relevant for interventional PASS. The search function provides a tool for regulators to monitor MAH compliance with the recommendations of GVP module VIII, particularly for imposed noninterventional PASS. MAH are also expected to register all noninterventional PASS included in an EU RMP under the respective study category. For newly registered studies requested by a regulatory authority, funded by a pharmaceutical company, and conducted in at least one EU country, the EMA notifies the national competent authorities of all EU Member States by providing a link to the EU PAS Register study record (EMA, 2016b).

Since its launch in 2010, the rate of study registration has increased over time with a significant rise in the years 2013 and 2014, following the implementation of the EU pharmacovigilance legislation and enacting the GVP requirements for PAS. By September 2016, the EU PAS Register contained 895 studies, 459 (51%) of which were requested by an EU and/or non-EU regulatory body. About 84% of these studies were noninterventional, 11% clinical trials, and 4% classified as active surveillance studies. Among the noninterventional studies, 32% included risk assessments, 22% drug utilization, 19% evaluation of risk minimization activities, and 9% disease epidemiology.

Approximately half of the studies were registered with the status "ongoing," 23% "planned," and 27% "finalized." Since July 2016, the EU PAS Register requires the assignment of an EU RMP category in line with GVP modules V and VIII (EMA, 2014, 2016a). As of October 2016, there were 39 studies registered that are imposed as a condition of marketing authorization (Category 1), 11 studies that are imposed as a specific obligation of marketing authorization under exceptional circumstances (Category 2), and 159 studies are requirements in the EU RMP (Category 3). These are prevalent figures based on 40% of registered studies given that the EU RMP category is a recently added feature of the EU PAS Register, and not all studies have been updated retrospectively. Table 2.1.3 in Chapter 2.1 provides an overview of these study categories.

Over the last decade, we have seen a shift toward well-designed pharmacoepidemiological PAS (both PASS and PAES) becoming a recognized tool for regulators and pharmaceutical industry as they allow for the earlier authorization of new medicinal products tackling unmet medical needs or orphan diseases or to monitor whether risk minimization measures are effective under normal conditions of use. Such recognition is largely based on trust in the results of noninterventional/observational research, and the EU PAS Register plays a key role to this effect, allowing stakeholders to verify study information, and investigators to promote their scientific independence and adherence to best methodological standards, potentially using different data source and analytical strategies. Patients, health-care professionals, and regulators are provided with a tool to compare real-world evidence and acknowledge the value of well-designed PASS, which help regulators to reliably assess the performance of medicinal products after launch. With the increasing number of electronic longitudinal data sources and data from patient registries, noninterventional PASS will continue to gain importance.

References

Engel, P., 2016. Three Years of EU Post-authorization Safety Studies: Design Expectations and Trends. Pink Sheet Pharma Intelligence. Available from: https://pink.pharmamedtechbi.com/PS118870/ Three-Years-Of-EU-PostAuthorization-Safety-Studies-Design-Expectations-And-Trends.

European Medicines Agency (EMA), 2014. Guideline on Good Pharmacovigilance Practices (GVP) Module V - Risk Management Systems (Rev. 1) (EMA/838713/2011). Available from: http://www.ema.europa.eu/docs/en_GB/document_library/Scientific_guideline/2012/06/WC50 0129134.pdf.

European Medicines Agency (EMA), 2016a. Guideline on Good Pharmacovigilance Practices (GVP) Module VIII - Post-authorisation Safety Studies (Rev. 2) (EMA/813938/2011). Available from: http://www.ema.europa.eu/docs/en_GB/document_library/Scientific_guideline/2012/06/WC50 0129137.pdf.

European Medicines Agency (EMA), 2016b. Guideline on Good Pharmacovigilance Practices (GVP) Module VIII - Addendum I — Requirements and Recommendations for the Submission of Information on Non-interventional Post-authorisation Safety Studies (Rev 2) (EMA/395730/ 2012). Available from: http://www.ema.europa.eu/docs/en_GB/document_library/Scientific_ guideline/2012/06/WC500129147.pdf.

European Network of Centres for Pharmacoepidemiology and Pharmacovigilance (ENCePP), 2010. Guide on Methodological Standards in Pharmacoepidemiology (Revision 5) (EMA/95098/ 2010). Available from: http://www.encepp.eu/standards_and_guidances/documents/ENCePP GuideofMethStandardsinPE_Rev5.pdf.

European Network of Centres for Pharmacoepidemiology and Pharmacovigilance (ENCePP), 2016. The ENCePP Code of Conduct (EMA/929209/2011). Available from: http://www.encepp.eu/ code_of_conduct/documents/ENCePPCodeofConduct_Rev3amend.pdf.

European Union (EU), 2001. Directive 2001/83/EC of the European Parliament and of the Council of 6 November, 2001 on the community code relating to medicinal products for human use. Official J. L311, 67—128.

European Union (EU), 2004. Regulation (EC) No 726/2004 of the European Parliament and of the council of 31 March, 2004 laying down community procedures for the authorisation and supervision of medicinal products for human and veterinary use and establishing a European Medicines Agency. Official J. L136, 1—33.

European Union (EU), 2012. Commission implementing regulation (EU) No 520/2012 of 19 June, 2012 on the performance of pharmacovigilance activities provided for in regulation (EC) No 726/2004 of the European Parliament and of the council and directive 2001/83/EC of the European Parliament and of the council text with EEA relevance. Official J. L159, 5—25.

European Union (EU), 2014. Regulation (EC) No 536/2014 of the European Parliament and of the council of 16 April, 2014 on clinical trials on medicinal products for human use, and repealing directive 2001/20/EC. Official J. L158, 1—76.

Goedecke, T., Arlett, P., 2014. A description of the European Network of Centres of Pharmacoepi-demiology and Pharmacovigilance as a global resource for pharmacovigilance and pharmacoepidemiology. In: Andrews, E.B., Moore, N. (Eds.), Mann's Pharmacovigilance, third ed. John Wiley & Sons Inc., Chichester, West Sussex, pp. 403—408.

Kurz, X., Blake, K., 2016. Drug utilisation research and the regulator's perspective in pharmacovigilance. In: Elseviers, M., et al. (Eds.), Drug Utilisation Research: Methods and Applications. John Wiley & Sons Inc., Chichester, West Sussex, pp. 408—416.

Schneeweiss, S., Avorn, J., 2011. Postmarketing studies of drug safety. Br. Med. J. 342, d342.

Index

'*Note*: Page numbers followed by "f" indicate figures and "t" indicate tables and "b" indicate boxes.'

A

ACR. *See* American College of Rheumatology (ACR)
Action Duchenne, 75
Activity trackers, 152
Acute physiology and chronic health evaluation (APACHE), 188
ADAPTABLE. *See* Aspirin Dosing: A Patient-centric Trial Assessing Benefits and Long-Term Effectiveness (ADAPTABLE)
Additional pharmacovigilance activities, 16–18
Additional risk minimization, 27–32
  tools for, 27–32
    controlled access systems, 30–32
    educational programs, 28–30
Additional risk minimization measures (aRMM), 22–23, 27
Adherence monitors, 152
Adjudication process, 55, 59
Administrative claims, 282–283
Administrative databases, 80
Adolescent immunizations, 296–297
Adverse events, 96, 209
AEE. *See* Average exposure effect (AEE)
AET. *See* Average exposure effect among treated (AET)
Age, 316–317
Agency for Healthcare Research and Quality, 74
Agreement form, 30–31

Alopecia, 69–70
Altos outpatient oncology clinic database, 71–72
American Academy of Pediatrics, 212
American College of Rheumatology (ACR), 228
Analytic methods, 273
Analytic platform, 88
Anemia, 69–70
Ankylosing spondylitis, 256
Annex III of Commission Implementing Regulation, 331
Anti-TNF alpha agents, 253
Anti-TNF biologics, 267–268
Anticoagulant agents, 136, 167–168
Antidiabetes medication, 167, 169–170
APACHE. *See* Acute physiology and chronic health evaluation (APACHE)
aRMM. *See* Additional risk minimization measures (aRMM)
"Artificial" treatment effect heterogeneity, 87
As-treated analysis, 143
Asian Pharmacoepidemiology Network (AsPEN), 210, 217–218
  example, 218
  governance and data, 217–218
Aspirin Dosing: A Patient-centric Trial Assessing Benefits and Long-Term Effectiveness (ADAPTABLE), 151

Association rule mining, 99
Atrial fibrillation, 167, 170
Average exposure effect (AEE), 186–187
Average exposure effect among treated (AET), 186–187

B

Baseline stroke, 56–57
Bayesian hierarchical model, 288–289
Behavioral modification, 37–41, 38t
Benchmarking, lack of, 35
Benefit information, 227–229
  presentation, 229
Benefit–risk assessments, 227–228, 230–232, 235–236
  PASS role, 236–237
Benefit–risk decision-making, 225
Benefit–risk evaluation frameworks, 4–5, 225
  benefit information, 227–229
    presentation, 229
  benefit–risk assessment, 235–236
    PASS role, 236–237
  ongoing benefit–risk evaluation, 237–238
  preferences and values, 233
  risk information, 229–232
    presentation, 231–232
  risk minimization measures, 233–234
  stakeholders, 226–227
    impact of uncertainty, 232

Bias, 186
  channeling, 271–272, 287
  healthy-vaccinee, 296
  information, 271, 272t
  selection, 113, 162, 270–271, 272t
Big data, 122, 210
  "bigness" creation, 81–85
  environment, 203–204
  example of combination of data
    sources through metaanalysis,
    84t
  methodological considerations,
    85–87
  modern methods for post-
    authorization safety studies
    employing, 87–88
  for post-authorization safety
    studies, 79–81
  sources, 80t
Biobanks, 151
Biologic and Biosimilars Collective
    Intelligence Consortium, 268
Biologic medicinal products, 253
Biologic products, 269
Biologics
  and biosimilars regulation,
    255–256
    timeline of overarching and
      product-specific biosimilar
      guidelines, 255f
  PASS designs for, 261–265
  regulation, 255–256
  safety concerns with, 256–258
  terminology, 254, 254t
Biosimilars
  methodological considerations,
    265–273
    comparator selection, 270
    exposure measurement,
      268–270, 271t
    outcome measurement,
      267–268
    research questions, 265–267
    validity considerations, 270–273,
      272t
  PASS, 266–267
    designs for biologics and,
      261–265

regulation, 255–256
  safety concerns with biologics and,
    256–258
  special considerations, 258–261
    interchangeability, switching,
      and substitution, 259t
Brochures and guides, 28–29

C
C-reactive protein (CRP), 228
Canadian Network for
    Observational Drug Effect
    Studies (CNODES), 210,
    215–217
  example, 216–217
  governance and data, 216
Cardiovascular risk
  factors for sildenafil, 114
  minimization measures for
    stronium ranelate, 22b
Cardioverter defibrillator (CD), 286
Case-centered designs, 310–311
Case-crossover approach, 122, 124f,
    126–129
  timeline of exposure and outcome
    for patients, 127f
Case–case–time–control design,
    134, 135f
Case–control designs, 308–309
Case–time–control design,
    133–134, 133f
CD. See Cardioverter defibrillator
    (CD)
CDAI. See Crohn's disease activity
    index (CDAI)
CDC. See US Centers for Disease
    Control and Prevention
    (CDC)
CDM. See Common data model
    (CDM)
"CE marking", 277–280
Centers for Medicare and Medicaid
    Services (CMS), 269
Channeling bias, 271–272, 287
Channeling phenomena, 112–113
Checklists, 28–29
Chemotherapy, 267
Chickenpox vaccine, 316–317

Chronic infections, 316–317
CISA network. See Clinical
    Immunization Safety
    Assessment network (CISA
    network)
Claims, 312–313
  analyses, 53
  claims-based post-authorization
    safety studies, 57–60
  data, 228
Claims databases, 49. See also
    Electronic medical records
    (EMRs)
  contents, 50–52, 50f
  open, 49–50
  strengths and limitations, 52–55
Class I devices, 277
Class IIa devices, 277
Class IIb devices, 277
Class III devices, 277
Clinical Data Interchange Standards
    Consortium, 284
Clinical Immunization Safety
    Assessment network (CISA
    network), 297–298
Clinical Practice Research Datalink
    (CPRD), 69, 116, 216
Clinical trials, 111
CMS. See Centers for Medicare and
    Medicaid Services (CMS)
CNODES. See Canadian Network
    for Observational Drug Effect
    Studies (CNODES)
Cohort designs, 112–113, 308
Cohort PASS, 308–309
Cohort studies, 139–144, 140f,
    305–306. See also Enriched
    studies
  cohort-event monitoring studies,
    114
  methodological considerations,
    142–144
"Combination" products, 278
PASS for
  analytical considerations,
    288–290
  methodological considerations,
    279–290

safety concerns with medical devices, 278–279
validity considerations, 284–290
Common data model (CDM), 204–205, 210–212
Communication plan, 29–30
Community-based choice, 225
Community-based decisions, 225
Comparator
  group, 185
  lack of, 34
Concurrent cohort, 191
Confounding, 271, 272t, 287–288, 322–324
  adjustment, 79
  control with DRS, 186
  by indication, 141, 169–171
Congenital malformations, 41
Consent form, 30–31
Construct validity, 37
Content validity, 37
Contraindications, 22b, 23, 39–41, 136–137, 294, 299, 317, 323
Controlled access systems, 30–32
Controlled dispensing and distribution, 32
Conventional passive surveillance methods, 302
Conventional pharmacy databases, 264
Copyright law, 100
Council for International Organizations of Medical Sciences, 95
Counterfactual theory, 183–184
Covariate balance, 191
Cox proportional hazards model, 146
CPRD. See Clinical Practice Research Datalink (CPRD)
Crohn's disease activity index (CDAI), 266
CRP. See C-reactive protein (CRP)
Cumulative incidence, 41
CYD tetravalent dengue vaccine, 304

D
Daily diaries, 152
DAS28. See Disease Activity Score (DAS28)
Data
  AsPEN, 217–218
  CNODES, 216
  extrapolation, 288
  linkage, 134–135
  Sentinels, 214
  transformation process, 207
  VSD, 211–212
Data analytic platforms
  CDMs and MAPs, 204–205
  limitations of data and analysis standardization, 207
  and transparency, 205–207
Data collection
  instrument, 36–37
  methods, 321, 321b
Data sources
  for DUS, 110–111
  for medical device, 281–284
    administrative claims, 282–283
    electronic medical record, 283–284
    registries, 281–282
DDN. See Distributed data network (DDN)
Dear Health Care Professional (DHCP), 30
Dengue, 318
Dependent variable, 133–134
Device exposure measurement, 279–281
Device PASS, 289–290
  claims data for, 282–283
  data sources for, 281–282
  EMR use for, 284
  UDI system for, 280–281
DHCP. See Dear Health Care Professional (DHCP)
DHPC. See Direct Healthcare Professional Communication (DHPC)
Diabetes, 167
Diagnosis codes, 51

Dipeptidyl peptidase-4 (DPP-4), 214–215
Diphtheria–tetanus–pertussis (DTP), 293–294
Direct Healthcare Professional Communication (DHPC), 30
Direct patient data collection methods, 314
Disease Activity Score (DAS28), 267–268
Disease registries, 41, 74–75
Disease risk scores (DRS), 182–183, 214–215
  development, 183–186
  empirical example, 190–192, 192t
  exposure propensity scores vs., 188–190
    limitations, 190
    strengths, 189–190
  future directions, 192–193
  historical disease risk scores estimation, 185–186
  methodological considerations, 186–188
  same-sample DRS estimation, 184–185
  stratification, 187f
Disproportionality analyses, 85
Distributed data network (DDN), 210, 268, 289
Distributed research network, 306
Double-masked placebo-controlled RCT, 197
DPP-4. See Dipeptidyl peptidase-4 (DPP-4)
DRS. See Disease risk scores (DRS)
Drug
  consumption, 39
  drug-eluting stents, 284–285
  exposures, 122–123
  Nordic, 110
  utilization, 155
Drug Safety and Effectiveness Network (DSEN), 215
Drug utilization studies (DUS), 107
  data source for, 110–111
  methodological considerations, 108–109

DSEN. *See* Drug Safety and Effectiveness Network (DSEN)
DTaP. *See* Diphtheria–tetanus–pertussis (DTP)
DTP. *See* Diphtheria–tetanus–pertussis (DTP)
Durham–Humphrey Amendments, 26
DUS. *See* Drug utilization studies (DUS)
Dystrophin gene, 75

E

EDC systems. *See* Electronic data capture systems (EDC systems)
Educational materials, 28
Educational programs, 28–30
Effectiveness, 242–243, 243t, 245. *See also* Post-authorization effectiveness studies (PAES)
  of medicinal product, 244
  of risk minimization, 32–41
    behavioral modification, 37–41, 38t
    models for risk minimization evaluation PASS, 33–41
    risk knowledge/comprehension, 36–37
    risk minimization tool coverage, awareness, and usage, 35–36
    safety outcomes, 41
Efficacy, 242, 243t, 245
Einheitlicher Bewertungsmaßstab system, 50–51, 282–283
Electronic data capture systems (EDC systems), 151, 313–314, 321
Electronic devices, 110–111
Electronic medical records (EMRs), 37, 63, 80, 108–109, 170, 182, 203, 209, 259–260, 280–281, 283–284, 296–297, 312–313, 332. *See also* Claims databases
  completeness of data in claims and EMR databases, 66f

  contents, 63–65, 64f
  data, 59–60
  EMR-based PASS, 68–70
  PASS using EMR linking to other data, 70–72
  strengths and limitations, 66–68
Electronic questionnaires, 314
Elekta/Impac Medical Systems, 69–70
Elements to assure safe use (ETASU), 27–28
EMA. *See* European Medicines Agency (EMA)
EMRs. *See* Electronic medical records (EMRs)
ENCePP. *See* European Network of Centers for Pharmacoepidemiology and Pharmacovigilance (ENCePP)
Enhanced passive safety surveillance (EPSS), 301, 303
  utility in seasonal campaigns, 302–304, 303b
  for vaccines, 300–304
Enriched PASS, 265
Enriched studies, 150–151. *See also* Cohort studies
  evaluation of secondary data sources for, 153
  methodological considerations, 154–156
  operationalizing enriched studies, 154
  strengths and limitations, 152–153
Enrollment dates, 55–56
Enrollment form, 30–31
EPS. *See* Exposure propensity scores (EPS)
EPSS. *See* Enhanced passive safety surveillance (EPSS)
Erectile dysfunction treatment, 114
Erythrocyte sedimentation rate (ESR), 228
Erythropoietin, 243–244
ESR. *See* Erythrocyte sedimentation rate (ESR)

ETASU. *See* Elements to assure safe use (ETASU)
EU. *See* European Union (EU)
EU PAS register. *See* European Union post-authorization study register (EU PAS register)
EUDRACT number, 333–334
European Medicines Agency (EMA), 3, 11–12, 74, 225–226, 246–247, 255, 260–261, 293, 329–330
  guidance, 22–23
European Network of Centers for Pharmacoepidemiology and Pharmacovigilance (ENCePP), 5, 329–330
European Pharmacovigilance Legislation, 2–3
European registries, 75–76
European regulatory, 109
European Union (EU), 2–3, 11–12, 20, 258, 278, 297, 329
  pharmacovigilance legislation, 230, 245, 247
  pharmacovigilance practices, 74
European Union post-authorization study register (EU PAS register), 5–6, 329
  monitoring compliance, 333–335
  registering studies, 332
  regulatory requirements for post-authorization safety studies, 331
  searching, 332–333
  study information in, 333t
Event-dependent exposures, 136–137
Exploring and Understanding Adverse Drug Reactions project, 70
Exposure, 183–184
  device exposure, 279–281
  drug, 122–123
  effect, 122
  event-dependent, 136–137
  "exposure-indexed" design, 125–126

long-term follow-up, 76–77
measurement, 268–270, 271t
population trends, 132–134
probability of, 123–124
propensity scores, 188–190
Exposure propensity scores (EPS), 167–168, 182–183, 188–190, 214–215, 288
    applications, 175–178
        matching, 176–177
        modeling, 177–178
        restriction, 176
        stratification, 176
        weighting, 178
    confounding by indication, 169–171
    development, 171–173
    strengths, 173–175
    transparency, 179–180
External comparators, 270

F

Facebook, 92–95
Fatigue, 69–70
FDA. *See* United States Food and Drug Administration (FDA)
FDA Amendments Act (FDAAA), 204
Final study report, 331–332
Fit-for-purpose technology, 313–314
Food, Drug, and Cosmetic Act (1938), 26
Frequency categories of adverse events, 1, 2t

G

GBS. *See* Guillain–Barré syndrome (GBS)
Geisinger Health System EMR database, 71
General Electric Centricity EMR database, 68–69
Global Vaccine Safety Blueprint, 304
Glucagon-like peptide-1 (GLP-1), 216–217
Glycosylated hemoglobin (HbA1c), 168–169, 246–247

Good pharmacovigilance practices (GVP), 2–3, 22, 331
Governance, 83
    AsPEN, 217–218
    CNODES, 216
    Sentinels, 214
    VSD, 211–212
Granulocyte-colony stimulating factors, 267–268
Group monitoring methods, 85
Guillain–Barré syndrome (GBS), 298
GVP. *See* Good pharmacovigilance practices (GVP)
GVP Module XVI, 27–28, 33–34, 36

H

Hawthorne effect, 37
Hazard ratios (HR), 191
HbA1c. *See* Glycosylated hemoglobin (HbA1c)
HCP. *See* Health-care professionals (HCP)
HCPCS. *See* Health Care Common Procedure Coding System (HCPCS)
hd-PS. *See* High-dimensional propensity scoring (hd-PS)
Health Care Common Procedure Coding System (HCPCS), 269
Health insurance administrative claims, 49, 282
    claims-based post-authorization safety studies, 57–60
    cohort selection and time periods for claims analysis, 56f
    contents of claims databases, 50–52
    databases, 49
    decision tree, 58f
    methodological considerations, 55–57
    strengths and limitations of claims databases, 52–55
Health-care
    cultures, 109

data, 203
databases, 123, 182
providers, 267
utilization, 120
Health-care professionals (HCP), 23
Health-seeking behaviors, 285–286
Healthcare Common Procedure Coding System, 50–51
Healthy-adherer bias. *See* Healthy-user bias
Healthy-user bias, 285–286
Healthy-user/sick-quitter effects, 134–136
Healthy-vaccinee bias, 296
Healthy-vaccinee effect, 323
Hemoglobin, 266
HES. *See* Hospital Episode Statistics (HES)
High-dimensional propensity scoring (hd-PS), 86
Hilfsmittelpositionsnummer, 282–283
Hip arthroplasty systems, 279–280
Historical cohort, 191
Historical comparators, 270
HL model. *See* Hosmer–Lemeshow model (HL model)
HLA-B*5701 allele, 30–31
Horizontal pooling, 81, 82t
Hosmer–Lemeshow model (HL model), 191
Hospital Episode Statistics (HES), 70–71
HPV infection. *See* Human papillomavirus infection (HPV infection)
HPV vaccine (HPV4), 310
HR. *See* Hazard ratios (HR)
Human papillomavirus infection (HPV infection), 294–295
Hybrid designs, 159–160

I

ICD. *See* International Classification of Diseases (ICD)
ICH. *See* International Conference on Harmonization (ICH)
Identifiable patient, 95
Identifiable reporter, 95

IMI-PROTECT. *See* Innovative Medicines Initiatived—the Pharmacoepidemiological Research on Outcomes of Therapeutics by a European Consortium (IMI-PROTECT)
Immortal-time bias, 286–287
Immunization programs, 293, 299–300
Immunogenicity, 257
Incidence rate, 41
Independent variables, 133–134
Infliximab, 256, 263
Infliximab biosimilar, 256, 261, 264
Infliximab-dyyb, 261
Influenza, 318, 323–324
    vaccine, 211–212, 285–286, 316
Information bias, 271, 272t
Ingenix Research Database, 59
INN. *See* International nonproprietary name (INN)
Innovative Medicines Initiatived—the Pharmacoepidemiological Research on Outcomes of Therapeutics by a European Consortium (IMI-PROTECT), 225–226
Instrumental variables (IVs), 197
    analyses, 288
    limitations of, 200
    methodological considerations, 198–200
    in noninterventional PASS, 198
Intention-to-treat (ITT), 142–143, 142f, 197
Interchangeability, 258–259, 259t
Interchangeable biologic products. *See* Biosimilars products
International Classification of Diseases (ICD), 50–51
    ICD-9 to ICD-10 codes, 54–55
International Conference on Harmonization (ICH), 4, 13, 21, 225–226, 229–230
International Consortium of Cardiovascular Registries, 282

International Consortium of Orthopaedic Registries, 282
International nonproprietary name (INN), 257
Interrupted time series design, 39, 40f
Interventional PASS, 262–263
Interventional studies, prospective, 158–160
Inverse probability of treatment weighting (IPTW), 178
Ipilimumab cancer immunotherapy, 247
IPTW. *See* Inverse probability of treatment weighting (IPTW)
Isotretinoin, 217, 234
ITT. *See* Intention-to-treat (ITT)
IVs. *See* Instrumental variables (IVs)

J

Japan Classification and Coding for Clinical Laboratory Tests (JLAC10), 50–51

K

Kefauver–Harris Amendments, 26

L

Labeling and pack design, 25
Laboratory tests, 69–70
Laboratory-based event assessments, 69–70
Large simple trials (LST), 158–159
Lenalidomide, 31b
Lexical approach, 98–99
License, 233–234
Licensed indication, 314–315
Lifestyle factors, 142
Line programming, 88
LinkedIn, 92
Live attenuated vaccines, 316
Logical Observation Identifiers Names and Codes, 64–65
Long-term follow-up of rare exposure, 76–77
Lot identification codes (lot IDs), 296–297

Lot identifications, 312, 317
LST. *See* Large simple trials (LST)

M

M-PEMS. *See* Modified PEMS (M-PEMS)
MAA. *See* Marketing authorization application (MAA)
Machine learning, 98–99
MAH. *See* Marketing authorization holders (MAH)
Manufacturing variability, 257
MAP. *See* Modular analysis programs (MAP)
Marketing authorization application (MAA), 1
Marketing authorization holders (MAH), 2–3, 11–12, 235, 331
Marketing of medicinal products, 107
Mass immunization, 295
Matching on EPS, 176–177
Maximum sequential probability ratio test, 85
MCV4. *See* Meningococcal conjugate vaccination (MCV4)
Measles, mumps, and rubella vaccine (MMR vaccine), 295
Measurable outcomes, lack of, 34–35
Medical devices, 277
    analytical considerations, 288–290
    methodological considerations, 279–290
        data sources, 281–284
        device exposure measurement, 279–281
    safety concerns with medical devices, 278–279
    validity considerations, 284–290
        confounding, 287–288
        healthy-user bias, 285–286
        immortal-time bias, 286–287
        provider-level factors, 284–285
Medicare claims, 59–60
Medication errors, 108

Medicinal products, 11, 20–21, 107–108, 139–140, 167, 253
Medullary thyroid carcinoma registry (MTC registry), 77
MedWatcher Social digital data-mining platform, 101
Meningococcal conjugate vaccination (MCV4), 306
MF59 adjuvant influenza vaccine, 314
MMR vaccine. *See* Measles, mumps, and rubella vaccine (MMR vaccine)
Moderate gastrointestinal effects, 231
Modified PEMS (M-PEMS), 114–116, 115t
Modular analysis programs (MAP), 204–205, 205t, 206f
Modular program, 215
MONICA. *See* Multinational Monitoring of Trends and Determinants in Cardiovascular Disease (MONICA)
"Monitored release", 111
MTC registry. *See* Medullary thyroid carcinoma registry (MTC registry)
Multinational Monitoring of Trends and Determinants in Cardiovascular Disease (MONICA), 160–161
Multivariate confounder score, 183
Myocardial infarction analysis, 53–54

N
National databases, 52–53
National Drug Code (NDC), 269
National Joint Registry, 281
National mortality data, 70–71
Natural language processing (NLP), 98
NCSP. *See* NOMESCO Classification of Surgical Procedures (NCSP)

NDC. *See* National Drug Code (NDC)
Nested case–control studies, 139, 144–147
    methodological considerations, 146–147
    selection of cases and controls, 144–146, 145f
Neutralizing antibodies, 257
Neutropenia, 69–70
NLP. *See* Natural language processing (NLP)
NOMESCO. *See* Nordic Medico-Statistical Committee (NOMESCO)
NOMESCO Classification of Surgical Procedures (NCSP), 50–51
Non-Hodgkin's lymphoma, 267
Nonhomogeneous Poisson process, 124–125
Noninterventional PASS, 179–180, 198, 263–265, 268, 322
Noninterventional studies, 160–161, 304–305
Nonstandard tests, 64–65
Nonsteroidal antiinflammatory drugs (NSAIDs), 70
Nordic countries, 55, 75–76
Nordic drug, 110
Nordic Medico-Statistical Committee (NOMESCO), 50–51
NSAIDs. *See* Nonsteroidal antiinflammatory drugs (NSAIDs)

O
Observational Health Data Sciences and Informatics (OHDSI), 204
Observational Medical Outcomes Partnership (OMOP), 204
Observational studies, 152
Odds ratio (OR), 127, 146
OHDSI. *See* Observational Health Data Sciences and Informatics (OHDSI)

OMOP. *See* Observational Medical Outcomes Partnership (OMOP)
On-treatment analysis, 143
Open claims databases, 49–50
Operationalizing enriched studies, 154
Operationen und Prozedurenschlüssel coding system, 50–51, 282–283
OR. *See* Odds ratio (OR)
Oral anticoagulant agent, 190
Orphanet, 76
OTC products. *See* Over-the-counter products (OTC products)
Outcome indicators, 33–34
"Outcome-indexed" design, 125–126
Over-the-counter products (OTC products), 26, 68

P
PAES. *See* Post-authorization effectiveness studies (PAES)
Paper questionnaires, 314
PARENT joint action initiative, 76
PAS. *See* Post-authorization studies (PAS)
PASI. *See* Psoriasis area severity index (PASI)
PASS. *See* Post-authorization safety studies (PASS)
Patient
    alert cards, 28–29
    diaries, 28–29
    enrollment, 320
    factor, 168
    registry, 74
    retention, 320–321
    safety, 22–23
Patient Enrollment and Consent Form, 30–31
Patient Package Insert (PPI), 23
Patient-reported outcomes (PRO), 313–314
Pattern matching approach, 99
PBRER. *See* Periodic benefit–risk evaluation reports (PBRER)

PCT. *See* Pragmatic clinical trials (PCT)
PEMS. *See* Prescription-event monitoring studies (PEMS)
Periodic benefit—risk evaluation reports (PBRER), 235, 237—238
Person-time
  before outcome, 123—124
  after outcome, 124—125
Personal choice, 225
Personal decisions, 225
Personalized effectiveness, 242—243, 243t
Perspective and preference, 233
Pharmacodynamics, 122
Pharmacoepidemiology, 88, 150, 173
  developments, 114
  studies, 182—183
Pharmacokinetics, 122—123
Pharmacovigilance, 108, 130—131, 257, 294
  social media and, 94—95
Pharmacovigilance plan, 14—18, 300
  additional pharmacovigilance activities, 16—18
  regulatory classification of post-authorization safety studies, 17t
  routine pharmacovigilance activities, 15—16
Pharmacovigilance Risk Assessment Committee (PRAC), 3, 25, 302
Pharmacy
  benefits management system record, 259—260
  dispensations of products, 110—111
  record, 259—260
PHARMO database, 71—72
PMC. *See* Postmarketing commitments (PMC)
PMCF studies. *See* Postmarket clinical follow-up studies (PMCF studies)

PML. *See* Progressive multifocal leukoencephalopathy (PML)
PMR. *See* Postmarketing requirements (PMR)
PMSS. *See* Postmarketing safety studies (PMSS)
Pneumococcal pneumonia, 323—324
Poisson regression, 308
POM. *See* Prescription only medicine (POM)
Population trends in exposure over time, 132—134
Population-based databases, 268
Population-level approaches, 281
Positive benefit—risk assessments, 236—237
Post-authorization effectiveness studies (PAES), 1, 17—18, 74, 237—238, 242—243
  benefit management for medicinal product, 244f
  in Europe, 244—246
  examples, 246—247
  future directions, 247—248
  in United States, 246
Post-authorization safety studies (PASS), 1—3, 12, 49, 63, 74, 79, 98, 107, 120, 139, 150—151, 158, 170, 182, 209, 226, 236—238, 243, 248, 256—257, 262, 293, 295—296, 307. *See also* Proactive safety surveillance programs (PSSP)
  big data for, 79—81
  for biologics and biosimilars, 261—265, 262t
    interventional PASS, 262—263
    noninterventional PASS, 263—265
  using EMR linking to other data, 70—72
  of medical devices, 289—290
  models for risk minimization evaluation, 33—41
  regulatory classification, 17t
  regulatory requirements for, 331
  role, 236—237

Post-authorization studies (PAS), 1, 329
Postlicensure Rapid Immunization Safety Monitoring (PRISM), 297—298, 312
Postmarket clinical follow-up studies (PMCF studies), 278—279
Postmarketing commitments (PMC), 3
Postmarketing requirements (PMR), 3
Postmarketing safety studies (PMSS), 161
PPI. *See* Patient Package Insert (PPI)
PPP. *See* Pregnancy Prevention Programs (PPP)
PRAC. *See* Pharmacovigilance Risk Assessment Committee (PRAC)
Pragmatic clinical trials (PCT), 159, 262—263
Pragmatic trials, 151, 158—159
Preauthorization phase, 1
  limitations of preauthorization studies, 2t
Preferences, 233
Pregnancy Prevention Programs (PPP), 32
Prescriber Enrollment and Agreement Form, 30—31
Prescriber factor, 168
Prescription only medicine (POM), 26
Prescription-event monitoring studies (PEMS), 111—114, 112b
  M-PEMS, 114—116
  operational characteristic in England, 113t
Pretesting, 37
Primary data collection, 110
PRISM. *See* Postlicensure Rapid Immunization Safety Monitoring (PRISM)
Privacy, 83
Privacy-preserving methods for multivariate analysis, 84

PRO. *See* Patient-reported outcomes (PRO)
Proactive safety surveillance programs (PSSP), 209. *See also* Post-authorization safety studies (PASS)
  AsPEN, 217—218
  CNODES, 215—217
  sentinels, 213—215
  VSD, 210—213
Probability of exposure, 123—124
Procedure coding systems, 50—51
Procedure-specific registries, 282—283
Process indicators, 33, 33t
Product information, 23
Product registries, 74—75
Product safety, 216—217, 295, 304—305
Prognostic balance, 184
Prognostic balancing scores, 182—183
Prognostic scores technique, 182—183
Progressive multifocal leukoencephalopathy (PML), 231
Propensity balance, 184
Prospective cohorts, 110
Prospective studies, 158
  methodological considerations, 146—147
  prospective interventional studies, 158—160
  prospective noninterventional studies, 160—161
PROTECT project, 236
Protocol-based assessment, 214—215
Provider-level factors, 284—285
Proxies, 285—286
Psoriasis area severity index (PASI), 266
Psoriatic arthritis, 256
PSSP. *See* Proactive safety surveillance programs (PSSP)
Public trust, 294—295

Q
Quantitative bias analysis, 273
Quasiexperimental designs, 34
Questionnaire-based survey PASS, 37

R
R "meta" analysis software package, 83
Random sampling, 281
Randomized clinical trials. *See* Randomized controlled trials (RCT)
Randomized controlled trials (RCT), 158—159, 175, 227—228, 232, 238, 242, 261—262, 280, 295—296
Randomized database studies (RDS), 158—159
Rapid-cycle analytics, 205
RCT. *See* Randomized controlled trials (RCT)
RDS. *See* Randomized database studies (RDS)
Real-world data, 203—204
Recorded release, 111
Reference medicinal product, 254
Registered release, 111
Registering studies, 332
Registries, 32, 74, 281—282
  data source, 281—282
  disease, 41, 74—75
  European registries, 75—76
  MTC, 77
  patient, 74
  procedure-specific, 282—283
  product, 74—75
  registry-based post-authorization safety studies, 76—78
  registry-based randomized trials, 158—159
  vaccination, 313
Regression
  discontinuity design, 39, 40f
  models, 182

Regulatory
  agencies, 1
  authorities, 23
  guidelines, 2—3
  requirements for post-authorization safety studies, 331
Reimbursement for biologic products, 261
Relative risk (RR), 142—143
Reliable unique identifier, lack of, 83
REMS. *See* Risk evaluation and mitigation strategies (REMS)
Renal anemia, 266
Reporting rates, 41
Restricted medical prescription, 26
Restriction, 176
Retrospective assessment of drug safety, 111—112
Retrospective cohort study, 306
Retrospective PASS, 264
Retrospective studies, 142
Rheumatoid arthritis, 267
Rheumatology diseases, 256
Risk assessment
  components of European risk management plan, 13t
  pharmacovigilance plan, 14—18
  safety specification, 13, 14t
Risk evaluation and mitigation strategies (REMS), 21—23, 230, 236—237
  document, 27—28
Risk information, 229—232
  presentation, 231—232
Risk interval designs, 310
Risk knowledge/comprehension, 36—37
Risk management, 4—5, 20, 21t
Risk management plan (RMP), 11, 300, 331
  for vaccines, 295
Risk management system (RMS), 11, 230
Risk minimization, 233
  additional, 27—32

Risk minimization (*Continued*)
  cardiovascular risk minimization
      measures for stronium
      ranelate, 22b
  EMA and FDA regulatory tools for,
      24t
  methods, 22–32
  program for preventing fetal
      exposure to lenalidomide, 31b
  routine, 23–26
Risk Minimization Action Plan
    (RiskMAPs), 21
Risk minimization measures
    (RMM), 4–5, 233–234
Risk Minimization Plan (RMiP), 11
Risk outcome, 233
Risk positivity, 188
Risk quantification and
    characterization, 20–21
Risk-based monitoring, 321
RiskMAPs. *See* Risk Minimization
    Action Plan (RiskMAPs)
Rituximab, 253
RMiP. *See* Risk Minimization Plan
    (RMiP)
RMM. *See* Risk minimization
    measures (RMM)
RMP. *See* Risk management plan
    (RMP)
RMS. *See* Risk management system
    (RMS)
Robotic-assisted surgery, 284–285
Rofecoxib, 213
Rotavirus, 323–324
Routine pharmacovigilance
    activities, 15–16
Routine risk minimization, 23–26.
    See also Additional risk
    minimization
RR. *See* Relative risk (RR)
Rule-out codes, 54–55

S
Safety outcomes, 41
Safety Report Card (SRC), 301
Safety specification, 13, 14t
Same-sample estimation, 184
  DRS estimation, 184–185

SAS. *See* Statistical Analysis System
    (SAS)
SAVR. *See* Surgical aortic valve
    replacement (SAVR)
SCCS. *See* Self-controlled case series
    (SCCS)
SCEMS. *See* Specialist cohort-event
    monitoring studies (SCEMS)
Score, 177–178
Screening procedures, 30–31, 59
SCRI. *See* Self-controlled risk
    interval (SCRI)
Seasonal diseases, 318
Seasonality of vaccine-preventable
    illnesses, 323–324
Secondary data sources evaluation
    for enriched studies, 153
Selection bias, 113, 162, 270–271,
    272t
Self-controlled case series (SCCS),
    131–132, 310
Self-controlled risk interval (SCRI),
    122, 129–132, 308, 310
Self-controlled studies
  assumptions and data
      requirements, 121–125
  across approaches, 121–123
  approaches using person-time
      after outcome, 124–125
  approaches using person-time
      before outcome, 123–124
  methodological considerations,
      132–137
  event-dependent exposures,
      136–137
  healthy-user/sick-quitter effects,
      134–136
  population trends in exposure
      over time, 132–134
  self-controlled design types,
      125–132, 126t, 128f
  case-crossover, 126–129
  self-controlled case-series,
      131–132
  self-controlled risk interval,
      129–130
  sequence symmetry analysis,
      130–131

Sentinels, 213–215, 306
  DDN, 298
  example, 214–215
  governance and data, 214
  system, 213, 289
Sequence symmetry analysis,
    130–131
Sequential probability ratio test
    method (SPRT method), 306
Sequential study design, 214–215
Shingles vaccine, 316–317
Signal
  confirmation, 86
  detection, 214
  detection algorithms, 85
  management, 15–16, 15f
Silver surfers, 96–97
Single-arm designs, 309
Site selection, 319–320
Site-specific EMR databases, 65
SKS-klassifikationerne code, 282–283
2SLS. *See* Two-stage least squares
    (2SLS)
Smaller platforms social media, 92
SmPC. *See* Summary of Product
    Characteristics (SmPC)
SMR. *See* Standardized mortality/
    morbidity ratio (SMR)
Social media, 92
  challenges with social media
      listening, 95–98
  ethical considerations, 99–102
  example of lexical diversity of social
      media posts, 97t
  methodological considerations,
      98–99
  and pharmacovigilance, 94–95
  sources, 93–94
Sodium valproate, 108–109
Special medical prescription, 26
Specialist cohort-event monitoring
    studies (SCEMS), 114,
    116–117
Specific medication, 96
Spontaneous reporting systems
    (SRS), 209

SPRT method. *See* Sequential probability ratio test method (SPRT method)
SRC. *See* Safety Report Card (SRC)
SRS. *See* Spontaneous reporting systems (SRS)
Stakeholders, 226–227
Standardization, 178
Standardized mortality/morbidity ratio (SMR), 178
Statistical Analysis System (SAS), 87
Statistical process control rules, 85
Stevens–Johnson syndrome, 41
Stratification, 176
Stronium ranelate, cardiovascular risk minimization measures for, 22b
Study protocol, 332
Substitution, 258–259, 259t
Summary of Product Characteristics (SmPC), 23
Supervised machine learning, 99
Surgical aortic valve replacement (SAVR), 288
Switching, 258–259, 259t
Switching phenomena, 112–113

T

TAVR. *See* Transcatheter aortic valve replacement (TAVR)
Teratogenic effect, 161
Tetanus, diphtheria, and acellular pertussis vaccine (Tdap vaccine), 305, 316–317
Thalidomide, 234
The Health Improvement Network database (THIN database), 71–72
Time-on-treatment (TOT), 142–143, 142f
Time-sequential screening method, 85
Time-trend analyses, 39
Time-varying confounding, 120–121
TNF. *See* Tumor necrosis factor (TNF)
TOT. *See* Time-on-treatment (TOT)
Training materials, 28–29

Transcatheter aortic valve replacement (TAVR), 288
Transparency, 5–6, 179–180, 205–207, 329–331
Trastuzumab, 253
Treated or on-treatment analysis. *See* Time-on-treatment (TOT)
Tree-based scan method, 85
Trimming EPS, 176
True treatment effect heterogeneity, 87
Tumor necrosis factor (TNF), 267–268
Twitter, 92, 93–95
Two-stage least squares (2SLS), 199

U

UDIs. *See* Unique device identifiers (UDIs)
Uncertainty about interpretation, 35
Uncertainty impact, 232
Uncontrolled before–after design, 39
Unique device identifiers (UDIs), 279–280, 282–283
Unique study identifier, 333–334
United States Food and Drug Administration (FDA), 3, 255, 297
  Sentinel modules, 88
  Sentinel Program, 150, 268
United States Package Insert (USPI), 23
University of Minnesota claims-based algorithm, 59
Unmeasured confounding, 172
US Centers for Disease Control and Prevention (CDC), 210, 297
US Department of Veterans Affairs EMR database, 71–72
USPI. *See* United States Package Insert (USPI)

V

VA. *See* Veterans Affairs (VA)
Vaccination, 313
  registries, 313

Vaccine
  administration setting, 317–318
  dosing schedule, 293
  formulation, 315–316
  indication, 314–315
  PASS for, 293
    background event rates, 322
    case definition, 322
    claims and electronic medical record, 312–313
    cohort and case–control designs, 308–309
    confounding, 322–324
    considerations for vaccine exposure measurement, 314–318, 315t
    data collection methods, 321, 321b
    data sources for vaccine PASS, 312
    designs, 304–318, 307t
    EPSS for vaccines, 300–304
    patient enrollment, 320
    patient retention, 320–321
    primary data collection, 313–314
    public trust, 294–295
    regulatory requirements for vaccine PASS, 298–300
    seasonal and regional considerations, 318–319
    signal detection, 305–306
    signal evaluation, 307–308
    site selection, 319–320
    special considerations for vaccine PASS, 295–297
    vaccination registries, 313
    vaccine safety surveillance programs, 297–298
    vaccinee-only designs, 310–311
  recommendations, 316
  vaccine route, lot, and expiration date, 317
Vaccine Adverse Event Reporting System (VAERS), 211, 297, 306

Vaccine Adverse Event Surveillance and Communication consortium (VAESCO), 297
Vaccine Safety Datalink (VSD), 210–213, 297–298, 306, 312
  example, 212–213
  governance and data, 211–212
Vaccinee-only designs, 310–311
  vaccine-only designs in vaccine PASS, 311f
VAERS. *See* Vaccine Adverse Event Reporting System (VAERS)
VAESCO. *See* Vaccine Adverse Event Surveillance and Communication consortium (VAESCO)

VAESCO-GBS case–control study, 309
Validation, 37
Values, 233
Varian Medical Systems, 69–70
Varicella Zoster Virus Identification Program, 301
Venous thromboembolism, 141–142
Vertical linkage, 81–82, 82t
Veterans Affairs (VA), 151
VSD. *See* Vaccine Safety Datalink (VSD)

W

Warfarin, 136, 171, 190
Wearable sensors, 152
Wearables, 151
"Web crawlers" of companies, 99–100
"Web scraping" exercise, 98
Weighting method, 178
World Health Organization (WHO), 107, 255, 304

Z

Zika, 318